Immunological and Molecular Aspects of Bacterial Virulence

Immunological and Molecular Aspects of Bacterial Virulence

S. PATRICK

M. J. LARKIN

The Queen's University of Belfast, Belfast, Northern Ireland, UK

JOHN WILEY & SONS

Chichester · New York · Brisbane · Toronto · Singapore

Published 1995 by John Wiley & Sons Ltd,
    Baffins Lane, Chichester,
    West Sussex PO19 1UD, England

        Telephone: National   Chichester (0243) 779777
                     International +44 243 779777

Other Wiley Editorial Offices

John Wiley & Sons, Inc., 605 Third Avenue,
New York, NY 10158–0012, USA

Jacaranda Wiley Ltd, 33 Park Road, Milton,
Queensland 4064, Australia

John Wiley & Sons (Canada) Ltd, 22 Worcester Road,
Rexdale, Ontario M9W 1L1, Canada

John Wiley & Sons (SEA) Pte Ltd, 37 Jalan Pemimpin #05–04,
Block B, Union Industrial Building, Singapore 2057

Library of Congress Cataloging-in-Publication Data

Patrick, S.
  Immunological and molecular aspects of bacterial virulence/S. Patrick
and M. J. Larkin.
      p.   cm.
  Includes bibliographical references and index.
  ISBN 0-471-95251-6
  1. Virulence (Microbiology)—Immunological aspects. 2. Virulence
(Microbiology)—Molecular aspects. I. Larkin, M. J. II. Title.
  QR175.P38   1995
  616'.014—dc20   94-24433
                                                             CIP

ISBN 0 471 95251 6

British Library Cataloguing in Publication Data

A catalogue record for this book is available from the British Library

Typeset by Photo·graphics, Honiton
Printed and bound in Great Britain by Redwood Books, Trowbridge, Wiltshire

To our children and in memory of Praful Shirodaria (1939–1994),
Lecturer and colleague at The Queen's University of Belfast

Contents

Preface

This book has evolved from lectures given in Bacterial Pathogenesis, Bacterial Genetics and Immunology courses to Honours year General Microbiology, Medical Microbiology, Genetics and Molecular Biology Students at the Queen's University of Belfast. Our intention is to provide material for the stronger student and hopefully to stretch, rather than confuse, other students. The book should also be of use to students in specialist postgraduate courses as well as post-graduates embarking on research into bacterial virulence. We hope that this text will fill the gap between excellent general texts such as *Mechanisms of Microbial Disease* (Eds Schaechter M., Medoff G., Eisenstein B. I., 2nd Edn, Williams and Wilkins) and more specialist texts such as *Molecular Basis of Bacterial Pathogenesis* (Eds Iglewski B. H., Clark V. L., Academic Press) and *Molecular Biology of Bacterial Infection* (Eds Hormaeche C. E., Penn C. W., Smyth C. J., Cambridge University Press). Our intention is to bring virulence into the context of both the host's immune response and the genetic systems which have evolved in bacteria, by considering molecular interactions. To this end the book covers the host's response to bacterial infection first, before the virulence determinants of bacteria, and ends with the genetic mechanisms which control the expression of bacterial virulence determinants. It is assumed that the underlying infections and pathogenesis of disease caused by individual bacteria are already familiar to the reader, as are fundamental aspects of microbiology, immunology, genetics, biochemistry and cell biology. Although biased towards human pathogens many of the general principles are equally applicable to veterinary pathogens.

Acknowledgements

We are very grateful to the following who took the time to read the manuscript, in whole or in part, and make critical comment: Gerry Collee, Tom McNeill, Susan McNerlan, Charles Penn, Ian Poxton and John Quinn. We accept responsibility for any errors and would welcome any comments from readers.

1 Pathogenic Bacteria in Context: An Overview

Bacteria are major recyclers on this planet; they degrade organic matter, solubilise inorganic compounds such as clay, contribute to the weathering of rock and degrade toxic pollutants generated by the industrial world. In short, bacteria as a group are capable of a wider range of chemical and metabolic activity than any other group of living organisms. The diversity of bacteria is exemplified by the range of environments that they can inhabit. They can inhabit environments with extremes of temperature, salinity and pressure as well as habitats devoid of oxygen. They have been isolated from environments with temperatures near to freezing and from lakes with both high salinity and temperatures of 44 °C. Thermophilic bacteria grow optimally between 55 and 75 °C; their habitats include naturally occurring hot muds and compost heaps. Some groups of bacteria utilise inorganic compounds as an energy source, some also photosynthesise in the absence of oxygen, while others conduct anaerobic respiration. It could be argued that this is due to the genetic diversity and plasticity of bacteria. Only mankind has matched their ability to survive in such extreme environments, in this case largely due to the evolution of the human brain rather than to the metabolic diversity that is exhibited by bacteria. In all these diverse environments, the resistance of the ecological niche to colonisation (which relates to the degree of adaptation required by the organism) is passive. The environment may be subject to rapid physical and chemical change, but the changes are not brought about by active participation of the environment. The only 'active' competition is from other species competing for the same niche. Bacterial colonisation of an ecological niche inside other living organisms is, however, another matter. Most multicellular organisms have evolved mechanisms to resist colonisation by microbes and this has culminated in the evolutionary splendour of the mammalian immune system; thus in colonising the living host the bacterium is faced with an environment which is actively dedicated to the prevention of its colonisation. Bacteria that can survive within this specialist niche are said to have 'determinants of virulence'; these are the attributes which allow them to survive. Those bacteria which cause abnormalities in the host as a result of colonisation are '**patho**logy **gen**erators' or pathogenic.

A large number of bacteria, the commensal flora, inhabit animals without being pathogenic. All animals have a commensal flora, which in the case of humans is estimated at 10^{14} microbial cells per person. In fact each human is inhabited by more bacteria than there are humans on the planet. In man, bacteria inhabit the skin, intestine, upper respiratory tract and genito-urinary tract and can be considered technically to be outside the host. The commensal bacteria do not multiply to the detriment of the host, provided they remain in the appropriate ecological niche. Indeed the commensal flora is considered to be largely beneficial to the host and may even be essential for its normal function. Where the commensal bacteria cross the boundaries of these habitats and enter into the host, under what could be considered abnormal conditions (for example as a result of mechanical injury to the host), they may have the potential to become pathogens.

The commensal bacteria and the truly pathogenic bacteria are part of the group of bacteria involved largely in the recycling of organic material and can be nutritionally classified as chemo-organotrophs: organic compounds are their major carbon source and energy is obtained from degradation of organic compounds rather than inorganic compounds or from light. Of this large group of bacteria only a minority are pathogenic and can multiply at the expense of a living host and cause disease. Therefore in the context of the general ecology of the planet and the bacteria which populate it, the pathogenic bacteria could be considered a curiosity; however, in the context of their potential to inflict damage on the human population, they represent a major threat to mankind. It is therefore not surprising that much time and effort has been invested in trying to understand the nature of virulent bacteria, thus enabling the development of means to prevent them from inhabiting this particular ecological niche. With the advent of clean water supplies, safe sewage disposal, successful antimicrobial therapy in the form of antibiotic treatment and vaccination programmes there was a brief per-iod of complacency in the western world when it seemed that bacterial infections were no longer a large threat to the human population. In the context of the whole world, however, the bacterium *Mycobacterium tuberculosis* still kills approximately 3 million people each year, more than any other single infectious disease. Even in the western world bacterial diseases remain a problem. For example in the United States of America sexually transmitted disease caused by *Chlamydia trachomatis* is thought to affect 3 million people annually and gonorrhoea is still the most frequently reported of the officially notifiable diseases, even though AIDS is also officially notifiable.

The study of pathogenic bacteria and an understanding of how they evolve and adapt should lead to better management of disease and more successful targeting of therapy. To do this requires knowledge of a number of areas which relate to both the bacterium and host. The biochemical con-stituents of the bacterium and the host are the starting point. An under-standing of bacterial genetics and the regulation of bacterial gene expression within the host is also essential, as is an understanding of the interaction of the bacterial constituents with the host cells and systems. The bacteriologist studying virulence has therefore to be an amalgam of biochemist, geneticist, cell biologist and immunologist. With the recent advances in understanding in all these areas, and of the molecules involved in the workings of biological systems in general, bacterial pathogenesis has become an exciting and fast-moving area of study. To date the molecular basis of bacterial virulence is known in part for only a few bacteria and these are by and large the simpler systems where one key characteristic of the bacterium, for example production of a toxin, can be clearly correlated with virulence. For most pathogenic bacteria many different characteristics or factors contribute to virulence and these may vary depending on the stage of infection; virulence is said to be 'multifactorial'. As the pathogenic process cannot be removed from the bacterial interactions with the host, it is very difficult to relate characteristics of the bacterium growing in culture media to virulence in the natural infection. Therefore studies of virulence have two essential requirements: firstly a suitable model system which mimics as closely as possible the natural infection so that putative virulence determinants can be identified; and secondly it is necessary to confirm that putative virulence determinants are expressed by the bacterium during the course of a natural infection. Thus clinical material must also be investigated. One of the most exciting models now being used to identify bacterial genes necessary for virulence which may be expressed **only** in response to host stimuli is in vivo expression technology (IVET). Regions of the bacterial chromosome are isolated, enzymically cut, modified and are inserted back into the genome in such a way that genes which are switched on in vivo can be identified.

As we more clearly understand molecular biology, both in the broad sense of all biological molecules and in the sense of manipulation of deoxyribonucleic acid (DNA), so our understanding of the fascinating co-evolution of pathogenic bacteria and the mammalian immune system will increase. In the long term this should lead to a further reduction of the large impact this minor group of bacteria has on human history.

FURTHER READING

Barinaga M. 1993. New technique offers a window on bacteria's secret weapons. Science 259, 595.

Drasar B. S., Duerden B. I. 1991. Anaerobes in the normal flora of man. In: Anaerobes in human disease (Eds B. I. Duerden, B. S. Drasar). E. Arnold: Sevenoaks, UK. Chapter 11, p 162–179.

Falkow S. B. 1990. The 'Zen' of bacterial pathogenicity. In: Molecular basis of bacterial pathogenesis (Eds B. H. Iglewski, V. L. Clark). Academic Press, London. Chapter 1, pp 3–9.

Finlay B. B., Falkow S. 1989. Common themes in microbial pathogenicity. Microbiological Reviews 53, 210–230.

Mahan M. J., Slauch J. M., Mekalanos J. J. 1993. Selection of bacterial virulence genes that are specifically induced in host tissues. Science 259, 686–688.

Mims C. A. 1987. The pathogenesis of infectious disease (3rd Edn). Academic Press, London.

Mitchison A. 1993. Will we survive? As host and pathogen evolve together; will the immune system retain the upper hand? Scientific American September, 102–108.

Morbidity and Mortality Weekly Report, Centers for Disease Control and Prevention, Atlanta, USA.

Penn C. W. 1992. Chronic infections, latency and the carrier state. In: Molecular biology of bacterial infection. Current status and future perspectives. Society for General Microbiology Symposium 49 (Eds C. E. Hormaeche, C. W. Penn, C. J. Smyth). Cambridge University Press, UK. pp 107–125.

Schaechter M., Medoff G., Eisenstein B. I. 1993. Mechanisms of microbial disease (2nd Edn). Williams and Wilkins, Baltimore, USA.

Smith H. 1989. The mounting interest in bacterial and viral pathogenicity. Annual Review of Microbiology 43, 1–22.

Smith H. 1990. Pathogenicity and the microbe in vivo. Journal of General Microbiology 136, 377–383.

Trends in Microbiology; Virulence, Infection and Pathogenesis, Elsevier Trends Journals, Cambridge, UK.

Part I

HOST DEFENCE: THE IMMUNE SYSTEM

The biggest problem in understanding how the mammalian immune system reacts to, or recognises, the foreign molecules of the bacterial cell is our lack of a detailed knowledge of large parts of the workings of the immune system. The recognition of small regions (or epitopes) of the bacterial surface molecules by specific binding of the host's immunoglobulins and T-cell receptors is now well understood. This part of the immune system probably represents the evolutionary 'state of the art' of immune recognition. There is the potential for clonal amplification of the cells which produce immunoglobulin and T-cell receptors (Figure I.1, overleaf), the generation of increased specificity during the amplification process by somatic mutation within the antibody producing B-cells and the ability to retain cellular memory of the specificity (see Chapter 3).

The plethora of other molecular interactions which occur between the immune system and the bacterial cell are, unfortunately, less well understood. Many of these are probably more primitive in evolutionary terms. A general term which can be used for these more primitive or non-clonal recognition events is **immunomodulation** whereby bacterial molecules trigger and interfere with the complex cellular and biochemical interactions of the immune system (Chapter 2). This triggering of the 'alarm bells' of the immune system constitutes an important first step in immune response to bacterial infection and inflammation. The interaction of bacterial molecules with the immune system can either result in an enhancement of the immune response, termed immunopotentiation, or depression of the immune response, termed immunosuppression. The underlying molecular mechanisms and the nature of the molecules which trigger immunomodulation are just beginning to be understood, although the effects, for example fever, have been known for centuries. Included in this initial host recognition stage is the 'acute phase' response which can occur within a few hours of infection. The concentration of a number of serum proteins, synthesised by hepatocytes in the liver,

_ continued

continued

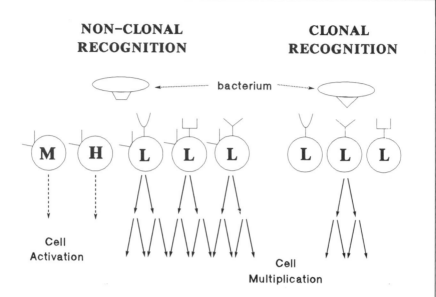

Figure I.1 Clonal versus non-clonal recognition of foreign molecules. Non-clonal recognition can result in the activation of a variety of cells of different lineage (M: macrophage; H: hepatocyte; L: lymphocyte). In lymphocytes the recognition may induce mitosis of cells which do not carry T-cell receptors or immunoglobulin specific for the foreign molecule. In many cases details of the molecular trigger or signal are not known. Clonal recognition, on the other hand, only involves the activation and multiplication of lymphocytes which recognise a specific epitope of the foreign molecule by either T-cell receptor–antigen or immunoglobulin–antigen interactions

increases by up to 1000 times. This is a direct consequence of the up-regulation of the genes which encode for the acute phase proteins. Some of these acute phase proteins bind specifically to bacterial surface molecules. For example the lipopolysaccharide (LPS) binding proteins recognise and bind to bacterial LPS.

Bacteria have undoubtedly evolved to counter the antimicrobial mechanisms of the host. Therefore older mechanisms of host resistance, in evolutionary terms, may now appear to confer no obvious advantage to the host and indeed may be detrimental. This moving picture of bacterial versus host evolution makes it difficult to untangle host recognition of the bacterium from bacterial interference with the host, particularly with respect to immunomodulation.

Recognition alone is insufficient to deter the invader; therefore, a variety of mechanisms for killing bacteria have evolved. The host, however, shows an evolutionary economy in that one type of recognition event, for example binding of specific antibody, can trigger more than one type of killing mechanism, for example both complement mediated and phagocytic killing. These aspects of the immune system are considered in Chapter 4.

2 Non-clonal Recognition and Immunomodulation

INTRODUCTION

Many bacterial molecules modulate the immune system, either by increasing (also known as the adjuvant effect) or decreasing its activity. They are therefore termed immunomodulators. Their activity constitutes a complex interplay between host recognition of the bacterium and bacterial virulence. It is likely that stimulation by bacterial components in the commensal flora is necessary for the development of the immune system in an individual not only in the first instance but also for it to function optimally thereafter.

One of the best known immunomodulators is complete Freund's adjuvant (from the Latin, *adjuvare*; to help). This has been known since the 1930s to enhance the immune response to antigens when injected along with the antigen in an oil–water emulsion. It contains a complex mixture of the components of the cell envelope of *Mycobacterium tuberculosis*. C. Janeway calls adjuvants such as Freund's the immunologist's 'dirty little secret'. For many years the consensus among immunologists was that as the immune system could produce specific antibodies to practically any molecule, there was no necessity for the molecule to be derived from a pathogenic microorganism. The conclusion made at that time was that the immune system was not selectively recognising infectious agents. This cast doubts as to whether the ability to generate specific antibody had evolved in response to infection. The theory was based on the work of Landsteiner on the generation of antibodies to aniline dyes. This theory, unfortunately, did not take into account the immunologist's 'dirty little secret'. Adjuvant, derived from bacteria, was necessary for a detectable immune response to the aniline dye. Thus, for an **efficient** response, the immune system does require modulation by molecules derived from an infectious agent.

A clear understanding of immunomodulation at a molecular level has not yet been reached, with the exception perhaps of the superantigens (see below); however, many of the molecules involved have been characterised and much is known about interactions at a cellular level. Table 2.1 lists bacterial molecules with known immunomodulatory activity.

Immunomodulators can have effects on cells such as **T- and B-lymphocytes** and **macrophages** which are similar to those of the host's own messenger molecules, the **cytokines**. Some of the cytokines involved in the

Table 2.1. Immunomodulatory molecules of bacteria

Peptidoglycan
Peptidoglycolipids
Muramyl dipeptide (a subcomponent of peptidoglycan)
Lipopolysaccharide
Lipid A (a subcomponent of lipopolysaccharide)
Teichoic acids and lipoteichoic acids
Exotoxins, including enterotoxins and pyrogenic toxins

---

immune system and their main functions are listed in Table 2.2. Their major activities are to cause cells to become activated, proliferate and differentiate (Figure 2.1). Activation occurs when a cell moves from the resting cell in the G_0 phase of the cell cycle into G_1. This is usually coupled with enlargement of the cell, RNA synthesis, the expression of new cell surface glycoproteins such as transferrin receptors for iron uptake and the release of further cytokines. Proliferation of the cell may then follow. The exceptions are cells such as macrophages and **neutrophils** which, although they become activated, do not proliferate. Cells which do proliferate, such as T- and B-lymphocytes, move in a cyclical manner through S phase, where DNA is synthesised, and G_2 and M phases, when the cell divides by mitosis. During this proliferation the cell may differentiate into a more mature form. For example a B-cell becomes a plasma cell which is effectively an antibody producing factory. Although immunomodulatory molecules trigger these events, it is thought that they act in concert with the cytokines of the host.

The major cytokines released in response to bacterial molecules are **interleukin 1** (IL1), **interleukin 2** (IL2), **interleukin 6** (IL6), **tumour necrosis factor** (TNF) and **prostaglandins**. These mediators can have multiple effects on the immune system as well as on other host functions (Table 2.2), in

Table 2.2. Normal activities of cytokines associated with bacterial induced modulation of the immune system

Activity	Cytokine			
B-cell activation	TNF,	IL1,		
proliferation	TNF,	IL1,	IL2,	IL4
differentiation	IL1,	IL2,	IL6,	IL4
T-cell activation	IL1,	IL2,	IL6	
proliferation	TNF,	IL1,	IL2,	IL6
differentiation	IL2,	IL6		
Pyrogenicity	IL1,	IL2		
Septic shock	TNF,	IL2,	IL6,	γIF

Key: TNF, tumour necrosis factor (synonyms TNF α, cachectin); IL1, interleukin 1 α and β; IL2, interleukin 2; IL4, interleukin 4; IL6, interleukin 6; γ IF, γ interferon.

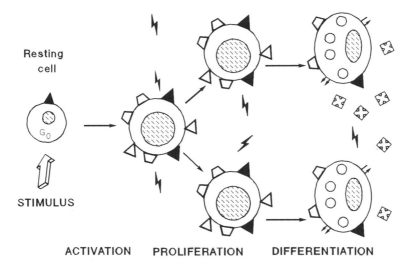

ACTIVATION   PROLIFERATION   DIFFERENTIATION

Key: ▲◻△||, surface glycoproteins; ⌇✧, secreted molecules

Figure 2.1. Cell activation, proliferation and differentiation. In response to a stimulus, such as a cytokine, foreign molecule or a combination of both, cells move out of resting stage (G_0) and produce new cell surface glycoproteins and secreted factors (activation). The secreted molecules may include more cytokines and in the case of B-lymphocytes, immunoglobulin. In cells such as T- and B-lymphocytes activation is followed by mitosis (proliferation). During mitosis the cells may mature, becoming more specialised (differentiation). The range of cell surface and secreted molecules will alter with differentiation. For example, B-lymphocytes may become plasma cells, committed to the generation of quantities of antibody of a particular isotype and specificity. Mixtures of different cytokines will influence the maturation of the cell as it progresses along the activation/differentiation pathway

that they can both up- and down-regulate cell functions. They are probably largely responsible for the modulatory activities associated with the bacterial molecules. Their activities will be discussed in more detail below.

The mitogenic activity of immunomodulators causes T- and B-cells to proliferate. This is an example of polyclonal activation and proliferation, as opposed to antigen specific activation of T- and B-cells which only affects one or a few clones of cells (see Figure I.1). The result is a shot-gun production of immunoglobulin with the possibility that some of the immunoglobulin may be specific for the infecting agent. Although potentially wasteful and not specifically targeted, such an increase in immunoglobulin production is fast and may be sufficient to prevent infection at an early stage, particularly if the infecting organism is one to which the host has already been exposed. Immunomodulators may influence the mobility of cells, in particular the phagocytic cells of the immune system. For example the migration of macrophages may be inhibited.

Immunomodulatory molecules may therefore enhance or potentiate the immune response at many levels. Problems can arise, however, where immunomodulatory molecules persist in the tissues, leading to chronic stimulation of the immune system and the destruction of the host by its own defences. In extreme cases this can result in arthritis or other autoimmune diseases. Indeed, molecules derived from bacterial cell envelopes, such as peptidoglycan, are used to create animal models of autoimmune disease. Many of these bacterial immunomodulators are also termed biological response modifiers as they have more general effects on systems of the body other than the immune system. These include the induction of fever (pyrogenicity), effects on the blood clotting system and effects on the levels of salt and iron (see Chapter 5) in the body.

As a result of the complex evolutionary inter-relationship between the pathogenic bacterium and the host it may never be possible to differentiate between host recognition and bacterial virulence in the context of immunomodulation.

IMMUNOMODULATORY MOLECULES: THE BACTERIAL CELL ENVELOPE

The specific molecules of the bacterium known to be involved in immunomodulation include many of the polymers of the bacterial cell envelope as well as excreted molecules originally identified as being toxic to the host, such as enterotoxins. In this section immunomodulatory components of the cell envelope will be considered. Details of the composition of bacterial cell envelopes and the molecular structure of components can be found in the Appendix.

Peptidoglycan and peptidoglycolipids

Preparations of peptidoglycan from both Gram negative and Gram positive bacteria and the related peptidoglycolipids of mycobacteria, are known to have immunomodulating activity (Figure 2.2). The minimal unit of the peptidoglycan molecule which retains immunopotentiating activity is N-acetyl-muramyl-L-alanine-D-isoglutamine, also known as **muramyl dipeptide** (MDP). Thus, both the sugar backbone and the cross-linking amino acids of the molecule are involved in its activity and the active unit is repeated throughout the molecule. The induction of polyarthritis in rats is one of the few immunomodulating activities which is not induced by synthetically produced MDP. In this instance the number of repeating N-acetyl muramic acid and N-acetyl glucosamine disaccharide units of the peptidoglycan is important; fractions with five or more disaccharides are more effective inducers of polyarthritis than those with only two or three. Therefore subtle changes in the size of the peptidoglycan molecule may change its activity

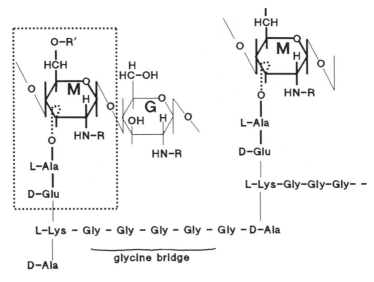

Figure 2.2. Peptidoglycan: muramyl dipeptide. Polysaccharide chain of repeating units of N-acetyl muramic acid (M) and N-acetyl glucosamine (G) cross-linked by peptides. R is either hydrogen or an acetyl group, R' is either hydrogen or a linkage point with teichoic acid. The peptide formation is non-ribosomal and involves only enzymic reactions. The amino acids vary with different bacteria, for example L-lysine may be replaced by diamino pimelic acid and may link directly to D-alanine without the poly-glycine bridge. Note that some of the amino acids are D-isomers, while amino acids in mammalian proteins are all L-isomers. The minimal unit of immunomodulatory activity is N-acetyl muramyl-L-alanine-D-isoglutamine or muramyl dipeptide (box)

from being advantageous to the host by increasing the activity of systems involved in clearing the infection, to an unwanted over-stimulation, which may be detrimental.

The question arises as to how these molecules might be present naturally during the course of an infection. The peptidoglycan surrounding both Gram positive and Gram negative cells is an insoluble 'bag-like' single molecule (see Appendix). Both the host and the bacterium are potential sources of enzymes which will degrade the peptidoglycan. In order to enlarge the cell envelope prior to cell division, the bacterium has to be able to break the existing covalent bonds in the peptidoglycan molecule and release new growing points. The enzymes responsible for this are termed autolysins. There are four common types classified according to the particular peptidoglycan bond broken (Figure 2.3). These enzymes have been commonly detected in Gram positive bacteria where they may be very active. For example, when growing *Enterococcus faecalis* cells are suspended in a buffer containing isotonic sucrose (0.5 mol/l) the cell walls are completely

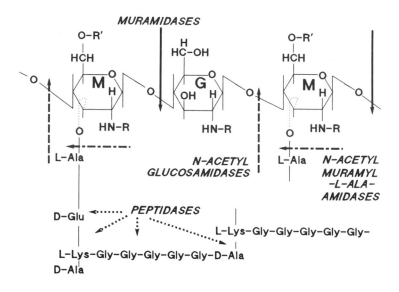

Figure 2.3. Peptidoglycan: sites of action of autolytic enzymes. Bacterial autolytic enzymes are necessary for the growth of the bacterial cell. Host derived enzymes such as lysozyme which is a muramidase (solid arrow) can have similar activities

digested within 6 hours at 37 °C. These autolytic enzymes normally remain associated with the cell wall and it is thought that their tight binding to teichoic acids (see Appendix) normally regulates their activity. The four types of enzyme are:

1. The lysozyme-like enzymes or muramidases. These enzymes hydrolyse the β(1–4) linkage in the peptidoglycan backbone, ultimately releasing disaccharide units, which may or may not be cross-linked to another disaccharide molecule. This releases the free-reducing groups of N-acetyl muramic acid. Host derived lysozyme, present in serum, tears and saliva as well as in the lysosomes of phagocytic cells, has similar activity.
2. The β-N-acetyl glucosamidases also release disaccharides. In this instance the free reducing group of N-acetylglucosamine is released.
3. N-acetylmuramyl-L-alanine amidase removes the peptide side chains by hydrolysing the bond between L-alanine and the peptide chain.
4. A range of different peptidases, which hydrolyse peptide bonds in the peptide side chains and cross-linkages, are also produced.

The action of autolysin is coincidentally important in the bactericidal effect of the β-lactam antibiotics, thus producing another means by which these molecules may be released in a form in which they can immunomodulate.

Autolysin expression in *Bordetella pertussis*, which causes whooping cough, is controlled by the bordetella virulence gene (*bvg*). Genes such as these respond to environmental stimuli (see Chapter 9) and in *B. pertussis bvg* coordinately regulates the expression of a large number of virulence genes. A number of genes encoding for virulence determinants are switched on by the environment in vivo. The genes encoding for the peptidoglycan autolytic enzymes are, however, down-regulated in vivo. This suggests that repression of autolysin activity in vivo confers a selective advantage on the bacterium, possibly by reducing the quantities of immunomodulatory sub-components of peptidoglycan which induce an inflammatory response. In an animal model of *Streptococcus pneumoniae* meningitis, bacterial strains which lacked autolysin activity produced a cryptic relapsing infection whereas those with autolytic activity produced an acute inflammatory response. As the different breakdown products of peptidoglycan can have different immunomodulatory activities, a knowledge of the particular auto-lysins that are active during bacterial growth in vivo may help us to under-stand better the course of bacterial infection.

Teichoic and lipoteichoic acids

The second major class of polymers of the Gram positive envelope includes the teichoic acids and lipid associated lipoteichoic acids (see Appendix). As is the case with peptidoglycan, these molecules may have either immuno-suppressive or immunopotentiating activity. Teichoic acids from both *Staphylococcus aureus* and *Streptococcus pyogenes* at high concentrations may suppress antibody formation, but at present there is little detailed infor-mation on the immunomodulatory activities of components of these poly-mers.

Endotoxin and lipopolysaccharide

The major component of the Gram negative envelope, lipopolysaccharide (LPS) has a very similar range of activities to peptidoglycan and may also have lethal effects. Indeed, LPS can affect practically every inflammatory and defence mechanism of the host. Mortality from **endotoxin shock** induced by the presence of quantities of endotoxin in the blood stream is of the order of 20–70%. Two of the major sources of the endotoxin are infection of the blood by Gram negative bacteria (septicaemia) and the escape of the gut flora as a result of injury. The toxicity is largely caused by interference with the host systems.

The terms endotoxin and LPS are frequently used synonymously; how-ever, LPS should only be used for the purified LPS molecule and endotoxin for LPS and any associated outer membrane proteins released from the cell surface. The term **endo**toxin, meaning bacterial associated toxin, was

initially used to distinguish endotoxin from the other protein toxins
secreted by bacteria, the **exo**toxins (see Chapters 5 and 6). Endotoxin is,
however, released from the bacterial cell surface in the form of outer membrane vesicles or blebs. This occurs during normal growth of bacteria both
in vivo and in vitro (Figure 2.4). Thus, LPS may function at a distance from
the focus of infection.

The molecular basis of LPS activity is still not completely understood
(see next section), although the molecular structure is known in detail. The
outer region of the molecule, in relation to the bacterium, consists of polymerised di- to penta-saccharide repeating units whose composition will
vary within a species or strain. The inner region is generally conserved
within a single genus, and consists of a core oligosaccharide linked by the
sugar 2-keto-3-deoxy-D-manno-octonate (KDO) to a disaccharide backbone

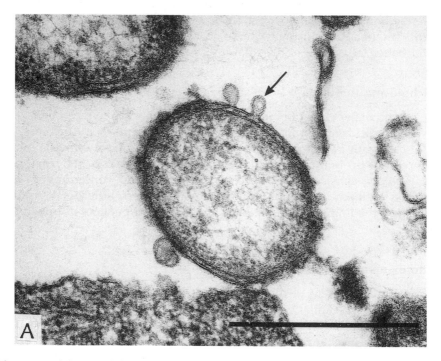

Figure 2.4. (*above and facing page*) Outer membrane vesicles. The outer membrane
of lipopolysaccharide and associated proteins can bud off from the surface of Gram
negative bacteria, thus releasing endotoxin into the surrounding environment. Electron micrographs of outer membrane vesicles (arrows) in *Bacteroides fragilis*. A.
Ultrathin section of vesicle budding from the outer membrane. B. Ultrathin section
of formed vesicle with associated capsular material. C. Negatively stained whole
cells of *Bacteroides fragilis* which have been labelled with a monoclonal antibody
specific for the lipopolysaccharide and a secondary antibody conjugated to gold
particles (black dots). Note that the outer membrane vesicles are labelled. Scale bar
= 0.5 μm

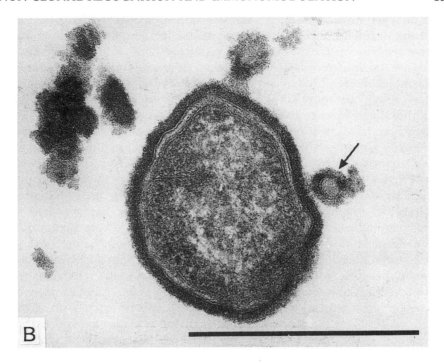

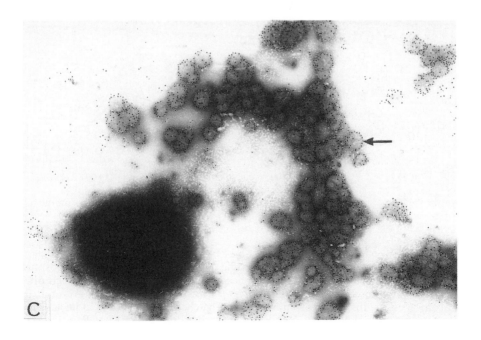

with attached long chain fatty acids, the lipid A (see Appendix for details). By using purified lipid A it has been possible to show that this component is responsible for much of the biological activity of the molecule. By purifying the lipid A molecule and making synthetic lipids the components of the molecules required to confer the greatest biological and immunomodulatory activity are now known; namely a glucosamine disaccharide, a bis phosphorylated lipid A and an acyl-oxyacyl group on the fatty acid chain (Figure 2.5). The loss of only one of these components, for example a phosphate group, reduces the activity of the molecule. LPSs from different genera of bacteria vary in their immunomodulating activity and studies of the fine structure of the molecules have begun to show very subtle differences. For example LPS from *Bacteroides* spp. is apparently less active in some of the tests for endotoxin activity than LPS from enteric bacteria. This was initially thought to be related to a lack of KDO in the core region of the LPS molecule; however, more sensitive detection methods have shown that KDO is present, but in a slightly modified form with an added phosphate group. Other differences in the LPS were found when the fatty acids from these two types of bacteria were compared. *Escherichia coli* has six fatty acid chains (or acyl groups) per diglucosamine backbone each with a chain length of 12–14 carbon atoms. Included in the acyl groups is 3-hydroxy tetradecanoic acid (3-OH-C14:0) which is absent in bacteroides strains. In

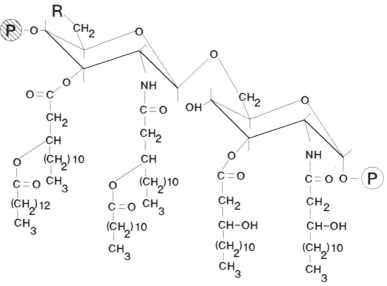

Figure 2.5. Lipid A molecule. A glucosamine disaccharide with attached phosphate and 6 acyl (fatty acid) groups. Different bacteria may have fatty acids which differ in complexity and chain length. *Bacteroides fragilis* lacks a phosphate group at the 4′ position on the distal glucosamine residue (hatched P) and differs in its activities from enterobacterial lipid A. The core oligosaccharide is attached at R

contrast, *Bacteroides fragilis* has 4–5 fatty acids of chain length 15–17 carbons per diglucosamine and has branched 3-hydroxy fatty acids. Studies of synthetic lipids have confirmed that reduced biological activity relates to fewer fatty acid chains.

Mouse strains have been bred which respond poorly to lipid A from enteric bacteria. Interestingly, *Bacteroides* spp. LPS will activate and is mitogenic for B-cells taken from the spleens of these mice, although it has a low activity with B-cells from normal mice.

The polysaccharide components of LPS from *Bordetella pertussis*, *Haemophilus influenzae* and *Bacteroides* spp. will activate B-cells. The evidence from studies with *Bacteroides fragilis* suggests that the polysaccharide of the LPS activates the B-cells indirectly by first triggering the macrophages and that this is the mechanism which occurs in the mice hyporesponsive to enterobacterial LPS, whereas the lipid A moiety triggers B-cells directly. Therefore different parts of the same molecule seem to interact with different types of host cell. There is also evidence which suggests that the immunopotentiating activity of a glycopeptide produced by mycobacteria is dependent on the saccharide residues of the molecule.

The outer membrane proteins associated with LPS in endotoxin preparations may themselves immunomodulate and there is evidence for direct effects on the immune system, that is without interleukin 1 acting as an intermediary. This suggests that prokaryotic molecules may mimic cytokine activity. This point will be returned to in relation to the mode of action of these immunomodulatory bacterial molecules.

LPS can also affect the expression of surface receptors, such as reducing the levels of receptors for the C5a component of complement (see Chapter 4) on polymorphonuclear leukocytes. Therefore LPS is apparently directly affecting gene expression in an unknown way.

Mode of action

With the exception of the superantigens (see below), molecular immunology research into the mode of action of these immunomodulatory molecules is still at an early stage of development; however, a number of possible routes of action can be speculated upon.

There is no obvious chemical group or moiety common to all these molecules which is responsible for their immunomodulating activity; however, one common feature is that they are amphiphiles, with both a hydrophobic part capable of dissolving in lipid membranes and a hydrophilic part which can remain in the water phase. Therefore a possible first step of molecular interaction is one between the amphiphilic molecule and the mammalian cell surface either by ionic binding, hydrogen bonding or hydrophobic interaction. The bacterial molecule may be inserted into the mammalian membrane by its hydrophobic moiety, or attach to membrane receptors with the hydrophilic moiety or through charge effects. Such interaction may then have the equivalent action of a host controlling molecule resulting in signal transduction and triggering of the cell. The immunomodulatory molecule may also mimic host molecules sufficiently to bind to host cell receptors and trigger cellular events. This interaction of bacterial molecules with host cell surface glycoproteins and glycolipids is well documented in relation to bacterial attachment to and entry into host cells (Chapters 7 and 8) and the action of bacterial toxins (Chapter 6).

Almost certainly much of the immunomodulating activity of many of these bacterial molecules is indirect and stems from the release of host mediators. There is growing evidence that the cytokines IL1, tumour necrosis factor (TNF; also called TNFα and cachectin) and IL6 are involved. The activities of these cytokines are described below and summarised in Table 2.2. As our knowledge and understanding of cytokines improves, so will our understanding of immunomodulation. It is probable that the activities of some of the more recently described cytokines such as IL10 and IL12 will also be modulated by infectious agents.

E. coli LPS will induce TNF and IL1 production in mice, and this in turn results in high levels of IL6. IL6 is known to be present in high levels in patients with a number of infectious diseases and in septic shock. LPS derived from Salmonella minnesota stimulates human endothelial cells to secrete IL6, as does IL1 and TNF. MDP increases the expression of the IL6 gene in human monocytes apparently independently of either IL1 or TNF, although addition of TNF enhances this expression.

The activities of **IL6** include regulation of the terminal stage of differentiation of B-cells to produce immunoglobulins, enhancement of the synthesis of acute phase proteins by hepatocytes, induction of a higher body temperature, synergistic action with IL1 on activation of T-cells. Together with IL3, it will also enhance proliferation of multi-potential haematopoietic progenitors, that is increase the number of stem cells from which the leukocytes develop.

IL1 (which exists in two forms alpha and beta) has many different functions which include: stimulation of the production of prostaglandin and proteases by fibroblasts; induction of synthesis of IL2 and expression of IL2 receptor in T-cells; effects on endothelial cells which result in vasodilation and leukocyte adhesion by inducing and increasing the expression of leukocyte adhesion molecules such as intercellular adhesion molecule (ICAM) 1 and 2 and E-selectin; and leukocyte recruitment by inducing the release of chemotactic factors such as IL8.

TNF is known to be involved in the induction of the catabolic state which often accompanies infection, and which if continued unchecked results in wasting and death (cachexia). The name, tumour necrosis factor, is slightly misleading as it refers to only one of the many activities of this cytokine, which overlaps with most of the activities of IL1 listed above, and the effects of the two cytokines may be additive. TNF may play a central role in the lethality of LPS as experimental results have shown that animals given a normally lethal dose of *E. coli* along with monoclonal antibodies which neutralise TNF survive. This indicates that death was caused by the host's over-reaction to the infection and not the infection or direct toxicity of the LPS. The activation of neutrophils by this cytokine is probably responsible for much of the morbidity and, along with the activation of epithelial cells, tumour necrosis activity. The mechanism by which LPS triggers TNF release from monocytes and macrophages is beginning to be understood. LPS-binding glycoproteins of about 60 kDa have been identified in elevated levels in serum during an acute phase response to challenge with LPS. This glycoprotein is synthesised in hepatocytes as a single 50 kDa polypeptide chain and has a binding site for lipid A. The **LPS binding protein** (LBP) contains sequences which are homologous with a protein from human plasma which is involved in transport of cholesterol ester. This suggests that both these molecules may be part of a family of molecules which transport amphipathic or hydrophobic molecules in aqueous environments. LBP will attach to Gram negative bacteria or free LPS and will mediate attachment to macrophages. The macrophage membrane receptor for the binding protein has been identified as CD14, a 55 kDa glycoprotein. The CD14 receptor molecule only recognises LBP when it is bound to LPS. The recognition of the LPS–LBP complex may either directly trigger TNF release, or hold the complex at the host cell surface in such a way that other host cell surface molecules trigger TNF release. LBPs also act as opsonins (Chapter 4), as do the other acute phase proteins which recognise bacterial surface molecules, C-reactive protein (CRP) and the mannan-binding proteins (MBP). They therefore form part of the non-clonal, but specific, recognition of bacteria which occurs within a matter of hours rather than the days required for clonal recognition by immunoglobulin. Interestingly, LBP shares regions of homology with bactericidal/permeability increasing (BPI) protein which is involved in the oxygen independent killing by phagocytic cells. BPI protein is lethal to some Gram negative bacteria (see Chapter 4).

Another intriguing possibility is that parts of the bacterial molecules may mimic host mediators directly. For example, MDP could have growth factor activity similar to that of IL1 or it could decrease or alter IL1 activity by binding to IL1 receptors. There is evidence that bacterial capsular polysaccharides may mimic the activity of IL1. The bacterium *Haemophilus actinomycetemcomitans*, which is associated with periodontal disease, produces an extracellular polysaccharide which apparently has some of the biological properties of IL1. MDP also resembles a sleep promoting glycopeptide, factor S, which is composed of glutamic acid, alanine, diaminopimelic acid and muramic acid. There is, however, some doubt as to whether factor S is truly a host product or derived from the peptidoglycan of commensal bacteria, as biosynthesis of muramic acid has not been detected in mammals. Fragments of peptidoglycan from *Neisseria gonorrhoeae* will induce slow-wave sleep in rabbits. It could therefore be speculated that the sleepiness associated with infections is caused by the infectious agent rather than a host response and that increased activity of gut commensal flora and leakage of MDP molecules from the gut contributes to the need for a postprandial snooze. It has also been suggested that MDP, although not synthesised by the host, is essential for its normal functions, in much the same way as vitamins are essential. It may be that the relationship between the host and the commensal flora is more complex than we realise at present.

The production of enzymes such as endoglycosidases and neuraminidases by bacteria (Chapter 5) could potentially modify any host molecule function in which oligosaccharides are involved. This could result in not only immunomodulation but the modification of the functioning of many systems within the body. Most cytokines and their receptors are glycoproteins, often with quite a large proportion of the molecule being composed of sugar residues. It seems that one of the possible functions of these sugar residues is regulation of the activity of the glycoprotein, akin to fine control tuning. This is the case for tissue plasminogen activator (tPA), a serum protease which induces fibrin clot lysis by converting plasminogen to plasmin. The activity of the hormone human chorionic gonadotrophin is dependent on the sugar residues of the glycoprotein, as when these are removed the hormone becomes inactive. So it is possible to speculate that, in the future, examples of molecules involved in the regulation of the immune system will be found where the oligosaccharide moieties are necessary for activity. Another area where sugar residues play an important role is in cell surface glycoprotein interactions which involve protein–carbohydrate recognition. Some of these are listed in Table 2.3. In the recircu-

Table 2.3. Host cell interactions mediated by carbohydrate–protein recognition

Recognition site on:	
Protein	Oligosaccharide
L-selectin on lymphocytes, neutrophils and eosinophils	50 kDa glycoprotein on high endothelial venules
E-selectin on microvascular endothelial cells	Glycoconjugate on neutrophils, monocytes and memory T-cells
P-selectin on platelets and endothelial cells	Glycoconjugates on neutrophils and monocytes
IgE receptor on B-cells, macrophage and eosinophils	IgE

lation and recruitment of leukocytes in the body the carbohydrate-recognising protein domains of glycoproteins of one cell bind specifically to the oligosaccharides of glycoconjugates on another type of cell. These recognition events control, for example, the movement of bloodborne lymphocytes into lymphoid organs. Specific recognition occurs between the lymphocyte and specialised cells in the wall of the blood vessel, known as high endothelial venules (HEV). The effect of the cleavage of sialic acid from oligosaccharides by neuraminidase enzymes on lymphocyte movement is considered in Chapter 5.

As a clearer understanding of cellular interactions is obtained, particularly with respect to the workings of the immune system, our understanding of bacterial immunomodulatory mechanisms should progress.

IMMUNOMODULATORY MOLECULES: TOXINS AND SUPERANTIGENS

It is now clear that a number of bacterial molecules, initially characterised as toxins, mediate their toxic effects by immunomodulation. The effect is not therefore simply one of direct toxicity to host cells, as in for example the ADP-ribosylation of intracellular control molecules (see Chapter 6), but an indirect stimulation of the immune system. Some toxins, such as the ADP-ribosylating toxins, with direct activity on host cells **also** act as immunomodulators. It is likely that this immunomodulatory activity is due, in some instances, to the binding of the toxin to host cell surface receptors and is separate from the toxic enzymic activity on host cell molecules (see Chapter 6). For example, cholera toxin has long been known for its adjuvant effect when inoculated along with another antigen. There is now evidence that it has direct effects on differentiating B-cells which cause the alteration of gene expression and this may be responsible for its activity as an adjuvant. Under normal conditions, B-cells switch from the production of one type of immunoglobulin, or isotype, to another as they differentiate under the influence of cytokines such as IL4 (see Chapter 3). Cholera toxin enhances the switch to the expression of the isotype IgG1 over and above the normal activity of IL4 alone. Thus IgG1 secreting B-cells are produced at the expense of IgM or IgG3 producing B-cells. This activity is related to the binding subunits of the toxin and not the enzymatically active subunit.

The toxicity of another group of bacterial toxins, including pyrogens, staphylococcal enterotoxins and toxic shock syndrome toxin, is thought to be mediated by immunomodulation. These are called the 'superantigens' because of the molecular basis of their immunomodulatory activity. Table 2.4 illustrates the range of bacteria which produce superantigens. Many of these are also referred to as the pyrogenic toxins because fever is frequently associated with intoxication. Most of these protein toxins fall into the

Table 2.4. Bacterial superantigen toxins

Bacterium	Molecular mass (kDa)	Toxin
Streptococcus pyogenes	25,29,24	Pyrogenic exotoxins A,B and C (SPE; scarlet/rheumatic fever toxins)
Staphylococcus aureus	22	Toxic shock syndrome toxin 1 (TSST1)
	12,18	Pyrogenic exotoxin A and B
	27–28	Enterotoxin A,B,C1–C3, D and E (SE)
	27	Exfoliatin toxin A and B (ET)
Pseudomonas aeruginosa	66	Exotoxin A
Mycoplasma arthritidis	?	Arthritis inducing toxin in rats

approximate molecular weight range of 20–30 kDa and many show signifi-
cant DNA sequence homology.

The enterotoxins of *Staphylococcus aureus*, designated A, B, C, D and E,
cause a rapid form of toxic food poisoning if food containing toxin is
ingested. Examination of the intestinal epithelium does not reveal any
associated damage, as would be the case for an ADP-ribosylating toxin,
such as cholera (see Chapter 6). Instead numerous T-cells are observed in
the underlying tissue. Investigations of the effect of enterotoxin on T-cells
showed that a small amount of entertoxin, less than that required for the
mitogenic effect of, for example concanavalin A or phytohaemagglutinin,
would trigger proliferation of as many as one in five T-cells, whereas normal antigen recognition triggers proliferation of about 1 in 10 000. (Normal
antigen, as opposed to superantigen, recognition by T-cells is described in
Chapter 3, Figures 3.2 and 3.3). T-cells which proliferate in response to
normal antigens carry T-cell receptors (TCR) specific for the antigen; those
which proliferate in response to superantigens do not. Superantigen-
induced T-cell proliferation requires presentation of antigen by antigen-
presenting cells, but in most instances no processing of the antigen. The
response time is therefore faster than with normal antigens which require
cellular processing of the antigen before presentation at the cell surface
in association with major histocompatibility group (MHC) molecules (see
Chapter 3). Antigen is presented to the T-cells not in the peptide groove

or cleft of the MHC Class II molecule, where antigen is normally presented, but at a different binding site on the MHC (Figure 2.6). Staphylococcal enterotoxins A and B bind at the same site on MHC Class II HLA-DR molecules. The enterotoxin then also binds to the variable region of the beta chain (V_β) of the TCR (Figure 2.6). Each individual has about 30 different types of V_β chain and the superantigen can only bind specifically to perhaps two or three of these, but as the V_β can be from a TCR of any **antigenic** specificity, far more T-cells will be affected than with a conventional antigen. The effects of this recognition are multiple and also dependent on the T-cell which is stimulated. T-cells carrying either the CD4 or CD8 cell surface glycoprotein recognise, or are recognised by, superantigens although binding is restricted to the MHC Class II molecule on the antigen-presenting cell. This is different from T-cell recognition of antigen in the MHC peptide groove, when MHC Class II only associates with CD4+ T-cells and MHC Class I with CD8+ T-cells (Chapter 3, Figure 3.1). If the recognition event occurs with a CD8+ cytotoxic T-cell, cytolysis of the antigen-presenting cell may ensue. The bacterium has therefore evolved a mechanism for the cytolysis of host cells which are highly efficient antigen presenting cells. This has the potential to destroy specific MHC Class II dependent

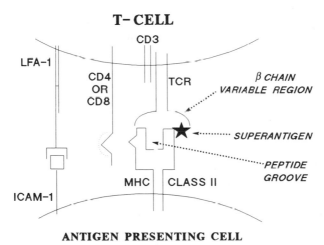

Figure 2.6. Recognition of superantigens. The superantigen (star) binds to the major histocompatibility group (MHC) Class II molecules, but not in the peptide groove where most antigens bind (see Figure 3.1). The superantigen also binds to the variable region on the β chain of a number of T-cell receptors (TCR). The T-cell does not need a CD4 molecule, which is normally required for MHC Class II–TCR interactions (see Figure 3.3) as CD8 positive T-cells are also reactive. Attachment of leukocyte functional antigen 1 (LFA-1) to immune cell adhesion molecule 1 (ICAM-1) is necessary. Where binding is to a CD4 positive T-cell, the cytokines IL2, IL4 and γ interferon are released from the T-cell, IL1 is released by the antigen-presenting cell and T-cell multiplication ensues. Binding to a CD8 positive T-cell, on the other hand, results in lysis of the antigen-presenting cell by the cytolytic T-cell

recognition. Binding of leukocyte function associated antigen (LFA) 1 (CD11a/CD18) on the cytotoxic T-cell to ICAM-1 (CD54) on the antigen presenting cell is necessary for this recognition event to take place. Stimulation and proliferation of CD4+ helper T-cells, on the other hand, will result in massive over-production of cytokines. It appears that it is these cytokines, in particular IL2, which are responsible for the symptoms associated with intoxication, for example vomiting, diarrhoea and fever. In the case of enterotoxins ingested in food the effects are transitory; however, where the toxin is produced by an infecting bacterium, the continued release of cytokines has a far more severe systemic effect. This is the case in toxic shock syndrome which is sometimes associated with the use of vaginal tampons. The clinical symptoms of toxic shock syndrome include diarrhoea, fever, renal failure and cardiac and pulmonary dysfunction, all of which may lead to death.

Immunosuppression is another possible outcome of superantigen activity, particularly where clones of T-cells stimulated by the superantigen either become inactivated or are deleted. The effects on T-cells will also influence the activities of B-cells which come under T-cell control, in particular where the B-cell is the antigen-presenting cell. Staphylococcal enterotoxin (SE) D induces IgM and IgG secretion when it cross-links B-cells and T-cells, whereas SEC induces T-cell proliferation but not immunoglobulin secretion. Other superantigens include the minor lymphocyte stimulating (Mls) antigens which are encoded by a mouse mammary tumour retrovirus that has integrated into the mouse germline DNA.

It is likely that SEA, SED and SEE are derived from a common ancestral gene as examination of the amino acid sequences of these superantigens has revealed striking similarity. SEB, SEC1–3 and streptococcal pyrogenic exotoxin (SPE) A can also be grouped together on the basis of amino acid similarity. Regions of DNA homology can also be identified amongst the other streptococcal and staphylococcal superantigens which have been sequenced. These include TSST-1, staphylococcal exfoliative toxin and SPEC.

It is now apparent that the genes encoding some of the superantigens are capable of both moving within the bacterial genome and transferring between bacteria. This genetic mobility is common to a number of bacterial virulence genes. The details of the genetic mechanisms involved are discussed in Chapter 9. The gene for TSST1, *tst*, is encoded on a mobile genetic element which is capable of insertion at a number of sites on the bacterial chromosome. The expression of the *tst* gene is under the trans-acting regulation of the accessory gene regulator (*agr*; designated *exp* by some workers), which also controls the expression of staphylokinase and haemolysins (see Chapters 5 and 9). The genes encoding the staphylococcal enterotoxins (SE) are also encoded on mobile genetic elements. The *entB*, *entC* and *entD* genes may be present on either plasmids or the chromosome.

It seems likely that movement of these genes (*tst* and *entB*, *entC* and *entD*) is dependent upon a hitchhiking transposon. As the expression of some of these toxins is mutually exclusive it is likely that the transposon has a limited number of integration sites within the bacterial chromosome. The *entA* gene which encodes SEA is located on a phage which can integrate at several chromosomal loci. The genes for streptococcal pyrogenic toxins A and C (*speA* and *speC*) are also carried by phage. *SpeA* is located on the lysogenic phage T12, which is thought to have originally acquired the *speA* gene as a result of abnormal excision of the phage. This may explain why a number of virulence determinants are phage encoded and raises the possibility of phage transfer of any virulence gene which maps close to a phage attachment site. The genetic mobility of other bacterial virulence determinants is considered in Chapter 9.

CONCLUSION

Immunomodulation can be seen from two different perspectives. From the point of view of the host it can act as a rapid recognition that the body has been invaded; this sets in motion all the systems of the body which have evolved to defend it. The bacterium then has the opportunity to interfere with the regulation of these systems and potentially use this to its own advantage. Immunomodulation may therefore either aid the clearance of bacterial infection or, if over stimulation occurs, may be potentially harmful to the host.

FURTHER READING

General

Baumann H., Gauldie J. 1994. The acute phase response. Immunology Today 15, 74–80.
Janeway C. A. 1989. Approaching the asymptote? Evolution and revolution in immunology. Cold Spring Harbor Symposia on Quantitative Biology 54, 1–13.
Owen P., Foster T. J. 1988. (Eds). Immunochemical and molecular genetic analysis of bacterial pathogens. Elsevier, Amsterdam, NL.
Steel D. M., Whitehead A. S. 1994. The major acute phase reactants: C-reactive protein, serum amyloid P component and serum amyloid A protein. Immunology Today 15, 81–88.
Stewart-Tull D. E. S., Davies M. (Eds). 1985. Immunology of the bacterial cell envelope. J Wiley & Sons, Chichester.

Cell envelope

Doyle R. J., Sonnefeld E. M. 1989. Properties of the cell surfaces of pathogenic bacteria. International Review of Cytology 118, 33–92.

Harvey W., Kamin S., Meghji S., Wilson M. 1987. Interleukin-1 like activity in capsular material from *Haemophilus actinomycetemcomitans*. Immunology 60, 415–418.

Holtje J-V., Tuomanen E. I. 1991. The murein hydrolases of *Escherichia coli*: properties, functions and impact on the course of infections *in vivo*. Journal of General Microbiology 137, 441–454.

Klasen I. S., Kool J., Melief M. J. 1992. Arthritis by autoreactive T cell lines obtained from rats after injection of intestinal bacterial cell wall fragments. Cellular Immunology 139, 455–467.

Raedmacher T. W., Dwek R. A. 1989. The role of oligosaccharides in modifying protein function. Carbohydrate recognition in cellular function. Ciba Foundation Symposium 145. J Wiley & Sons, Chichester. pp 241–256.

Schumann R. R., Leong S. R., Flaggs G. W. *et al.* 1990. Structure and function of lipopolysaccharide binding protein. Science 249, 1429–1431.

Stoolman L. M. 1992. Selectins (LEC-CAMs): lectin-like receptors involved in lymphocyte recirculation and leukocyte recruitment. In: Cell surface carbohydrates and cell development (Ed M. Fukuda). CRC Press. Chapter 3.

Wright S. D., Ramos R. A., Tobias P. S. *et al.* 1990. CD14, a receptor for complexes of lipopolysaccharide and LPS binding protein. Science 249, 1431–1433.

Superantigens

Gohach G. A., Fast D. J., Nelson R. D., Shlievert P. M. 1990. Staphylococcal and streptococcal pyrogenic toxins involved in toxic shock syndromes and related illnesses. Critical Reviews in Microbiology 17, 251–272.

He X., Goronzy J., Weyand C. 1992. Selective induction of rheumatoid factors by superantigens and human helper T cells. Journal of Clinical Investigation 89, 673–680.

Johnson H. M., Russell J. K., Pontzer C. H. 1992. Superantigens in human disease. Scientific American April, 42–48, 73.

Misfeldt M. L. 1990. Microbial superantigens. Infection and Immunity 58, 2409–2413.

3 Clonal Recognition: Antibodies and T-cell Receptors

INTRODUCTION

Clonal recognition occurs when specific molecules on a clone of host cells fit onto one small part, or epitope, of a foreign molecule resulting in stimulation of the host cell. This fitting of the host cell surface molecule to a single bacterial epitope will in some instances trigger cell proliferation and therefore enlargement of the clone. This will normally occur concomitantly with non-clonal activation where host cells specific for different epitopes are stimulated by a different type of signal (see Figure I.1). This recognition of foreign molecules can occur in two ways. Some bacterial components are recognised directly. Others are recognised only after host cells have processed the bacterial molecules and compared them with the molecules which identify the host as self.

The host molecules involved in these recognition processes are the major histocompatibility group (MHC) molecules, the T-cell antigen receptors (TCR) and the B-cell antigen receptors, the immunoglobulins (Ig). All of these recognition molecules have some degree of gene sequence homology and are thought to be related in evolutionary terms. They belong to what is called the immunoglobulin superfamily of molecules. We will now consider their involvement in specific recognition of bacteria.

MAJOR HISTOCOMPATIBILITY GROUP MOLECULES

Human cell surface glycoprotein molecules encoded by genes in the MHC region of chromosome 6 are the markers which identify cells as self. The MHC molecules are low affinity receptors for processed antigens, usually short peptides. These are produced as a result of degradation or processing of protein antigens, either from the host cell or from, for example, the degradation of a bacterial cell or other foreign protein within the host cell. After this, fragments of the molecules (peptides of usually between 8 and 24 amino acids long) are presented on the cell surface, associated with the MHC molecule in such a way that the presented peptide fragment is ensconced in a 'groove' on the surface of the MHC (Figure 3.1). The mode of presentation of the antigen has been likened to the sausage in a hot-dog bun. The small amount of information available about the processing of

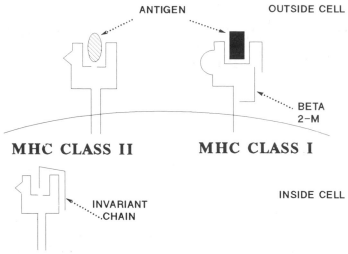

Figure 3.1. Major histocompatibility group (MHC) molecules Class I and II. MHC Class I molecules are composed of a single chain to which β-2 microglobulin (β 2-M) is non-covalently associated. MHC Class II molecules are composed of two chains, α and β. Antigen is presented to T-cells at the cell surface in the peptide groove. In the cytosol the groove of MHC Class II molecules is occupied by a host derived peptide known as the invariant chain

polysaccharide antigens is described below under 'T-cell Help and Immunoglobulin Production'.

The affinity of the MHC molecule for the presented antigen is not as great as it would be between, for example, the antigen and its specific T-cell receptor or immunoglobulin. The part of the antigen involved in this association may differ for different MHC molecules present in the one cell; therefore different epitopes may be presented on the same cell. Once at the cell surface the MHC glycoprotein–antigen complex is 'inspected' by T-cells. These processed pieces of foreign molecules are recognised by T-cell receptors (TCRs) specific for a part of the peptide antigen which is different from that which associates with either the MHC molecule or immunoglobulins.

The MHC glycoproteins come in two types (Figure 3.1): Class I and Class II.

The Class I antigens are subdivided into types A, B and C and are present on all nucleated cells and platelets. These are single transmembrane glycoproteins and are associated non-covalently with a molecule known as β-2 microglobulin which is also a member of the immunoglobulin superfamily. In normal host cells part of all of the proteins produced by that cell will be present on the host cell surface in association with the MHC Class I.

The Class II antigens are subdivided into types DP, DQ and DR and are only found on B-lymphocytes, monocytes, macrophages, dendritic cells, melanoma cells, some activated T-cells and possibly some epithelial cells. They consist of two non-covalently associated glycoproteins (α and β) and are also inserted into the plasma membrane. A third glycoprotein, known as the invariant chain, may be associated with the α and β chains from the time of synthesis in the rough endoplasmic reticulum, until the Class II MHC associates with the peptide which it subsequently presents at the cell surface. It is thought that two MHC Class II heterodimers interact together, possibly allowing interaction with two TCRs at the same time.

These Class I and II antigens are also sometimes referred to as human lymphocyte antigens (HLA), although their expression is not confined to lymphocytes. MHC molecules can also be detected free from cells in body fluids, although it is the membrane associated molecules which are involved in antigen presentation.

The variation (or polymorphism) in the genes which encode for the MHC glycoproteins leads to, in an out-bred population, variations in regions of these molecules between individuals. For example, there may be as many as 70 different possible Class I B molecules within the human population. As these glycoproteins mark the host cell as self and the host carries more than one type of identifying molecule, this reduces the probability of a bacterium successfully mimicking all the identity markers of an individual. Therefore variation in the host's identity molecules within individuals, and also between individuals in and out-bred population, may help to indirectly limit the extent of infectious diseases. The higher susceptibility of the cheetah to viral epizootics, when compared with other big cats, is thought to be caused by a lack of diversity in the MHC locus in this animal.

ANTIGEN PRESENTATION

In relation to infection, the MHC group Class I and II molecules are involved in the presentation of both host derived and foreign antigen at the host cell surface. Parts of practically all the peptides produced within a host cell are presented at the surface in association with MHC group Class I molecules. T-lymphocytes are thought to only recognise foreign antigen when it is associated with MHC molecules.

Figures 3.2 and 3.3 summarise the presentation of molecules by either Class I or II MHC and the consequences of this. During biosynthesis of Class II molecules an 'invariant' peptide chain associates with the α and β chains. The term invariant is used as the gene encoding for this peptide and the corresponding amino acid sequence do not vary between individuals, as does the MHC (i.e. the gene is not subject to allelic polymorphism). The invariant chain is thought to direct the movement of the MHC Class II molecules from the endoplasmic reticulum to the endocytic vesicles of the host cell. The presence of the invariant chain probably also prevents the association of Class II molecules with the same peptides as the Class I mol-

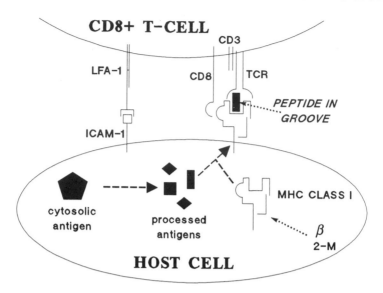

Figure 3.2. Antigen presentation by MHC Class I molecules. All host cells carry MHC Class I molecules, which normally present molecules derived from the cytosol of the cell at the cell surface. If the cell is infected by a microorganism, parts of the microorganism will be presented at the cell surface, instead of parts of the cell. These will then be recognised by T-cells which carry the CD8 glycoprotein and the infected cell will usually be destroyed by the T-cell

ecules. Class II molecules associate with antigens which are synthesised outside the host cell, such as whole bacteria which may have been taken up by the host cell by phagocytosis, or parts of bacteria which may be taken up by either phagocytosis or endocytosis (see Chapter 4). After being subjected to degradation by host cell enzymes, or processed, the fragments of molecules associate with the MHC molecules in the endocytic vesicles. It is thought that the low pH of endocytic vesicles favours the dissociation of the invariant chain from the MHC Class II molecule, thus allowing binding of the processed peptide which is subsequently presented at the host cell surface.

Therefore **exogenous** antigens are processed by the antigen-presenting cells and presented to T-cells in association with Class II molecules. Hence molecules from bacteria growing in the extracellular matrix and body fluids are presented in this way. These foreign antigen–Class II combinations are recognised by the T-cell receptors of T-cells which express the CD4 glycoprotein (called L3T4 in mice). These MHC Class II restricted T-cells subsequently become activated. This forms the most important aspect of specific recognition of bacteria which are free-living (i.e. not intracellular) by T-

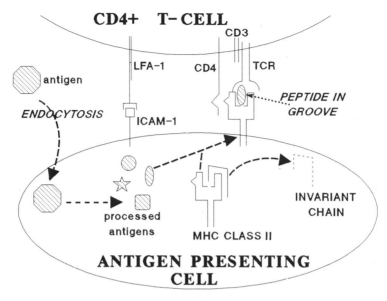

Figure 3.3. Antigen presentation by MHC Class II molecules. MHC Class II molecules are only present on a restricted range of host cells, for example monocytes/macrophages, B-cells and other specialised antigen-presenting cells such as dendritic cells. Antigens which enter into the cellular vacuoles by either endocytosis or phagocytosis are broken down or processed. The processed parts displace the host-cell derived invariant chain and are presented at the cell surface by the MHC Class II molecule. The antigen is recognised by T-cells which carry the CD4 glycoprotein. CD4 positive T-cells release cytokines (T-cell help) which will have multiple effects on other cells in the area as well as the antigen-presenting cell

cells. Upon activation of the T-cells cytokines are released (termed T-cell help) which enhance and control the activity of other cells of the immune system. The activity of these cytokines is particularly important in the activation of macrophages, recruitment of phagocytic neutrophils to the site of infection and in the control of B-cell differentiation and antibody production.

Class I molecules are known to be associated with the presentation of antigens which are formed within the cell, either by the host cell itself or by intracellular bacteria such as *Listeria monocytogenes* and *Mycobacterium leprae* and also viruses. Molecules to be presented are thought to be selectively transferred from the cytoplasm into the endoplasmic reticulum by permease-type enzymes present in the membrane. The molecular fragments associate with the MHC in the endoplasmic reticulum, not in endocytic vesicles as with Class II molecules, and then move to the host cell surface. The host cell is therefore normally decorated with fragments of its own molecules and, if it is being parasitised by a bacterium, also fragments of the bacterium. Associations of Class I molecules with foreign antigens are recognised by the T-cell receptors on T-cells which express the CD8 molecules (called Lyt 2 in mice). The process of recognition then triggers these T-cells to lyse the cells presenting the foreign antigen. The induced lytic activity is therefore very specifically restricted. This will be considered in relation to the cytolytic activity of T-cells below.

The relationship between expression of either the CD4 or CD8 glycoprotein and T-cell function is not, however, always clear-cut. Although normally the CD4 molecule interacts with MHC Class II and CD8 with MHC Class I, the activities triggered in the T-cells are not **always** those of T-cell help and T-cell cytotoxicity respectively. CD4 bearing cytotoxic T-cells and CD8 positive T-helper cells have been described. Also, both CD8 and CD4 bearing T-cells have been reported to release cytokines which suppress the immune system, although at present less is known about the activities of this type of cell. These cells are sometimes referred to as T-suppressor cells; however, it is likely that the types and activities of cytokines released from T-cells can vary depending on the environment surrounding the cell and that a T-helper may become a T-suppressor cell with varying external conditions.

T-CELL HELP AND IMMUNOGLOBULIN PRODUCTION

The antigen-presenting cells which constitutively express the Class II MHC molecules (e.g. B-lymphocytes, macrophages, dendritic cells) are all involved in the processing of foreign molecules and the presentation of parts of these molecules to T-cells as discussed in detail above.

Presentation to a subset of T-cells, known as **T-helper** (T_h) cells which normally carry the CD4 cell surface glycoprotein, is important for the subsequent production of highly specific immunoglobulin by B-cells. This section deals with the mechanisms by which the host produces this specific antibody, while the next section covers the activities of the immunoglobulin molecules.

Molecules are taken up by the antigen presenting cells probably by endocytosis and whole bacteria by phagocytosis. Parts of the bacteria are then processed or degraded by enzymes in endosomes and lysosomes as discussed above.

Most of our knowledge of antigen presentation involves protein and polypeptide antigens. It is not yet known if carbohydrate antigens are processed and presented in a similar way. Some of the polysaccharides of the bacterial envelope, for example lipopolysaccharides and peptidoglycans, are readily degraded in phagocytic cells by the action of enzymes such as lysozyme or lipases; however, it is less likely that degradative enzymes for the many different types of extracellular capsular polysaccharides are present in mammalian cells. Also, there is no strong evidence that carbohydrate specific T_h cells exist. This may be to prevent T-cells from reacting against the carbohydrate moieties of the mammalian cell surface glycoproteins. T-cell help for production of anti-carbohydrate antibody may therefore be dependent on T-cells which recognise non-carbohydrate bacterial molecules and release cytokines in the area of the host where the infection is occurring. T-cells specific for the glucose polymer, dextran, have been described. These T-cells suppress B-cell activity, probably by releasing inhibitory rather than stimulatory cytokines. Thus, the production of IgG specific for dextran is suppressed and the accumulation of dextran specific memory B-cells is controlled. What role, if any, these carbohydrate specific T-cells might play in combating bacterial infection remains to be elucidated, as does the fine detail of how the imune system deals with carbohydrate and lipid antigens.

Antigen presentation enables the host, through the T-cell receptor and associated molecules, to compare the foreign antigen with self. Where the T-cell receptor of a T_h cell is specific for the bacterial component, the T-cell becomes activated, resulting in the release of 'help' in the form of cell growth and stimulatory factors (cytokines such as IL1, IL2, IL4, IL6, γ IF). As only T-cells which recognise or are specific for an individual epitope are affected, the recognition event is clonal. These cytokines can act on cells provided they are expressing the appropriate cytokine receptor, activating them, in turn, and also causing further proliferation and differentiation. As yet specific attraction between a cell presenting a particular antigen and T- and B-cells specific for epitopes on the same antigen has not been demonstrated.

The activities of the cytokines of T-cell help include the growth and expansion of the T-cell clone itself. This is termed autocrine stimulation of the T-cell. The cytokines may also attract and activate macrophages at the site of infection. This is an essential part of the defence against intracellular bacterial parasites where specific antibodies, although useful in preventing bacterial attachment to host cells by interfering with attachment mechanisms (see below), may not be effective in clearing an established intracellular infection such as those caused by *Mycobacterium tuberculosis*, *Neisseria gonorrhoeae* and *Listeria monocytogenes*. Cytolytic T cells may also be involved in combating infection with intracellular bacteria, providing a more specific killing mechanism than the macrophages (see below).

T-cell help is also required for the full range of the B-cell response to infection. The B-cell response involves an initial activation or priming of the B-cell by specific recognition of a foreign molecule by surface membrane associated **immunoglobulin** (sIg). As only B-cells with some specificity for the foreign molecule are activated, the recognition is again clonal. The part of the molecule or epitope, recognised by the B-cell will be different from that recognised by the T-cell receptor. Under the influence of the T-cell derived cytokines, the activated B-cells proliferate and the expression of

Class II antigens and sIg is increased. B-cells then become efficient antigen presenters as the uptake of antigen occurs specifically through sIg. That is the B-cell takes up antigen by sIg, processes it and presents it in association with Class II molecules to the T-cell which in turn secretes cytokines which help the B-cell to multiply and differentiate. Precursor B-cells originate in the bone marrow in adults and each has the potential to undergo a series of changes which results in mature B-cells. The differentiation process involves gene rearrangements to enable production of immunoglobulin with different specificities; the generation of diversity. One of several hundred gene segments coding for the variable region of the immunoglobulin is recombined with the other gene segements necessary to form the complete immunoglobulin molecule. Somatic mutation of these genes also occurs during B-cell development (see below). Further gene rearrangements occur at a later stage of B-cell development which generate different classes of immunoglobulin, while retaining the same antigenic specificity. B-cells at an early stage of development express surface immunoglobulin classes M and D. The class of an immunoglobulin is determined by the heavy chain component of the antibody molecule, all classes of immunoglobulin having either κ or λ light chains associated with them (see Appendix for structure of antibody molecules). After primary stimulation with antigen, IgM is secreted. Secondary stimulation with more antigen results in further gene rearrangements and either IgG, IgA or IgE antibodies being expressed and secreted.

IgG and IgA can also be divided into subclasses which, in some instances, seem to be associated with particular antigens (see below). This change in the type of antibody produced as the B-cell matures is termed 'class switching'. IgM is therefore the primary antibody produced in response to infection and raised levels in serum can be used to monitor infection. The secondary stimulation of B-cells results in the formation of different classes or subclasses of antibody with the same specificity as the IgM. IgG is also present in quantity in circulating serum, and is an **opsonising antibody**. This means that when attached specifically it renders the bacterium more susceptible to phagocytic uptake (see Chapter 4). Normally only the IgM and IgG subclasses 1 and 3 trigger the classical complement pathway (Chapter 4). **IgA** is present in serum in low concentrations, but is the predominant antibody present in mucosal secretions on for example oral, bronchial, respiratory, intestinal, urinary and genital epithelial surfaces. The binding of IgA to antigen does not initiate the lytic activity of complement as this would potentially damage the mucosal surface. In relation to the host defences, IgA production is in the front line, as it protects the host from the challenge of both inhaled and ingested microorganisms. About 5–15 g of IgA are secreted at mucosal surfaces each day and this accounts for more than 60% of all immunoglobulin produced daily. The function of IgA in relation to host defence and mucosal immunity will be discussed again later in this chapter (Figure 3.6).

IgE antibody is not involved in defence against bacterial infection. It is found in very small amounts in serum and is largely involved in defence against infection of the gut by helminthic worms. Components of the worm infecting the gut cross the gut epithelium and this stimulates an IgE response in the gut associated lymphoid tissue. Mast cells become coated with the specific IgE as they mature and subsequently migrate to the gut mucosa. When they come into contact with the worm they degranulate and release mediators which increase vascular permeability and attractants for cells such as eosinophils which carry Fc receptors for IgE. The eosinophils kill worms that are coated with specific IgE. This mechanism, which has evolved to defend us against parasitic worms, has an unfortunate side effect. In some individuals quantities of IgE specific for innocuous antigens such as pollen are produced. This leads to inappropriate immune responses known as allergies (Type 1 hypersensitivity reactions) where the immune response can damage the host. Examples include asthma, hay fever and eczema.

There is growing evidence that **subsets** of **T-helper** (T_h) cells in mice regulate the class of immunoglobulin expressed by secreting different lymphokines. A T_h cell, termed T_h2, secretes IL4 and IL5 which induce the expression of IgG1, IgE and IgA in B-cells. The T_h1 subset does not secrete IL4 but does secrete γ IF and IL2 which induces the expression of mouse IgG2a and antibody. Other cells such as dendritic cells may also be involved in the control of class switching of antibody types. It therefore seems likely that the mixture of cytokines in the micro-environment surrounding the B-cell controls the switch to an appropriate class of immunoglobulin in a particular tissue, for example IgA in the gut mucosa.

Gene rearrangements can also result in **somatic hypermutation** of the immunoglobulin genes coding for the variable region of the immunoglobulin molecule, which is present on both the heavy and light chains. This means that rearrangements of the DNA occur without meiosis and interchange of chromosomes between cells. The mutation events occur in the region of the gene coding for the variable part of the immunoglobulin, the V region and tend to be localised at particular regions within this gene or 'hot-spots'. These frequently contain palindromic sequences of DNA.

By a process of clonal selection not yet clearly understood, B-cells producing higher affinity immunoglobulin for the original antigen are selected for, possibly because of the way in which they interact with the antigen. If the interaction with the antigen is of high affinity the B-cells receive some sort of 'survival signal'; if it is not high affinity, there is no survival signal and the B-cells die by controlled cell death, or apoptosis.

The B-cells then either become long-lived memory cells, which retain the ability to produce high affinity immunoglobulin and persist in the lymphoid organs such as the spleen, or terminally differentiate into plasma cells which are specialised immunoglobulin producing 'factory' cells. This process is central to specific adaptive immunity of the host whereby the host can improve on its inherited or 'naive' B-cell repertoire by generating a 'memory' B-cell repertoire, capable of producing immunoglobulin of higher affinity. In other words the host has a 'memory' of an encounter with a foreign molecule which allows it to produce high affinity immunoglobulin if it encounters the same foreign molecule at a later date.

A number of bacterial molecules activate B-cells independently of T-cells. These are termed **T-independent** (T_{ind}) **antigens** and are generally polymeric in nature. Extracellular polysaccharides such as levan and dextran, LPS and flagella which are composed of protein polymers have all been shown to be T_{ind} in mice. It is thought that the cross-linking of the surface immunoglobulin by the polymers is involved in activation of the B-cell clone involved. Some of these molecules may also act directly as mitogens after binding specifically to the surface immunoglobulin. At higher concentrations the bacterial molecules can act as polyclonal B-cell activators, stimulating B-cells not carrying immunoglobulin specific for their epitopes (Chapter 2). It is likely that although B-cell activation and proliferation may occur in a T_{ind} manner, some form of non-specific T-cell help, probably in the form of cytokine activity, is necessary for the production of antibody secreting cells. A subset of B-cells (carrying a surface molecule known as CD5 in humans and Ly-1 in mice) will react in this way and it is thought that these cells do not go through hypermutation of the immunoglobulin genes or go on to form memory cells (Figure 3.4). The antibody produced by these B-cells is therefore generally low affinity IgM and probably constitutes a rapid initial first line of defence, with the later production of high affinity immunoglobulin being necessary for successful elimination of the pathogen. The T_h cell dependence of B-cell memory production may be a way of avoiding the acquisition of auto-reactive B-cells, that is B-cells which produce immunoglobulin which is specific for host molecules, as a result of hypermutation. Auto-reactive T-cells are selected against an early stage of development in the thymus. As T-cells do not appear to undergo somatic hypermutation, recognition of an antigen by both the T-cell receptor and immunoglobulin may be an important way of selecting against any anti-self B-cell clones generated by hypermutation.

Studies of human serum samples have revealed that the pattern of **IgG subclass** produced relates to the antigen (Table 3.1). It is striking that the IgG subclasses 1 and 2 are the predominant serum immunoglobulins produced in response to polysaccharide antigens (top half of Table 3.1). The subclasses produced may also vary depending on how the individual is exposed to the antigen, that is whether by natural infection or immunisation. Another difficulty is that Ig subclass distribution in serum may differ from that measured at the site of infection. This was found to be the case

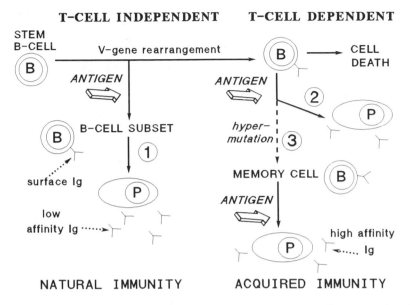

Figure 3.4. Routes of B-cell differentiation. B-cells (B) may differentiate by three pathways, each of which requires stimulation by antigen. 1. A small subgroup of B-cells, which in humans carry the CD5 surface glycoprotein, can differentiate into immunoglobulin (Ig) factory cells called plasma cells (P) without cytokine help from T-cells or their genes undergoing somatic mutation (T-cell independent). The immunoglobulin produced is of low affinity. 2. Plasma cells are produced from B-cells with T-cell help (T-cell dependent). 3. The immunoglobulin genes can undergo somatic mutation. Any B-cells in which mutations give rise to immunoglobulin of higher affinity for the antigen will be selected for. These can form memory B-cells, which may differentiate into plasma cells if exposed to the same antigen at a later date. As this involves the mutational evolution of genes encoding for altered immunoglobulin, under the selective pressure of antigen, this type of immunity is termed 'acquired immunity'. Reproduced, with permission from the *Annual Review of Immunology*, Volume 7, © 1989, by Annual Reviews Inc

for *Porphyromonas gingivalis*, which is associated with periodontal disease. Measurement of serum IgG antibody levels indicated that antibody specific for fimbrial protein was predominantly IgG1, 2 and 3. Antibody present in the gingival crevice was, however, predominantly IgG1 and IgG4. Age also plays a part in the IgG subclass repertoire as once maternal antibody levels decline, humans are not apparently capable of producing the full range of IgG subclasses until about the age of two. IgG2 levels, in particular, are low. This may have implications for the increased susceptibility of babies to infection by bacteria such as *Haemophilus influenzae* (Chapter 7) where the major virulence determinants are polysaccharides. Interestingly adults who are deficient in IgG2 production are more susceptible to infection by bacteria in which the polysaccharides are associated with virulence. The

Table 3.1. Immunoglobulin class production in response to various antigens

Antigen	Major immunoglobulin class					
	IgA1	IgA2	IgG1	IgG2	IgG3	IgG4
Normal Mucosa	+		u	u	u	u
LPS, e.g. *Salmonella* spp. *Shigella* spp. *Vibrio cholerae*		+	+	+		
Teichoic acid		+	+	+		
Streptococcus pneumoniae PS		+	+	+		
Haemophilus influenzae type b PS: infection	u	u	+	+		
vaccine			+	+		
Streptococcus pyogenes PS	u	u		+		
Streptococcus agalactiae PS	u	u	+	+		
Neisseria meningitidis PS	u	u	+	+		
Klebsiella pneumoniae PS	u	u	+	+		
Tetanus toxoid vaccine	u	u	+			+
Cholera toxin vaccine	u	u	+	+		
Pertussis toxin: infection	u	u	+	+		
vaccine	u	u	+	+		
Neisseria meningitidis OMP (vaccine)	u	u	+		+	
Staphylococcus aureus: TSST 1	u	u	+			+
α toxin	u	u	+			+
Porphyromonas gingivalis fimbriae	+		+	+	+	

u, Untested in the study; PS, polysaccharide; +, major specific immunoglobulin classes produced.

relevance of Ig subclass production to the virulence of individual pathogens and the disease process will perhaps become clearer as more studies are undertaken in which Ig is monitored at the site of infection as well as in peripheral blood (see Chapter 7, section on immunoglobulin-binding proteins).

ACTIVITIES OF IMMUNOGLOBULIN

The final outcome of all these complex interactions is immunoglobulin with high specificity for bacterial molecules present in the blood, tissue fluids and at mucosal surfaces. These can then interfere with and prevent bacterial colonisation and infection in a number of different ways (Figure 3.5). By producing one type of highly specific molecule, the immunoglobulin, which can be used to mediate the clearance or killing of the pathogen by more than one mechanism, the specific defence mechanism of the host exhibits a degree of economy. The specific molecule is used to target other less specific defence mechanisms. (Human immunoglobulin molecules are illustrated in the Appendix.)

One of the simplest functions of immunoglobulin is the prevention of bacterial colonisation of mammalian cell surfaces by binding to, and therefore masking, the molecules used by the bacteria to adhere. This may be one of the most important functions of secretory **IgA** (sIgA) which can prevent initial epithelial attachment and systemic invasion at mucosal sites such as the oral cavity, the urinary, genital, intestinal and respiratory tracts. This process is known as **immune exclusion** whereby antibody specific for bacterial adhesins such as fimbriae blocks attachment to the host cell's surface receptor. The mucosal immune system generates these large quantities of specific IgA by a cyclical process (Figure 3.6). Molecules which attach to specialised epithelial cells known as **M cells** are taken up into clathrin coated pits by endocytosis. Bacteria which attach may be taken up whole by a process of phagocytosis (see Chapters 4 and 8). M cells also take up small quantities of the external milieu into coated and uncoated vesicles. These 'samples' are released inside an epithelial pocket which contains antigen presenting cells and lymphocytes. Whole bacteria may then be subsequently phagocytosed and killed by macrophages. This movement of antigen across the M cells is termed transcytosis. As a result, B-cells which express IgA antibody specific for the antigens which have come effectively from the 'outside' are generated. B-cells at these mucosal sites are switched to IgA production as a result of the cytokines present. The B-cells then migrate to other mucosal sites and glands in the body and differentiate into plasma cells. The cycle is completed by the attachment of IgA to polymeric IgA receptors on epithelial cells. (Polymeric IgA is formed when two or more molecules of IgA are joined by a J (joining) chain.) This polymeric IgA binds to receptor molecules present at a wide range of sites, including the digestive, respiratory and genital tract and mammary, salival and lacrimal epithelium. Binding to the polymeric IgA receptor mediates the transport of IgA across the epithelium, inside cellular vesicles. During this intravesicular-transepithelial transport, the five immunoglobulin-like extracellular domains of the polymeric Ig receptor are cleaved off and join onto the polymeric IgA. These cleaved parts of the IgA receptor are termed the secretory component. The secretory component is thought to provide some protection from proteolytic attack on the IgA when the polymeric IgA and the associated secretory component are released into the lumen. Therefore as a result of sampling of antigen at one site, specific IgA antibody will be released at distant mucosal sites. Bacteria which are capable of an intra-

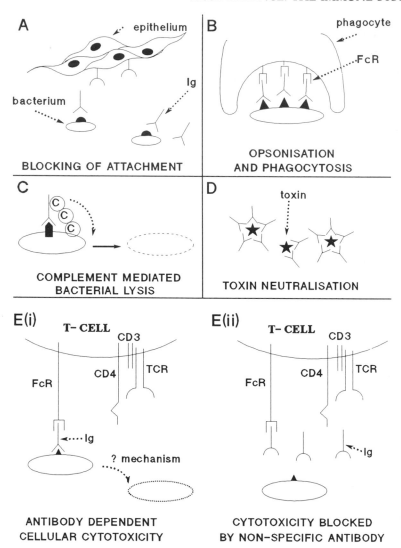

Figure 3.5. Activities mediated by immunoglobulin. The immunoglobulin molecule can target a number of activities of the host's defences. A. Blocking of attachment. Immunoglobulin (Ig) specific for bacterial molecules which mediate attachment to host cells (epithelium) will block attachment. B. Opsonisation and phagocytosis. Ig will enhance attachment to phagocytic cells which carry receptors for the Fc region of the Ig molecule (FcR) (see Chapter 4). C. Complement mediated bacterial lysis. The enzymic activities of the complement cascade (C) are triggered when Ig binds to the bacterial cell surface. This culminates in lysis of Gram negative bacteria (see Chapter 4). D. Toxin neutralisation. Ig binding of toxin can prevent interaction of toxin with host target molecules. E. Antibody dependent cellular cytotoxicity. (i) Interaction of Fc receptors on T-cells carrying glycoprotein CD4 with Ig attached to bacteria can trigger killing of the bacteria. (ii) Although the mechanism of killing is not understood it can be blocked if non-specific Ig binds to the FcR

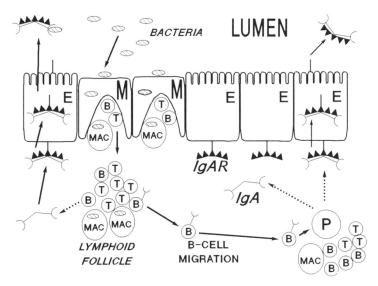

Figure 3.6. Generation of specific immunoglobulin A at mucosal surfaces. Whole bacteria or samples of the gut lumen contents are taken up into M-cells (M) in the mucosal epithelium. The antigen passes across the cell inside a vesicle (not illustrated) into the M-cell pocket where it contacts antigen-presenting cells such as macrophages (MAC). Antigen specific B-cells are generated at and immediately below the M-cells in lymphoid follicles such as Peyer's patches. The B-cells will switch to IgA secretion under the control of the cytokines present at these sites. B-cells will migrate to the other lymphoid follicles and glands, distant from the initial site, where they can differentiate into plasma cells (P) and generate more immuno-globulin. The IgA travels back into the gut lumen through other epithelial cells (E) which carry IgA receptors (IgAR) on their inner side (basolateral membrane). IgA which has docked onto a receptor moves through the cell within a vesicle (not illustrated) and out into the lumen, taking with it the terminal region of the IgAR known as the secretory component. The IgA can now block the adhesion of the bacteria to the epithelial cells.

cellular existence may use this as a way of gaining entry to the host and subsequently colonising other sites in the body (see Chapter 8). By the time that specific IgA, capable of blocking adhesion, is produced the bacteria are colonising other sites within the host. Polymeric IgA released into the mucous secretions is able to cross-link bacteria thereby blocking attachment to the epithelial surface. At this point non-specific defences against attach-ment such as the flow of mucous secretions and saliva, movement such as peristalsis in the gut and ciliary action play a crucial role in the physical removal of the pathogen from the host.

Specific immunoglobulin binding to a bacterial toxin may **neutralise** its toxic activity. For example, in *Vibrio cholerae* infection the enterotoxin binds to the ganglioside receptor GM_1 and ultimately causes fluid loss from the gut (Chapter 6). Specific immunoglobulin, probably sIgA, in binding to the toxin, neutralises its activity. Immunoglobulin is not generally directly toxic to the bacterial cell, although immunoglobulin specific for proteins involved in, for example, the transport of molecules into the bacterium could be detrimental to the bacterium. Immunoglobulin does, however, provide a way of specifically targeting other host mechanisms of killing; for example, the killing activity of the **complement pathway** and **phagocytosis**, where polymorphonuclear leukocytes and macrophages have surface receptors for the Fc region of the antibody molecule (see Appendix for immunoglobulin structure). Both the non-specific and specific immunoglobulin mediated activities of the complement pathway and mechanisms of phagocytosis are discussed in Chapter 4.

Antibody may also mediate killing of bacteria by a subset of T-cells carrying the surface markers CD4 and CD3, but not the CD8 molecule, and Fc receptors for IgG or IgA. This type of killing is termed **antibody dependent cellular cytotoxicity** (ADCC). The precise mechanism by which the bacteria are killed is poorly understood. Immunoglobulin of the same class, but not specific for the bacterium, will block the killing activity (Figure 3.5E). Hence the binding of immunoglobulin to the Fc receptors may trigger the killing in some way.

The specificity of each of the mechanisms discussed above is mediated by one type of molecule, the immunoglobulin.

NATURAL ANTIBODY

As well as the raised level of immunoglobulin which can be monitored in circulating serum as a result of infection, serum contains what is known as 'natural antibody' which is present throughout life. It is thought that this immunoglobulin is present as a result of the continuous immune stimulation by endogenous commensal bacteria. The antibody is probably derived from the subset of B-cells which carry the CD5 glycoprotein (see above) which constitute approximately 20% of peripheral blood B-cells in normal individuals. For example, IgG specific for the carbohydrate epitope Gal(α1–3)Gal accounts for 1% of circulating IgG and has been found to react with the lipopolysaccharide of *E. coli*, *Klebsiella* spp. and *Salmonella* spp. isolated from faeces. This epitope is also present on the surface of mammalian cells. This has possible implications in relation to malfunctioning of the immune system and the generation of autoimmune reactions.

RECOGNITION OF HEAT SHOCK PROTEINS

Another group of molecules, which are the **dominant antigens** recognised by the host in many infections caused by bacteria which grow within the host cells and may be involved in generation of autoimmune disease, are the molecular chaperone family of proteins, also known as stress or heat shock proteins. These are a family of proteins which are highly conserved in living systems and normally present in low levels within cells. Their major function is in the assembly and disassembly of polypeptides into oligomeric complexes and the translocation of some proteins across membranes. They are termed chaperones as they do not form part of the final protein. These chaperone molecules do not act like conventional enzymes as they do not catalyse changes in molecular bonding and remain associated with their target proteins for longer than an enzyme and substrate.

When living organisms are stressed, for example as a result of temperature or nutrient change, there is a dramatic increase in the production of some of these proteins which are thought to assist in the refolding of denatured proteins. The stress proteins of bacteria such as *Salmonella typhimurium, legionella pneumophila, Mycobacterium tuberculosis* and *Mycobacterium leprae*, which grow intracellularly, are the major antigens recognised by the immune response. Both specific T-cell receptors and immunoglobulin are produced. It seems likely that they are expressed in enhanced levels by the bacteria as a result of the stress of growing intracellularly (Figure 3.7). Such cross-reactions with the host's or self stress proteins and bacterial heat shock proteins (Figure 3.7), in particular those of mycobacteria, may play a role in autoimmune diseases such as rheumatoid arthritis.

CYTOLYTIC T-CELLS

Cytolytic T-cells (Tc) usually carry the CD8 cell surface glycoproteins. CD8 positive T-cells recognise foreign antigens associated with MHC Class I molecules which are present on host cells. It has generally been considered that only antigen which is produced within the host cell, that is **endogenous** antigen, is presented with Class I MHC molecules and it has long been thought that the induction of cytolytic activity in T-cells was only relevant to viral parasitism of host cells. Bacteria can, however, grow inside host cells other than those with the Class II molecule and it seems unlikely that the host would not have evolved some defence mechanism for recognising and dealing with such an invasion. There is now evidence, obtained from mice, that CD8 positive Class I restricted T-cells, which are specific for **intracellular pathogens** such as *Listeria monocytogenes, Mycobacterium tuberculosis, M. bovis, M. leprae, Rickettsia typhi* and *R. tsutsugamushi* will lyse host cells infected with the corresponding pathogen. This suggests that Class I MHC molecules can associate with antigen that is not synthesised by cellular machinery, although it is synthesised within the host cell. It also raises the intriguing questions of how bacterial molecules effectively become endogenous molecules and which bacterial molecules are involved. The cytolytic mechanism may be mediated by a number of factors. This includes both activity of secreted factors and membrane interaction, with-

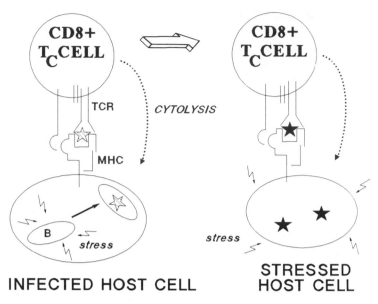

Figure 3.7. Recognition of heat shock proteins. Bacteria (B) growing intracellularly produce elevated levels of heat shock proteins (Hsp) in response to the stress of survival within the host cell. Parts of the bacterial Hsp (star) will be presented at the host cell surface in association with MHC Class I molecules. These will be recognised by specific T-cell receptors and results in lysis of the infected cell. The specific T-cells may cross-react with host derived Hsp which will be presented at the surface of host cells if they are stressed, resulting in autoimmune destruction. T$_c$ cell: cytolytic T-cell. From Kaufmann S.H.E. 1989. Immunity to bacteria and fungi. *Current Opinion in Immunology*, volume 1, pages 431–440. Reproduced by permission of Current Science, Ltd

out secretion. The mechanism of cytolytic T-cell and natural killer cell mediated killing is considered in Chapter 4.

As well as cytolytic activity, CD8 positive T-cells specific for *Listeria monocytogenes, Mycobacterium leprae* or *M. tuberculosis* will secrete γ interferon which is involved in macrophage activation. Macrophages will phagocytose debris of lysed infected cells, including any cell free bacteria which may be released (Chapter 4). It is interesting that both mice in which the gene which codes for γ interferon has been inactivated (knockout mice) and normal mice which have been treated with antibodies specific for γ interferon are particularly susceptible to infection with *L. monocytogenes* and mycobacterial infection. It seems that γ interferon is required by macrophages for the production of nitric oxide which is involved in macrophage killing mechanisms (Chapter 4).

In humans, evidence for cytolytic T-cells specific for bacterial antigens is dependent on identifying cells expressing the CD8 molecule. It is therefore difficult to distinguish the CD8 positive cytolytic T-cells from T-suppressor cells which also express CD8. CD8 positive T-cells are, however, observed associated with lepromatous lesions and in tuberculin positive individuals when challenged with *M. tuberculosis* antigen.

Cytolytic T-cells, with specificity for molecules of the intracellular bacteria, allow the host to lyse infected non-professional phagocytes, which, even under the influence of cytokine stimulation, are unable to kill the intracellular bacteria by themselves. It also allows the host a second method of attack on those bacteria which are resistant to the killing mechanisms of professional phagocytes. In the case of obligately intracellular bacteria this should result in the demise of the pathogen and, in the case of the facultatively intracellular pathogen, expose it to the other killing mechanisms of the immune system.

One adverse effect of such cytolytic activity may be the nerve destruction observed in leprosy patients, which probably results from the cytolytic destruction of the major habitat of *Mycobacterium leprae*, the Schwann cells which wrap around nerve cells to form a protective sheath. The facultatively intracellular bacterium with a range of virulence determinants for combating the host defence can use the lysis of the infected cells as a method of spreading through the host.

FURTHER READING

General

Roitt I., Brostoff J., Male D. 1993. Immunology. Mosby, London, UK.

Antigen presentation

Austin J. M. 1989. Antigen-presenting cells. IRL Press, Oxford, UK.
Hackett C. J. 1991. Antigen presentation: later for the rendezvous. Nature 349, 655–656.
Kaufmann S. H. E. 1990. Immunity to bacteria. Current Opinion in Immunology 2, 353–359.
Parham P. 1989. MHC Molecules: a profitable lesson in heresy. Nature 340, 426–428.
Ploegh J., Benaroch P. 1993. MHC class II dimer of dimers. Nature 364, 16–17.
Townsend A. 1992. Antigen processing: a new presentation pathway? Nature 356, 386–387.

T-cells

Barinaga M. 1993. Interfering with interferon. Science 259, 1693–1694.
Campbell P. A. 1990. The neutrophil, a professional killer of bacteria, may be controlled by T cells. Clinical and Experimental Immunology 79, 141–143.
Emmrich F. 1990. Do carbohydrate antigens stimulate human T-cells? Acta Pathologica Microbiologica Immunologica Scandinavica 98, 1–8.

Julius M ., Maroun C. R., Haughn L. 1993. Distinct role for CD4 and CD8 as co-receptors in antigen receptor signalling. Immunology Today 14, 177–183.

Kaufmann S. H. E. 1988. CD8+ T lymphocytes in intracellular microbial infections. Immunology Today 9, 168–174.

Mackay C. R. 1991. Lymphocyte homing: skin-seeking memory T-cells. Nature 349, 737–738.

Naor D. 1992. A different outlook at the phenotype-function relationship of T cell subpopulations: fundamental and clinical implications. Clinical Immunology and Immunopathology 62, 127–132.

B-cells

Callard R. E. 1989. Cytokine regulation of B-cell growth and differentiation. British Medical Bulletin 45, 371–388.

Jelinek D. F., Lipsky P. E. 1987. Regulation of human B-lymphocyte activation, proliferation and differentiation. Advances in Immunology 40, 1–59.

Antibodies

Casali P., Notkins A. L. 1989. CD5+ B lymphocytes, polyreactive antibodies and the human B-cell repertoire. Immunology Today 10, 364–368.

Childers N. K., Bruce M. G., McGhee J. R. 1989. Molecular mechanisms of immunoglobulin A defense. Annual Review of Microbiology 45, 503–536.

Heilmann C. 1990. Human B and T lymphocyte responses to vaccination with pneumococcal polysaccharides. Acta Pathologica Microbiologica Immunologica Scandinavica 98 (Supplement 15), 5–23.

Kocks C., Rajewsky K. 1989. Stable expression and somatic hypermutation of antibody V regions in B-cell developmental pathways. Annual Review of Immunology 7, 537–559.

Kraehenbuhl J-P., Neutra M. R. 1992. Transepithelial transport and mucosal defence II: secretion of IgA. Trends in Cell Biology 2 June, 170–174.

Neutra M. R., Kraehenbuhl J-P. 1992. Transepithelial transport and mucosal defence I: the role of M cells. Trends in Cell Biology 2 May, 134–138.

Proceedings of a workshop on 'IgG subclass deficiency: fact of fiction?' 1990. Pediatric Infectious Disease Journal 9 Supplement.

Quinti I., Velardi, A., LeMoli S. 1990. Antibacterial polysaccharide antibody deficiency after allogeneic bone marrow transplantation. Journal of Clinical Immunology 10, 160–166.

Tagliabue A., Villa L., De Magistris M. T. 1986. IgA-driven T cell-mediated antibacterial immunity in man after live oral Ty 21a vaccine. Journal of Immunology 137, 1504–1510.

4 Clearance Mechanisms: Complement, Phagocytosis and Cell Mediated Cytotoxicity

INTRODUCTION

The successful pathogenic bacterium has evolved ways of either avoiding or interfering with the destructive mechanisms of the host. Therefore, in order to understand the virulence determinants of bacteria which allow evasion of the host defence, it is necessary to have an understanding of these destructive mechanisms.

The host has developed three major mechanisms for killing bacteria and infected cells: complement mediated lysis, phagocytosis and cell mediated cytotoxicity. There is some overlap between these; for example, complement may in some instances enhance phagocytosis rather than kill the bacterium directly. As these mechanisms of destruction can potentially damage host tissues and cells, the tight control of their activities is essential. One of the ways the host does this is by specific recognition of the foreign antigen by T-cell receptors, immunoglobulin or some of the acute phase proteins which bind specifically to bacterial surface molecules. The activities of complement are essentially non-specific, in that it will bind to most molecules which have either a hydroxyl or amino group. The host control against complement activity therefore involves active defence by the host. This chapter considers each of these killing mechanisms.

COMPLEMENT

Complement is the general name given to a group of about 20 plasma glycoprotein molecules which act in concert. The term 'complement' was originally used because the action of these glycoproteins was initially defined as being complementary to that of antibodies. Complement glycoproteins have potential enzymic activity and act in a series of steps or pathway, each step being dependent on the previous one, in what is known as the complement cascade. Successful activation of the initial reactions results in subsequent amplification of these reactions, as regulation of the pathway involves positive feedback loops. These molecules play an important role in the clearance of invading bacteria and aggregates of antibody and antigen known as immune complexes. Complement is not, however, a mechanism for recognition of foreign antigens as it does not discriminate between self and non-self in the strict sense; rather host cell surfaces protect themselves from the activities of complement (see below). Neither does it discriminate between different foreign antigens.

The components or complement glycoproteins are denoted by numbers from C1 up to C9, the numbers relating in general to the order in which the molecules react. During the cascade of activation, the complement molecules are cleaved into smaller units by the enzymic activity of other complement components and these 'subunits' are designated by letters of the alphabet. For example C3 is split into C3a and C3b, C3b is split into C3c and C3d. The action of cleaving converts some of the molecules from proenzymes or zymogens, with potential enzymic activity, into active enzymes. An 'i' preceding the name as in iC3b indicates that the component has been subsequently inactivated. The activities of complement are controlled by a number of regulatory proteins, some of which are present in serum and some associated with the host cell membrane. The components and interactions of the complement molecules are illustrated in Figure 4.1. The regulation of the complement cascade and how bacteria subvert this is covered in Chapter 7 (Figure 7.7).

There are two ways in which complement functions can be triggered, named for historical reasons the **classical** and the **alternative** pathways. These form the branches of a central pathway which has the potential to damage membranes and lyse cells. In the alternative branch (alternative complement pathway; ACP), complement component C3, deposits and covalently attaches directly onto a cell surface, be it host or bacterial. The second mechanism of triggering complement activity (classical complement pathway; CCP) is usually initiated by the association of the C1, C2 and C4 molecules with immunoglobulin which is already attached to an antigen. For triggering of the CCP, IgM has to be bound to antigen at two of its possible binding sites or IgG has to bind in doublets, close enough together to allow bridging with C1q. Subsequently C3 is bound to the cell surface as in the ACP. The final stages result in the build up of C5–9, the **membrane attack complex** (MAC), on the membrane surface and the consequent disruption of the membrane.

With respect to defence of the host, complement activity has three separate effects on the invading bacterium. Firstly, C3b (the part of the C3 molecule which remains covalently bound to the bacterial cell surface) acts as an **opsonin**; this makes the bacteria more easily engulfed by phagocytic cells which carry surface receptors specific for C3b. This will be considered again in the section dealing with phagocytosis. Secondly, during activation of the complement enzymes, small fragments of the molecules are cleaved off and these lock onto specific receptors present on macrophages and polymorphonuclear leukocytes (PMNL) causing both **activation** of these phagocytic cells and **chemotaxis** to the site of infection. Finally, if the MAC inserts

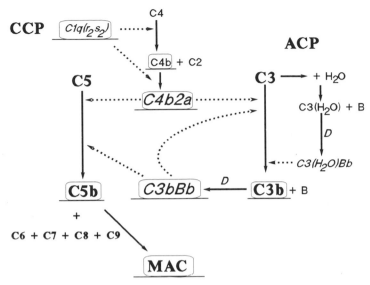

Figure 4.1. The complement cascade. The two arms of the complement cascade are the classical complement pathway (CCP), which is normally triggered by antigen–antibody complexes, and the alternative complement pathway (ACP), which is continuously triggered in the fluid phase at a low level, probably by water. Triggering of the pathway causes the formation of reactive molecules C3b, C4b and C5b, which attach to cell surfaces (boxes). These attached molecules form convertase enzymes (italics) on the cell surface with other factors (B and D). The enzymes amplify the production of the reactive molecules. C5b attached to the cell surface will bind complement molecules C6–9 at the cell surface to form the membrane attack complex (MAC) which causes membrane lysis. The molecules which control the complement pathway are not included in this diagram (see Chapter 7. Figure 7.7)

into the outer membrane of susceptible Gram negative bacteria, effectively forming a **transmembrane pore**, they will be killed. The MAC will also kill host cells if it inserts into the plasma membrane.

The reactivity of C3 hinges on the internal thiolester bond of the C3 glycoprotein (Figure 4.2). This thiolester bond, between a -COOH group on a glutamine residue and -SH group on a cysteine residue, is unstable and can be broken by an electron donor (nucleophile). This happens spontaneously at a very low rate where water molecules are present, the C3 being converted to C3 (H_2O), designated C3i. (C4b, generated by the action of the C1q (r_2s_2) enzymic complex also has an internal thiolester bond which attaches to -OH and -NH_2). The C3i has a binding site for a molecule, present in plasma, known as factor B which, after binding, is cleaved by factor D into Ba and Bb. The Bb remains associated with C3i and this two component molecule now has enzymic activity which can split or convert other C3 molecules into C3a and C3b. The thiolester bond of C3b is far more unstable than that of native C3 and will bind covalently to adjacent

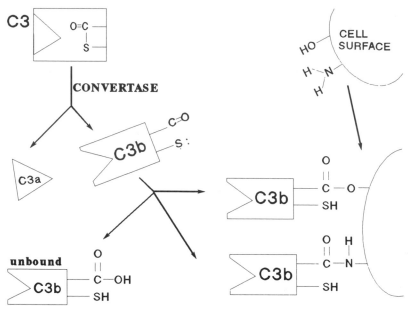

Figure 4.2. Binding of C3b to cell surface molecules. The convertase enzymes C3bBb, C3(H_2O)Bb and C4b2a split C3 into C3a and C3b. This exposes the internal thiolester bond of C3 which will potentially react with any adjacent hydroxyl or amide group or H_2O. If the hydroxyl or amide group is on a cell surface, bound C3b can react with factor B of the complement pathway and generate more convertase enzyme at the cell surface (see Figure 4.1)

hydroxyl or amide groups (Figure 4.2). This continuous low level activation of C3b can be considered as an engine idling, out of gear, which is effectively put into gear when C3Bb attaches onto an unprotected surface; the complement cascade then runs. The regulatory factors which down-regulate the enzymic activities of complement are effectively acting as the brakes. The molecules which regulate complement are considered in detail in Chapter 7 in relation to bacterial evasion of complement activity (Figure 7.7).

As C3 binding can occur indiscriminately to proteins or carbohydrates on host or bacterial cell surfaces, complement is not always capable of discriminating between self and non-self (i.e. between the host and the pathogen). It is therefore important for the host cells to protect themselves from further activation of complement. Molecules inserted in the plasma membrane effectively patrol the cell surface, as though they were looking for complement which has become attached. **Decay acceleration factor** (DAF) is one such molecule which prevents further association of the surface bound C3b with factor B, thus stopping the production of more C3 convertase and therefore amplification of the pathway. **Membrane cofactor**

protein (MCP) acts by binding to C3b and thus prevents its further activity. These two molecules belong to a family of regulatory glycoproteins, regulators of complement activation (RCA) whose genes are clustered at one chromosomal site. They have a common structure and the peptide components are composed of a single repeated 60 amino acid domain. The complement receptors present on PMNLs and monocytes, which interact with C3, C4 and their derivatives, also belong to this family.

For some reason complement does not successfully bind to some molecules. This may be related to the presence of particular neuraminic acids on the host or bacterial cell surface which affect the regulation of complement and prevent its activity. This point will be returned to in relation to bacterial resistance to complement activity (Chapter 7). The internal thiol-ester bonds of C3b and C4b do not interact equally with -OH and $-NH_2$ groups on different molecules. For example, C4b reacts with glycine, whereas C3 does not. As yet the reasons for these differences in specificity are unknown; however, it is possible that this may also have a bearing on the resistance of some bacterial molecules to complement.

When the complement cascade is successfully initiated, the few molecules which bind are soon followed by many more, resulting in amplification of the pathway. The CCP and ACP pathways converge with the formation of either a C4b2aC3b complex (CCP) or C3bBbC3b (ACP), both of which can enzymatically convert C5 to C5b. This initiates the final part of the reaction where the complement glycoproteins which form the MAC, C6, C7, C8 and oligomers of C9, are inserted into the outer membrane (OM) of Gram negative bacteria. The **MAC** consists of a 15–16 nm long, hollow cylinder with an internal channel of 10 nm which is embedded into the membrane. The molecular detail of how this kills the bacterial cell is unclear, but disruption of the OM and loss of molecules from the periplasm may be important. Lethal killing may be related to insertion of MAC at the points where the OM and the cytoplasmic membrane (CM) are joined. There are approximately 80 of these per bacterial cell and they are thought to be involved in the translocation of the components required for assembly of the outer membrane. Lysozyme activity, which will degrade the peptidoglycan between the OM and CM, is not essential for the bacterium to be killed. Complement activation may result in the release of lipopolysaccharide from the OM, even in the absence of C9 which is required for the completion of the MAC. Gram positive bacteria are not killed by the MAC as the thick layer of surface polymers (see Appendix Figure A6) prevents access to the CM; however, deposition of complement occurs, as it does to any unprotected surface, via the ACP and also after antibody deposition. The C3b molecules thus covalently bind and act as opsonins for phagocytic uptake.

The mechanisms by which Gram negative bacteria avoid the activities of complement are considered in Chapter 7.

PHAGOCYTOSIS

Phagocytosis probably evolved originally as means by which single celled phagocytes, such as the amoeba, obtained food. As a result of the digestion of prokaryotes, the eukaryotes could also compete successfully with prokaryotes which have the ability to multiply at a much faster rate and potentially use up the available nutrients. This 'primitive' phagocytosis may be interpreted in simple terms as 'eat your neighbour before it out-competes you'. Only more recently, in evolutionary terms, has phagocytosis become solely a defence policy. In the sophisticated world of the mammalian immune system there are two major types of phagocytic cell, the **polymorphonuclear leukocyte** phagocytic cells (PMNLs) and those which are derived from the mononuclear cell lineage and generally develop into **macrophages**. Both types of phagocyte are derived from similar precursor cells in the bone marrow, but will differentiate into the two cell types under the influence of different cytokines (Figure 4.3).

The major group of PMNLs involved are termed 'neutrophils' because of their neutral reaction when stained with the pH indicator dyes used for light microscopy. These provide the basic function of engulfing and killing

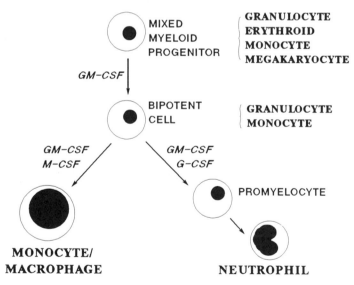

Figure 4.3. Differentiation of phagocytes. Stem cells (mixed myeloid progenitor) with the potential to form granulocytes, erythrocytes, monocytes or megakaryocytes become bipotent stem cells with the potential to form granulocytes or monocytes when exposed to the cytokine granulocyte-macrophage colony stimulating factor (GM-CSF). A combination of the cytokines GM-CSF and granulocyte-CSF (G-CSF) results in the production of neutrophils, whereas a combination of GM-CSF and macrophage-CSF (M-CSF) results in the production of monocytes/macrophages

the bacteria (Figure 4.4). Neutrophils are short-lived cells at the terminal stage of their cellular differentiation pathway. After release from the bone marrow they circulate in the blood for about 10 hours and then are thought to survive within the tissues for only about two days. These are the 'foot-soldiers' of the immune system which die in the 'front line', after engorging themselves with bacteria.

The second type of phagocytic cell are those of the mononuclear phagocytic system. Although they are derived from the same stem cells as the neutrophils, they diverge during differentiation within the bone marrow and can undergo further stages of differentiation within the tissues. Thus they are generally referred to as monocyte/macrophage cells, as circulating monocytes in the blood may differentiate into different types of macrophages in the tissues, e.g. peritoneal macrophages, Kuppfer cells in the liver, alveolar macrophages in the lungs. The monocyte/macrophages have a much more complex life history than the neutrophils and may live for months or possibly years. They play a central role in controlling many of the functions of the immune system and are akin to 'mobile command units'. Macrophages are one of the major groups of cells which process antigen and present it to T-cells in association with major histocompatibility complex (MHC) molecules (Chapter 3). Thus the destruction of the pathogen occurs in a carefully regulated and selective manner and, if antigen is successfully presented at the macrophage cell surface to a T-cell, will enhance the specific immune response. Macrophages also pass information on to other cells by their release of cytokines such as IL1 and TNF (see Chapter 2 for details of cytokine activity) and may be induced to secrete complement glycoproteins.

Chemotaxis of phagocytic cells

The engulfment of bacteria, by its nature, requires that the phagocytic cell is in close contact with the bacterium. Phagocytic cells are attracted to sites of infection by sensing either host-derived or bacterial molecules. One group of bacterial molecules which chemoattract phagocytic cells are unique bacterial products such as **formyl-methionyl-leucyl-phenylalanine** and related peptides. These peptides starting with N-formyl-methionyl are produced when bacteria initiate protein synthesis. If they are released from the bacteria in vivo, they are highly chemotactic for human phagocytic cells. Chemoattractant host products include the **C5a** component of complement, **thrombin** and fragments of **fibronectin, collagen** and **elastin**. A number of **cytokines** are reported to act as chemoattractants and these include tumour necrosis factor (TNF), granulocyte-macrophage colony stimulating factor (GM-CSF) and platelet-derived growth factor (PDGF). The lipid, **leukotriene B4** (LTB4), is a potent attractant of both neutrophils and monocytes. When neutrophils are stimulated, they release LTB4 in quantity. It is

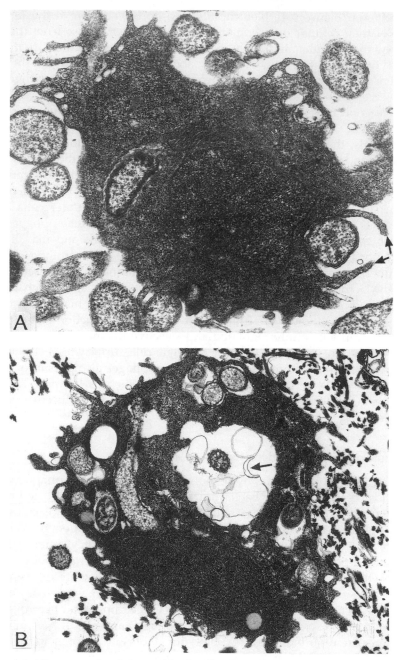

Figure 4.4. Phagocytosis of *Bacteroides fragilis*. Transmission electron micrographs: ultrathin sections of mouse neutrophils phagocytosing *Bacteroides fragilis*. Note pseudopodia surrounding bacterial cell (A; arrow) and degraded bacteria within vacuoles (B; arrow)

thought that release of LTB4 by neutrophils, which are usually present first at a site of infection, mediates the secondary infiltration of monocytes. Neutrophils have specific surface receptors for these molecules which are taken into the neutrophil by receptor mediated endocytosis. Receptor mediated endocytosis is triggered by the attachment of a molecule to a specific receptor and is different from phagocytosis. (The different routes of cellular uptake are considered in more detail below, in relation to toxin uptake in Chapter 6 and to intracellular growth of bacteria in Chapter 8). Endocytic uptake then triggers some of the activities of the neutrophil such as chemotaxis towards the attractant molecule, the release of digestive enzymes by exocytosis (granule enzyme secretion) and the generation of oxygen free radicals (see section below on phagocytic killing).

Phagocytic uptake

Once present at the site of infection the phagocytes must now make contact with bacteria. In general both the phagocyte and bacterial cell will have a net negative charge as a result of the surface polymers of the bacterial envelope and the oligosaccharides associated with lipids and proteins on the host cell. Non-specific physico-chemical interactions dependent on the net surface charge and hydrophobicity of the cell surfaces probably play some role in whether or not the bacteria become attached to the approaching phagocyte. Measurement of the relative hydrophobicity and hydrophilicity (or wettability) can be related to whether, or not, a bacterium is taken up by a phagocyte. If the bacterial surface is more hydrophilic than that of the phagocyte, it will not be phagocytosed unless the surface is modified by soluble proteins (see Chapter 7).

Specific molecular interactions which govern the phagocytic uptake of bacteria may be either directly between molecules on the bacterial and phagocytic cells' surface, or involve bridging molecules or opsonins. Examples of opsonins include specific immunoglobulin, C3b of complement and the acute phase proteins, such as C-reactive protein, which bind to specific components of the bacterial cell surface.

Direct interaction between molecules on bacteria and phagocytic cells normally involves binding between carbohydrates and protein lectins (i.e. polyvalent carbohydrate-binding proteins). This **lectinophagocytosis** may occur either way round, with the lectins either on the bacterium or the host cell. Known examples of bacterial protein lectins are the fimbriae (or pili; see Chapter 7) which enable bacteria to attach to host cells by binding to sugar residues on host cell surface glycoproteins and glycolipids. In many instances the ability to attach to host cells is thought to play an important role in the pathogenesis of bacterial infection, but it may also enhance phagocytosis of the bacteria. This point will be considered in relation to genetic control of bacterial variation (Chapter 9). The Type 1 fimbriae produced by some *E. coli* strains (see Chapter 7) are known to bind to mannose-containing oligosaccharides present on many host surface glycoproteins. This binding of bacteria can be blocked by adding excess mannose to assay systems. It has been shown that Type 1 fimbriae attach to glycoproteins of the same molecular weight as the α and β chains of the complement receptor 3 (CR3, also called MAC 1, for macrophage). This is the receptor for the iC3b component of complement and is a member of the integrin superfamily of cell adhesion molecules. Hence it may be that the bacterial fimbriae recognise the carbohydrate moiety and iC3b the peptide part of the same molecule.

Type 2 fimbriae of *Actinomyces viscosus* and *A. naeslundii*, which may be involved in causing dental caries and gingivitis, are specific for β-galactoside sugars such as lactose, galactosyl (β1–4) N-acetyl-D-glucosamine and galactosyl (β1–3) N-acetyl-D-galactosamine. Attachment of Type 2 bearing strains to human neutrophils occurs in the absence of serum and can be blocked by adding methyl β-galactoside and lactose to the assay system. There is also some evidence that P fimbriae of *E. coli* which bind to Gal(α1-4)Gal residues of the P blood group are involved in lectinophagocytosis. The role of fimbriae in attachment to host cells is discussed in Chapter 7.

Mammalian cells carry a number of surface lectins which bind to carbohydrates. These are known to be involved in the host-cell adhesion, recognition and development. A good example is the specific movement of lymphocytes where protein–carbohydrate binding can determine where in the body lymphocytes congregate (Chapter 2). It is likely that the lectins expressed on phagocytic cells mediate attachment of bacteria. For example, lipopolysaccharide (LPS) is thought to bind directly to receptors on the monocyte/macrophage cell surface. A number of surface glycoproteins have been suggested as possible receptors, although there is some controversy as to which particular receptors are involved. It has been suggested by some workers that some of the members of the leukocyte-cell adhesion molecule (L-CAM) family, namely, CR3 (composed of an α chain CD11b and β chain CD18), CR4 (p150, 95; CD11c/CD18) and leukocyte function associated antigen (LFA 1; CD11a/CD18), as well as CD14, have binding sites for the core sugar region of LPS. CR3 binds to the three amino acid sequence arginine-glycine-aspartic acid (RGD) of complement component iC3b (see below), but it is thought that the LPS binding site is distinct from this (see Appendix for diagram of LPS). There is also evidence that LPS may attach to monocytes through non-specific hydrophobic interactions. Macrophages such as Kuppfer cells and alveolar macrophages bear lectins which may react directly with bacterial surface polysaccharides and include: mannose-type lectins, which bind to mannose, glucose, L-fucose and N-acetyl glucosamine; galactose-type lectins which bind to galactose and N-acetyl glucosamine and finally lectins which bind to L-fucose. *Streptococcus agalactiae* (also known as Lancefield group B streptococcus) contains mannose and galactose in its surface polymers and is thought to attach to macrophages by this mechanism. Some strains of *E. coli* may be recognised through sugar residues in the LPS.

This process of lectinophagocytosis represents a primitive non-clonal recognition of bacteria. It is possible that opsonin mediated phagocytosis has evolved to deal with bacteria which have developed ways of avoiding lectin mediated interactions. Opsonins act as bridging molecules attached at one end to molecules on the surface of the phagocyte and at the other to molecules on the surface of the bacterium. Opsonising molecules found in circulating serum and lymph are summarised in Table 4.1.

The **acute phase proteins** C-reactive protein (CRP), mannose-binding protein (MBP) and LPS binding protein (LBP) are normally present only in trace amounts in serum, but in the acute phase of the inflammatory response their level increases up to 1000-fold (see Chapter 2). These proteins bind to molecules which may be present on invading microoranisms and constitute one facet of non-clonal immune recognition. Once bound, they can act as opsonins for phagocytosis. A general term sometimes used for these host proteins which bind to carbohydrates on microbial surfaces is **collectin**.

CRP binds to phosphorylcholine carbohydrates and was initially characterised by its ability to bind to what is called the C polysaccharide found on all strains of the Gram positive bacterium *Streptococcus pneumoniae*, hence C-reactive protein. The C polysaccharide is in fact a ribitol teichoic acid substituted with phosphorylcholine. CRP is a member of a conserved group

Table 4.1. Examples of opsonising molecules

Opsonin	Phagocyte receptor
Acute phase reactants	
Mannose binding protein	C1q receptor
Lipopolysaccharide binding protein	CD14
C-reactive protein + complement C3b	?CR1
Complement components	
C3b	CR1
iC3b	CR3, CR4
Immunoglobulin	
IgG1,3	Fc γ RII, III
IgG1,3,4	Fc γ RI
IgA	Fc α
Pulmonary surfactant proteins	
SP-A	C1q receptor
SP-D	?

Most of the receptors are expressed on both monocytes/macrophages and neutrophils. Fibronectin may also act as an opsonin.

of plasma proteins known as the **pentraxins** which are formed from a cyclic pentameric arrangement of subunits. Binding to carbohydrate is dependent on the presence of calcium ions. Another pentraxin, **serum amyloid P component** (SAP), may also be involved in opsonisation. After binding of CRP, complement is activated and C3b deposited at the surface of the bacterium may form the bridge to the phagocytic cell. The role of CRP in the host's defence is not yet proven. As yet, within the human population, no mutational deficiencies in the production of CRP have been identified which relate to a greater susceptibility to bacterial disease.

MBP binds to polysaccharides containing mannose and N-acetyl glucosamine. It was originally identified by its ability to bind to LPS and termed Ra reactive factor (RaRF). It is structurally related to C1q component of complement being a multimer consisting of collagen fibre stalks connected to globular heads which carry the lectin site, thus forming a structure which resembles a bunch of tulips. The deposition of MBP will activate the complement pathway. It may be that MBP effectively replaces C1q in the classical complement pathway. Individuals in the human population who carry a mutational defect in the gene for MBP are particularly prone to bacterial infection in the early years of life. In relation to bacterial recognition, it will opsonise bacteria with mannose in the O-antigenic region of LPS. An example is the O-antigen of some *Salmonella* spp. which have a repeating unit of one galactose and four mannose residues.

LBP is a glycoprotein of about 60 kDa which can be detected in serum about 24 hours after the initiation of the acute phase response. Binding to LPS is thought to occur in the region of the diglucosamine backbone of the lipid A component. Cell-free LBP, by binding specifically to LPS, acts as a bridge between the bacterium and the CD14 receptor present on macrophages.

Two other collectins, which may be involved in opsonisation of bacteria in the lungs, are the **surfactant proteins** (SP) -A and -D. These proteins are synthesised by non-ciliated alveolar epithelial cells and are specific to the lungs. SP-A is structurally similar to the bunch of tulips structure of MBP and C1q whereas as in SP-D the collagen stalks and globular heads form a cross. Both of these molecules will bind to sugars of LPS and will enhance phagocytosis by alveolar macrophages. They may therefore be an important part of the first line of defence against inhaled bacteria.

Fibronectin is a host proteoglycan (Chapter 5) with possible binding sites for a range of molecules, including those on the surface of phagocytes. The fibronectin binds to proteins with the amino acid sequence arginine-glycine-aspartic acid (RGD). Some streptococcal lipoteichoic acids will bind to fatty acid binding sites on fibronectin. This point is also considered in relation to bacterial attachment to host cells and tissues as a means of successful colonisation of the host in Chapter 7. Whether opsonisation with fibronectin enhances phagocytosis or not is still a matter of debate. There are also reports of a staphylococcal protein which binds to host fibrinogen. Fibrinogen, when activated, forms fibrin clots (Chapter 5).

The **complement molecules** are indisputably major mediators of opsonisation of bacteria. Phagocytes express the C3b receptor, complement receptor 1 (CR1), which belongs to the family of molecules involved in the regulation of complement activation. CR3 and CR4 are phagocyte receptors for iC3b. iC3b is generated by the cleavage of C3f from C3b by the controlling factor I. (Note that CR2, a receptor for C3d, is found on B-cells.) Interestingly the half-life of C3b when fixed to an antigen is approximately 90 s, whereas that of iC3b is about 35 min. This suggests that iC3b may be the more effective opsonin. Binding to CR1 and CR3 does not induce the release of reactive oxygen metabolites involved in bacterial killing (see below) and therefore seems to be a favoured route of entry for bacteria which subsequently grow inside the phagocytic cell (see Chapter 8).

Polymorphonuclear leukocytes and monocyte/macrophages also carry receptors for the Fc part of **immunoglobulin molecules** and can thus target their killing mechanism to 'clonally recognised' bacteria. Fc α receptor binds IgA, and IgG receptors of high, medium and low affinity (Fc γ receptors I, II and III) have been described.

Once attachment has occurred phagocytes are triggered to engulf the bacterium by surrounding it with pseudopodia (Figure 4.4). All host cells can take up small particles by endocytosis, in which parts of the cytoplasmic membrane bud inwards into the cell; however, under normal circumstances it is only the 'professional' phagocytes, the polymorphonuclear leukocytes and the macrophages, which actively surround the particle to be ingested (see Chapter 8 on intracellular growth and survival of bacteria). The movement of the pseudopodia around the bacterium probably involves actin-binding proteins, as the drug cytochalasin which stops polymerisation of actin also inhibits phagocytosis. It is thought that as the bacterium enters the phagocyte the opsonins on the bacterial surface lock onto the receptors on the phagocytic cell membrane in much the same way as a zipper locks together (Figure 4.5). The fusion of the phagosome to form a discrete vacuole is probably under the control of specific fusogenic proteins which as yet are not characterised, but may be related to the proteins involved in the entry of viruses into host cells. As yet, the precise molecular details of fusion are not known.

Once inside the vacuole, or phagosome, fusion with other intracellular vacuoles or granules (named after their granular appearance by microscopy) will take place. These granules are packages of enzymes and antibacterial molecules which are involved in killing the bacterium and also, in the case of macrophages, in processing of bacterial molecules for antigen presentation (Chapter 3). The phagocyte derived molecules with potential antibacterial activity are listed in Table 4.2. The bacterium may then be killed by either oxygen dependent or independent mechanisms.

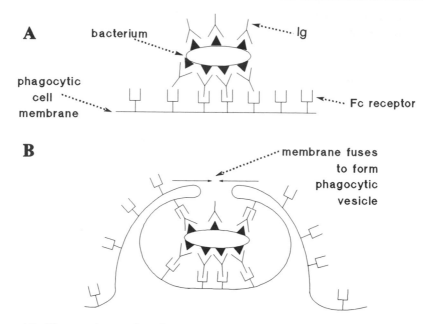

Figure 4.5. Phagocytic uptake of opsonised bacteria. The Fc region of immuno-globulin (Ig) coating a bacterium binds to the Fc receptors (FcR) on the phagocytic cell (A). This triggers the formation of pseudopodia around the bacterium (B). The pseudopodia finally fuse and the bacterium is enclosed within a phagocytic vesicle

Table 4.2. Phagocyte derived molecules with anti-bacterial activity

Hypohalous acids (generated by the action of myeloperoxidase and hydrogen
    peroxide)
Hydroxyl free radicals
Hydrolase enzymes (e.g. elastase, nuclease, glycosidase, lipase)
Lysozyme
Neopterin
Nitric oxide
Iron chelators (e.g. lactoferrin)
Bactericidal/permeability increasing protein (BPI)
Cationic proteins (e.g. defensins, cathepsin G, CAP 37, azurocidin)

Phagocytic killing

Oxygen dependent killing of bacteria is associated with rapid uptake of a large amount of oxygen by the phagocytic cell, termed the **respiratory burst**. This measurable uptake of oxygen is the end-result of the stimulation of the oxidase system by attachment of the bacterium to phagocytic cell receptors such as those discussed above. The oxidase system is effectively

an electron transport chain in which electrons move from glucose to nicotinamide adenine dinucleotide phosphate (NADPH) and finally oxygen
(Figure 4.6). The outcome of the addition of the electron to oxygen is the
formation of superoxide. Addition of subsequent electrons generates hydrogen peroxide and finally hydroxyl free radicals. Free radicals are unstable
as they are effectively looking for another electron to form a pair, and will
break other atomic bonds to obtain one. This creates radicals in the target
molecule and will generate a destructive chain reaction. The **hydroxyl free
radicals** are therefore toxic to all living cells as they have the potential to
oxidise the cellular macromolecules. In spite of this, it is unlikely that these
radicals are solely responsible for killing bacteria. The enzyme **myeloperoxidase** (MPO) is present in neutrophils and monocytes in quantity. MPO
catalyses the oxidation of chloride and iodide by hydrogen peroxide to free
chlorine and iodine, and their corresponding **hypohalous acids**. These products are reactive and highly toxic to cells as they will halogenate molecules
such as lipids, proteins and nucleic acids; this mix of toxic components has
been appropriately termed intraphagosomal bleach by G. A. W. Rook. The
halogenation of the bacterial molecules generates chloramines and amino
aldehydes, which, along with chlorine and hypochlorous acid, will affect
normal bacterial structure and metabolic function. These activities seem to
be limited to the inside of the phagocytic vacuole or outside the cell if they
are released into the extracellular environment. The phagocytic cells protect
themselves by having copious amounts of antioxidants (e.g. ascorbic acid,
vitamin E), catalase and superoxide dismutase which neutralise their
effects. It is likely that successful killing of the bacterium is dependent not

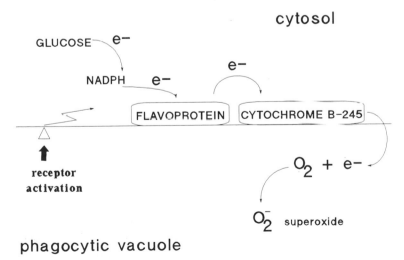

Figure 4.6. Generation of the respiratory burst. Electrons, from glucose, move along
the electron transport chain to generate superoxide

only on these oxygen dependent mechanisms, but also on other factors which are termed 'oxygen independent'.

Oxygen independent killing of bacteria within intracellular vacuoles occurs when the contents of intracellular granules fuse with the phagosome to form the phagolysosome. The granules contain a wide range of antibacterial molecules with varied activities, some of which are more specific than others. One type of granule, the lysosome, contains about 40 different acid **hydrolase enzymes**, including proteases such as elastase, nucleases, glycosidases, lipases, phospholipases and sulphatases with an optimal activity at about pH 5. As the pH of the cytosol of the neutrophils is at about 7.2 any enzymes which leak out will not be active. This explains their lack of destructive activity on their own cell. Another important enzyme in the lysosome is lysozyme (also called muramidase) which hydrolyses the β-1-4 link between the N-acetylglucosamine and N-acetylmuramic acid of the peptidoglycan molecule (see Chapter 2, Figure 2.3) and will kill some Gram positive bacteria in vitro such as *Micrococcus luteus* and *Bacillus megaterium*.

Macrophages release quantities of **neopterin** in response to γ interferon. In mammalian systems, dihydroneopterin triphosphate, a precursor of neopterin, acts as a cofactor in the production of dopamine and serotonin by oxidation of phenylalanine, tyrosine and tryptophan. How this relates to γ interferon induced release of neopterin is unclear, although neopterin is detectable in the urine and plasma of individuals with leprosy and tuberculosis. (This also occurs in parasitic infection with malaria and toxoplasmosis.) In bacteria neopterin is an intermediate in the conversion of guanosine triphosphate (GTP) to folic acid. One hypothesis which has been put forward for the anti-bacterial action of neopterin is that if the mammalian neopterin is oxidised it could inhibit the bacterial folate pathway. This would be similar to the action of sulphonamides. Therefore neopterin could effectively be considered to be a natural antibiotic.

Another macrophage product with the potential to damage bacteria is **nitric oxide**. It is now clear that nitric oxide (NO) plays a central role in a number of the systems of the body. It is a major biological messenger which is involved in the dilation of blood vessels and also acts as a neurotransmitter. On another level NO can be extremely toxic. In the macrophage, L-arginine is oxidised to produce NO which will rapidly decay to nitrite and nitrate in the presence of oxygen and water. It is the production of nitrates which allows for the measurement of NO production by macrophages. NO production may be triggered by, for example, γ interferon and LPS. As a free radical, NO is potentially a highly reactive molecule. In terms of toxicity to bacteria, NO will inhibit enzymes which contain iron and sulphur. It also causes loss of intracellular iron. There is evidence that with *Mycobacterium avium*, killing of the intracellular bacteria is dependent on NO generation rather than the reactive oxygen intermediates generated by the respiratory burst. Highly virulent *M. avium*, which can survive even

NO attack, produce a manganese containing superoxide dismutase (SOD) which appears to mop up the NO. Other strains of *M. avium* which lack this manganese containing SOD are less virulent.

Iron chelating agents such as lactoferrin and transferrin are present in granules of neutrophils and these may limit the growth of the bacteria and also aid in their subsequent destruction. These chelating agents trap any free iron, an essential nutrient required for bacterial metabolism and growth. Bacteria which produce their own chelating agents with a higher affinity for iron than the host's chelating agents may not be susceptible to this type of nutrient starvation (Chapter 5).

Another antibacterial molecule, which is active against Gram negative bacteria is **bactericidal/permeability increasing protein** (BPI). This protein has an apparent molecular mass of 60 kDa and is only effective against some Gram negative bacteria. For example, strains of *Escherichia coli, Salmonella typhimurium* and *Pseudomonas aeruginosa* are susceptible, but *Serratia marcescens* is not. This specificity is in some way related to the affinity with which the molecule binds to unknown components of the outer membrane of the bacteria. The longer the O-antigen chain of the lipopolysaccharide the lower the affinity of the BPI. After binding to the bacterial outer membrane, the outer membrane becomes more permeable and allows the entry of molecules which would normally be excluded because of their size. The colony forming ability of the susceptible bacterium can be lost within 15 seconds of exposure to BPI. BPI has no apparent effect on the cytoplasmic membrane and it is possible that the killing action is similar to that suggested for the membrane attack complex of the complement pathway (see above), with the BPI inserting at the adhesion points between the bacterial cytoplasmic and outer membranes. These junctions seem to be very important for the viability of the Gram negative bacterium.

The **defensins** are another major group of antibacterial components of the phagocytes. This family of cationic proteins are major components of the phagocytic cells and have been identified in both polymorphonuclear neutrophils and macrophages from a range of animal species including man and rabbits. They can comprise up to 5–7% of all cellular protein in human and 18% in rabbit polymorphonuclear neutrophils and are therefore major constituents of the phagocytic cell. They are short peptides of 29–34 amino acids in length with an apparent molecular mass of 3–4 kDa. All of the defensins examined to date have six conserved cysteine residues which form three intramolecular disulphide bonds and are rich in arginine to a varying extent. Three human neutrophil defensins have been characterised and a fourth is also known to exist. Crystallisation of these peptides and nuclear magnetic resonance spectroscopy show that the molecules are amphiphiles with distinct hydrophobic and charged regions. This may allow these peptides to insert into phospholipid membranes, probably causing membrane disruption. The activity of the defensins is not restricted to

Gram negative bacteria as Gram positive bacteria and some enveloped viruses are also susceptible to their killing action. Their mode of action is therefore less specific than the BPI molecule described above. It is not clear how the phagocytic cells are immune to the activities of the defensins. In relation to their antimicrobial activity, the defensins can be divided into two different types: those which require actively metabolising bacteria and are more cationic, and those which will kill bacteria which are not actively metabolising. For example, human neutrophil defensins 1 and 2 require glucose in the reaction mixture to kill *Staphylococcus aureus* and a nutrient medium to kill *Escherichia coli*, in vitro. On the other hand, two of the rabbit defensins, NP 1 and 2, will kill bacteria in buffer without added nutrients. The mechanism of the killing activity of the defensins is almost certainly related to the disruption of both the cytoplasmic and outer membranes. The formation of multimers of defensins at the membrane surface may be important for killing of the bacteria, but the fine detail remains to be elucidated. *Salmonella typhimurium*, an intracellular pathogen, is resistant to the microbicidal activity of defensins and a bacterial gene controlling this resistance has been identified. This, and other mechanisms by which bacteria successfully avoid intracellular killing by the host's phagocytes, are discussed in Chapter 8.

CYTOLYSIS

The major groups of host cells with lytic activity are the cytolytic T-cells (see Chapter 3) and the natural killer cells. The T-cell receptors of **cytolytic T-cells** recognise cells which display foreign antigen on their surface in association with the MHC Class I molecule, usually as a result of infection of the host cells by either a bacterium or virus. Some tumour cells and also transplanted tissue will also be recognised in this way.

Natural killer cells (also termed large granular lymphocytes) are lymphocytes which, unlike T- or B-cells do not rearrange either immunoglobulin or T-cell receptor genes. In terms of surface glycoprotein markers, these cells lack CD3 and T-cell receptors but carry CD16 and NKH-1. CD16 is a low affinity receptor for the Fc of IgG. Precisely how their cytolytic activity is targeted is not known, but they do not seem to require antigen to be presented in association with MHC Class I molecules. NK cells may use more than one mechanism for distinguishing self from non-self. For example, NK cells are one of the mediators of antibody-dependent cell mediated cytotoxicity (ADCC; see Chapter 3) by virtue of the CD16 Fc receptor (activated T-cells and monocytes/macrophages can also mediate ADCC). These NK cells are sometimes termed K cells. Others may recognise foreign antigen directly. It therefore seems that NK cells may recognise a variety of different structures on target cells. There is evidence that in bacterial infection the killing activity can be directed against both infected host cells and extracellular bacteria. Under the influence of interleukin 2 (IL2) some NK cells (termed lymphokine activated killer, LAK, cells) become activated and proliferate. These cells have been shown to kill monocytes infected with *Mycobacterium avium* or *Legionella pneumophila*. LPS from *Escherichia coli* and *Pseudomonas aeruginosa* and extracts from *Streptococcus* spp. stimulate NK cell cytotoxic activity. At present the role of NK cells in protection against bacteria is an unknown quantity. They may, however, play a central role in the early stages of the immune response to bacterial infection as circulating NK cells from healthy individuals do not require pre-activation and will lyse target cells within minutes of being triggered.

Although the recognition mechanisms of cytolytic T-cells and NK cells are different, the killing mechanisms share a number of features. Perforin (also called pore-forming protein, PFP), enzymes derived from intracellular granules (also called granzymes), lymphotoxin (also called tumour necrosis factor β) and natural killer cell cytotoxic factor may all be involved in the cytotoxic action of these cells. Perforin is a 70 kDa protein which forms pores on the target membrane and may mediate cell lysis in a similar way to the membrane attack complex of complement. The killing of infected host cells may be more complex than this as there is evidence, from virally infected cells, that the infected host cell dies by a process of programmed cell death, or apoptosis. The cell dies in an ordered manner under the control of an autocatalytic cascade. The nucleic acid is fragmented within the intact cell, which shrivels rather than bursting open. This type of cell death could be a type of 'induced suicide' of the cell, as the cell which dies takes an active part in controlling its own demise. The details of how bacteria are killed by these cells remain to be determined, although there is evidence that both Gram positive and Gram negative bacteria are susceptible to NK cell activity and that killing is mediated by soluble factors.

FURTHER READING

General

Gallin J. I., Goldstein I. M., Snyderman R. 1992. Inflammation: basic principles and clinical correlates (2nd Edn). Raven Press, New York.

Complement

Law S. K. A., Reid K. B. M. 1988. Complement. IRL Press, Oxford, UK.
Mollnes T. E., Lachmann P. J. 1988. Regulation of complement. Scandinavian Journal of Immunology 27, 127–142.
Muller-Eberhard H. J. 1986. The membrane attack complex of complement. Annual Review of Immunology 4, 503–528.
Volankis J. E. 1990. Participation of C3 and its ligands in complement activation. Current Topics in Microbiology and Immunology 153, 1–21.

Phagocytic uptake

Couturier C., Haeffner-Cavaillon N., Caroff, M. *et al.* 1991. Binding sites for endo-toxins (lipopolysaccharides) on human monocytes. Journal of Immunology 147, 1899–1904.

Ezekowitz R. A. B. 1991. Ante-antibody immunity. Current Biology 1, 60–62.

Ezekowitz R. A. B. 1992. Antigens coming to a sticky end. Current Biology 2, 147–149.

Holmskov U., Malhotra R., Sim R. B., Jensenius J. C. 1994. Collectins: collagenous C-type lectins of the innate immune defense system. Immunology Today 15, 67–73.

Kaufmann S. H. E., Reddehase M. J. 1989. Infection of phagocytic cells. Current Opinion in Immunology 2, 43–49.

Ofek I., Sharon N. 1988. Lectinophagocytosis: a molecular mechanism of recognition between cell surface sugars and lectins in phagocytosis of bacteria. Infection and Immunity 56, 539–547.

Schumann R. R., Leong S. R., Flaggs G. W. *et al.* 1990. Structure and function of lipopolysaccharide binding protein. Science 249, 1429–1431.

Steel D. M., Whitehead A. S. 1994. The major acute phase reactants: C-reactive protein, serum amyloid P component and serum amyloid A protein. Immunology Today 15, 81–88.

Wright S. D., Levin S. M., Jong, T. C. *et al.* 1989. CR3 (CD11b/CD18) expresses one binding site for Arg-Gly-Asp-containing peptides and a second site for bacterial lipopolysaccharide. Journal of Experimental Medicine 169, 175–183.

Wright S. D., Ramos R. A., Tobias P. S. *et al.* 1990. CD14, a receptor for complexes of lipopolysaccharide (LPS) and LPS binding protein. Science 249, 1431–1433.

Zembala M., Asherson G. L. (Eds). 1989. Human monocytes. Academic Press, London.

Killing mechanisms

Denis M. 1991. Tumour necrosis factor and granulocyte macrophage colony stimulating factor stimulate human macrophages to restrict growth of virulent *Mycobacterium avium* and to kill avirulent *M. avium*: killing effector mechanism depends on generation of reactive nitrogen intermediates. Journal of Leukocyte Biology 49, 380–387.

Elsbach P., Weiss J. 1992. Oxygen-independent antimicrobial systems of phagocytes. In: Inflammation: basic principles and clinical correlates (2nd Edn). (Eds. J. I. Gallin, I. M. Goldstein, R. Snyderman). Raven Press, New York. Chapter 30.

Ganz T., Selsted M. E., Szklarek D. *et al.* 1985. Defensins: natural peptide antibiotics of human neutrophils. Journal of Clinical Investigation 76, 1427–1435.

Klebanoff S. J. 1992. Oxygen metabolites from phagocytes. In: Inflammation: basic principles and clinical correlates (2nd edn) Eds. J. I. Gallin, I. M. Goldstein, R. Snyderman. Raven Press, New York. Chapter 28.

Lanier L. L., Philips J. H. 1992. Natural killer cells. Current Opinion in Immunology 4, 38–42.

Moncada S., Palmer R. M. J., Higgs E. A. 1991. Nitric oxide: physiology, pathophysiology and pharmacology. Pharmacological Reviews 43, 109–142.

Rook G. A. W. 1989. Intracellular killing of microorganisms. In: Human monocytes. Eds. M. Zembala, G. L. Asherson. Academic Press, London. Chapter 5.1.

Selsted M. E., Lehrer R. I. 1990. Defensins. European Journal of Haematology 44, 1–8.

Snyder S. H., Bredt D. S. 1992. Biological role of nitric oxide. Scientific American May, 28–35.

Trinchieri G. 1989. Biology of natural killer cells. Advances in Immunology 47, 187–376.

Young S. 1992. Life and death of the condemned cell. New Scientist 25 January, 34–37.

Part II

THE BACTERIAL INVASION

Having considered our understanding of how the host defends itself against bacterial infection, we will now consider the other side of the coin; how the pathogenic bacterium successfully colonises the living host and how bacteria have adapted to the specialised niche of the mammalian animal.

One of the first prerequisites for survival is a plentiful nutrient supply (Chapter 5). Compared with many of the non-living environmental niches occupied by bacteria, the living host appears on first appraisal to provide rich pickings for the bacterium, with a plentiful range of organic substrates in the form of cells and the extracellular matrix; host cell lysis having the potential to release many preformed metabolites. Indeed, many of the bacterial virulence determinants, defined as toxins because of their detrimental effects on the host, are cytolysins and therefore may play a part in bacterial nutrition. Certain nutrients essential for the survival of bacteria, such as iron, are, however, in very limited supply in the host. Bacteria have therefore to make use of nutrient scavenging mechanisms which perhaps originally evolved in bacteria able to cope with nutrient poor environments.

The selective advantage to the bacterium of generalised toxicity to the host, mediated by for example the neurotoxins and ADP-ribosylating enzyme toxins (Chapter 6), is not perhaps immediately obvious. Maybe as the activities of these toxins are elucidated their relationship with the evolution of the successful pathogenic bacterium will be better understood.

Unlike other environments colonised by bacteria, the host is not passive. The bacterium therefore has to survive not just a changing environment, but an environment which is **actively** trying to prevent colonisation. As the primary site of interaction between the bacterium and the host immune system is the bacterial cell surface, many of the bacterial surface molecules are involved in virulence (Chapter 7). To escape the antibacterial activities of the host a number of bacteria have opted for an intracellular existence, some even surviving within the host cells whose major function appears to be the eradication of the bacteria (Chapter 8). Central to the success of the pathogenic bacterium is the tremendous adaptability and genetic plasiticity of bacteria. The underlying genetic mechanisms involved in generating this diversity and variation are considered in Chapter 9.

5 Bacterial Nutrition: The Host as a Substrate

INTRODUCTION

A prerequisite for bacterial colonisation of any environment is the biochemical machinery necessary to obtain adequate nutrition. Bacteria are biochemically extremely versatile, far more so than eukaryotic organisms. This is reflected in the wide range of natural environments which they colonise. The bacteria which colonise humans can be broadly divided into two groups, the commensal flora and the pathogens. The opportunist pathogen which is also a member of the commensal flora may be in either group depending on circumstance. Many truly commensal bacteria tend to be less nutritionally versatile than the pathogens. For example the lactobacilli can be considered to be nutritionally handicapped in that they lack many biochemical pathways. This group of bacteria require many amino acids to be readily available as they lack the biochemical pathways necessary to produce their own. Many pathogenic bacteria are capable of utilising a wide range of substrates and have retained a biochemical adaptability which contributes to their success as pathogens. The substrates of the host can be divided into cells and their contents, the extracellular matrix which essentially holds the tissues together and molecules which are free in the body fluids. Some components may come into either category. For example immunoglobulin can remain cell associated or be free in serum and fibronectin can be either part of the extracellular matrix or free in body fluids. Many pathogenic bacteria either release enzymes or have cell associated enzymes which degrade all or some of these body components during active growth of the bacterium. This may benefit the bacterium by enabling it to spread through the host degrading for example the macromolecules of the extracellular matrix while taking up the released nutrients. These enzymes are also frequently directed at cells and molecules of the immune system which makes it difficult to classify them as either virulence determinants involved in avoiding the immune response, toxins, spreading agents or as purely playing a nutritional role. As many of these are expressed by the bacteria during exponential growth there is always the possibility that components of the degraded substrate may be taken up and utilised by the growing bacteria. Therefore these will be considered independently of other toxins which either do not have enzymic activity such as endotoxin (see

Chapter 2), or act intracellularly, have no obvious immediate nutritional benefit to the bacterium and are often produced as secondary metabolites (see Chapter 6).

Further problems have arisen in determining the precise nature and activities of these toxins as one bacterial type usually produces a variety of enzymes and toxins; the single toxin equating with virulence is the exception rather than the rule. Many of these molecules are multimeric and some require very specific conditions for activation. This makes it difficult to obtain the toxin in purified form. There is also the further complication that some of the infections in which these enzymes appear to participate are polymicrobial. For example in gas gangrene, infection results in the progressive pulping of muscle tissue. The causative organism may be *Clostridium perfringens* alone, or in combination with any of seven other clostridial species (e.g. *C. hystolyticum*, *C. oedematiens*, *C. sporogenes*).

Many of the bacterial toxins described in this chapter are designated by letters of the Greek alphabet. This usually relates to the order in which they were discovered and not necessarily to their relative importance as virulence determinants.

Types of bacteria where enzymic activities are probably related to virulence include *Staphylococcus* spp., *Streptococcus* spp., *Clostridium* spp., *Pseudomonas aeruginosa* and the non-spore forming anaerobes such as *Bacteroides* spp. and *Porphyromonas* spp. We will consider the range of substrates within the host which they are capable of acting on and how they go about degrading them. Unfortunately, although many studies have been done in which the presence or absence of degradative enzymes has been monitored, in many instances this has not been followed up with studies to determine how this might relate to either nutrition or virulence in vivo. Therefore, with a few exceptions, the true role of these toxins and enzymes in bacterial pathogenesis remains a matter for speculation.

One nutrient which is undoubtedly linked to virulence of bacteria is iron. Iron in the host is not readily available to the invading bacterium as it is sequestered to host molecules. There is clear evidence that this is one instance where the host is successfully controlling the growth of the invading microorganism as the list of pathogenic bacteria whose virulence and lethality are increased in animal models of infection if extra iron is provided is long and wide ranging. Species include: *Bacillus anthracis*, *Campylobacter jejuni*, *Clostridium perfringens*, *Escherichia coli*, *Listeria monocytogenes*, *Mycobacterium tuberculosis*, *Neisseria gonorrhoeae*, *Pasteurella multocida*, *Pseudomonas aeruginosa*, *Salmonella typhimurium*, *Staphylococcus aureus*, *Vibrio cholerae*, *Yersinia pestis*. From this it can be inferred that if the host did not restrict the availability of iron, the effects of these pathogens would be far more severe. Bearing in mind that most of these infections are limited, the bacteria have evolved specialised mechanisms for procuring iron. Some of these mechanisms appear to have evolved directly in response to the selective pressures of growth in vivo and involve highly specific interactions with host molecules. Other bacterial mechanisms for ion scavenging are of a more general nature and could be potentially useful to the bacterium in any nutrient poor environment.

HOST CELL LYSIS

Many pathogenic bacteria release enzymes with the potential to cause host cell death and destruction. Again it is not always possible to distinguish whether these activities of the pathogen contribute in a major way to virulence, or are largely nutrient scavenging mechanisms of the pathogen.

One of the most obvious and easily detectable activities of bacterial pathogens is the ability to lyse host cells by damaging the host cell membrane. This is easily demonstrated in the laboratory by incorporating blood cells into agar plates and observing the clear areas surrounding colonies where the blood has been lysed. Hence many of the bacterial enzymes with more general cytolytic activity are still called **haemolysins**, although strictly speaking they are **cytolysins**. As a result of the ease of detection of haemolytic activity, it has been used historically as a means of classifying pathogenic bacteria such as the streptococci.

Lysis of host cells could be advantageous to the invading pathogen in a number of different ways. Firstly it may be simply a way of releasing nutrients not otherwise readily available to the bacterium, such as intracellular iron (see below). For bacteria which have a requirement for the porphyrin ring of haem, lysis of red blood cells may be an important mechanism for obtaining this essential nutrient. Secondly, host cell destruction may allow the bacterium to spread through the tissues, in the same way that degradation of the extracellular matrix allows spreading. Finally, by lysing cells of the immune system, the bacterium may avoid the host's defence. This may in turn generate further cellular and tissue damage as a result of the release of the intra-cellular enzymes present within the host's lysosomal vesicles. Bacteria which are known to produce one or more cytolysin include a wide range of different species. Examples include *Escherichia coli, Proteus vulgaris, Streptococcus* spp., *Staphylococcus* spp. and *Clostridium* spp.

The mechanism of cell lysis may be specific for a given cell type and therefore probably involves recognition of a particular host cell receptor. Non-specific cytolysins, which have the potential to damage the membrane of any cell, are also produced by bacteria. Lysis is normally mediated by either the activity of lipase enzymes or the formation of pores (or ionophores) as a result of the insertion of the cytolysins in the host cell membrane. Some bacteria are profligate cytolysin producers and are capable of expressing a number of different types of cytolysin each with different activities (e.g. *Clostridium* spp. and *Staphylococcus* spp.). Other cytolysins (e.g. thiol-activated cytolysins and 'repeats-in-toxin' (RTX) cytolysins) with similar structures and activities are common to a wide range of bacteria.

Clostridial cytolysins

Clostridium spp. are a good example of bacteria which produce a range of different types of cytolysin.

The **phospholipase C** (also called lecithinase) enzyme or α toxin of the obligate anaerobe *Clostridium perfringens* is an example of a cytolysin whose activity is that of a lipase enzyme. This bacterium can cause septicaemia and anaerobic infection of muscle tissue known as gas gangrene. *Clostridium novyi* type D phospholipase C has similar activities and causes a frequently fatal disease of cattle. Phospholipase C, in combination with the collagenase enzyme also produced by these bacteria (see below), may have a lethal effect on the host. Other *Clostridium* spp. produce a phospholipase enzyme, but these do not seem to be the major virulence determinants. Why the phospholipase of *C. perfringens* has a different effect is unclear. *C. perfringens* also produces a number of other enzymes, such as elastase, hyaluronidase, neuraminidase and deoxyribonuclease, which degrade the host's extracellular matrix and cellular components. Exactly what contribution these enzymes make to virulence is not known, but they probably aid in the spread of infection.

The phospholipase C acts on two components of the host cell membrane: phosphatidyl choline (lecithin), which is hydrolysed to phosphorylcholine and a diglyceride, and sphingomyelin, which is hydrolysed to phosphorylcholine and ceramide. The site of action of phospholipase C is illustrated in Figure 5.1. This enzyme is therefore potentially lethal to a variety of different tissues and not specific for one type of cell. Its measureable activities include haemolysis of red blood cells and the enhancement of haemolytic activity of other bacteria such as *Staphylococcus aureus, Staphylococcus epidermidis* and *Serratia marcescens*. It will cause damage to the membranes of leukocytes, fibroblasts and muscle cells and causes platelets to aggregate and lyse. The enzyme has an apparent molecular mass of 43 kDa, contains zinc and is resistant to proteolytic degradation. Calcium or magnesium is required for its activity and is thought to be required to produce a positive charge on the surface of the phospholipid. The effects of the phospholipase C and the outcome of infection are dependent on the initial site of infection. *C. perfringens* is sometimes responsible for post-abortion septicaemia where it causes haemolysis on a large scale and renal damage, which may result in death. This is a rare example of the activity of a single molecule on a single substrate being largely responsible for the virulence of the bacterium; namely the phospholipase C acting on the membranes of the red blood cells and capillary epithelium. In contrast, in gas gangrene, where the bacterium colonises muscle tissue, again usually as a result of mechanical damage,

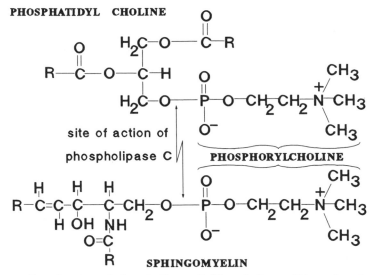

Figure 5.1. Site of action of phospholipase C. Phospholipase C is a phosphodiester-ase enzyme which cleaves phospholipids at the phosphodiester linkage (zigzag arrow). Phosphatidyl choline is split into phosphorylcholine and a diglyceride; sphingomyelin is split into phosphorylcholine and ceramide. R represents long chain hydrocarbons

the phospholipase is necessary to establish infection in the muscle tissue, but it does not enter into general circulation within the body. There is no large scale haemolysis and injection of anti-phospholipase C immuno-globulin into the infected muscle does not protect against the lethal effect of the infection. The activities of the collagenase enzyme which acts in con-cert with the phospholipase C are thought to be important in this instance (see above).

Perfringolysin (θ toxin) of *C. perfringens* also has general cytolytic activity. It belongs to the **thiol-activated cytolysins** (see below) which poly-merise on the host cell surface to form **pores** which apparently mediate cell lysis (see below).

Clostridium perfringens also produce a cytolysin which has **specific** activity against a restricted range of host cells, the **δ toxin** with a molecular mass of 42 kDa. It was initially described as being haemolytic towards a restricted range of animal species but is now known to be cytolytic for rabbit alveolar and peritoneal macrophages and human monocytes, but not thymocytes. This is in marked contrast to the non-specific lytic activities of the α toxin (or phospholipase C) described above. The specificity of the action of this toxin is determined by the host receptor to which it binds, namely GM_2 gangliosides or similar types of structure. These host cell surface glycolipids are mainly present on cells of the nervous system and are also found on cells of the immune system. For example thymocytes, lymphocytes, natural killer cells and macrophages can all carry gangliosides. Cell-free receptors are shed from some cells and lymphocytes and macrophages are known to have surface receptors for these molecules. It therefore seems that they play a role in cell-cell interactions, probably similar to that of interleukins. It is thought that the specificity of the molecule is related to the sialic acid-containing oligosaccharide moiety associated with the lipid and it is this to which the δ toxin binds. As the same oligosaccharide may be associated with different proteins and lipids on the one cell, the receptor should ideally always be defined in terms of the oligosaccharide part of the molecule. If erythrocytes carry a similar oligosaccharide this could explain the observed haemolytic activity of the δ toxin. This is one example of bacterial interaction with the host cell surface oligosaccharides. The oligosaccharides of gangliosides are also used by bacteria as receptors for some of the ADP-ribosylating toxins such as cholera toxin (Chapter 6). Bacterial molecules may also mimic the oligosaccharides of the host as in the striking similarity between *Neisseria meningitidis* type b capsular polysaccharide and ganglioside GM_1 (Chapter 7).

The specificity of δ toxin activity, in contrast with the more general activity of the α toxin, suggests that in relation to virulence the interaction of the δ toxin with host is more subtle than a simple nutrient scavenging mechanism. The δ toxin allows the bacterium to specifically interfere with the activities of cells of the immune system and may represent an evolutionary step-up from the crude cellular destruction.

Staphylococcal cytolysins

Staphylococcus aureus is another pathogen which produces host membrane damaging toxins which range from those with general activity to the very specific.

The *S. aureus* **α toxin** forms **pores** or transmembrane channels in a wide range of host cells. The channels consist of hexameric rings of 34 kDa toxin units, which alter the permeability of the host cell, causing cell lysis. The pores are homogeneous in nature, with an external diameter of approximately 8–10 nm and an internal pore of 2–3 nm diameter. Depending on the dose of toxin and the route of entry into the host this toxin can cause paralysis, neurotoxicity, necrosis or death. It is released from the bacteria during exponential growth and has a molecular mass of 33 kDa. Expression of the gene encoding the α toxin, *hly*, is under the control of the *agr* (*accessory gene regulator*; also called *exp*) gene which coordinately controls the expression of a number of extracellular proteins, including exfoliatin toxin, toxic shock syndrome toxin, α, β, δ toxins, enterotoxin b, lipases and nucleases (see Chapter 9).

The *S. aureus* **β toxin** is more restricted in its activity. It is a phospholipase which attacks sphyngomyelin in the cell membranes of erythrocytes, macrophages and platelets. Expression of the β toxin is controlled by the presence of bacteriophage in the staphylococcal genome. Two different phage are known to be involved. They are thought to stop β toxin production, either by inserting into the gene encoding for the toxin, *hlb*, or by encoding for molecules which repress production of the toxin. One of these phage encodes a gene for the staphylokinase enzymes (see below); therefore when the β toxin is switched off, staphylokinase is switched on.

The γ and δ toxins of *S. aureus* are also active against host cell membranes. The γ toxin is composed of two chains of 32 and 36 kDa but the mechanism of action is not known. The δ toxin is a much smaller molecule of only 3 kDa which lyses many cell types by solubilising the lipid of the membrane in a similar manner to a detergent.

The **leucocidin toxin** of *S. aureus* is **specifically** active against polymorphonuclear leukocytes (PMNLs) and macrophages. This toxin has two components, the F component of 32 kDa and S of 31 kDa. The S component binds specifically to ganglioside GM_1 and is followed by binding of the F component. Associated with the binding of the toxin there is an irreversible increase in the activity of the host cell membrane enzyme acyl-phosphatase and the activation of host cell phospholipase 2. The final outcome is lysis of the host cell. Host adenyl-cyclase activity is also increased but this is thought to be secondary to the other activities of the toxin. This toxin is therefore interfering in a very specific way with the normal activities of the host cell.

The **epidermolytic toxins** of *S. aureus* are another type of toxin with very **specific** activity. Two immunologically distinct molecular forms of this toxin are known, exfoliatin toxin A of 27 kDa and exfoliatin B of 27.5 kDa. Both toxins may be produced by the same strain and seem to have identical biological activity. These toxins may also behave as superantigens (see Chapter 2). Bacterial strains producing these toxins are responsible for the phenomenon known as scalded skin syndrome observed mostly in children, where the skin surface blisters and ultimately peels off, exposing the underlying epidermal layers. These toxins are specific for cells of the epidermis belonging to a layer known as the granular cell layer (Figure 5.2). The granular cell layer forms a narrow layer outside the prickle cell layer (named because the cell desmosomes appear as tiny prickles by light microscopy) and immediately beneath the dead flattened scales or squames, packed with keratin, which form the outermost layer of the skin. Exfoliatin does not strictly act on the cell membrane, but on the filaggrin group of proteins in intracellular keratohylin granules of cells of the granular layer. These granules are linked to the intermediate filaments of keratin which give structure to the cell and which extend across the inside of cells from the desmosomes. The desmosomes are the thickened regions of the cell membrane within tissues where cell adhesion molecules lock the cells together. After treatment with the exfoliatin toxin, the desmosomes split.

OUTSIDE

epidermal layer

- keratinised squames (dead cells)
- *granular cells*
- prickle cells
- basal cells (dividing cells)

INSIDE

Figure 5.2. The epidermal layer. Basal layer, the innermost layer of cells which divide and differentiate into the prickle cells, whose desmosomes appear as prickles on the cell surface by light microscopy. Granular cells, which are derived from the prickle cells, form a thin layer in which the cells are beginning to lose their nuclei and organelles. The granular layer is effectively the boundary between living cells and the layer of squames formed by dead cells packed with keratin. The squames form the outermost layer of the epidermis. Exfoliatin toxin acts specifically on the granular cells (italics)

As the cell adhesion molecules are specific for different tissue types, this may partly explain the specificity of the action of the exfoliatin toxin (Figure 5.3). Exfoliatin toxin A is encoded by a chromosomally located gene, *eta*, whereas the gene for toxin B, *etb*, is plasmid encoded. The genes for both toxins have been cloned and sequenced. They show remarkable similarity in the protein sequence, despite being immunologically distinct, with three major regions of close homology. It has been suggested that these regions may be important for the biological activity of the molecule. The *eta* gene is controlled by the *agr* gene regulator which is a member of the histidine-protein kinase response regulator superfamily (see Chapter 9).

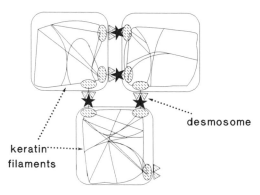

keratin filaments

desmosome

Figure 5.3. Schematic diagram of the granular cell layer. The intracellular keratin filaments extend across the inside of the cell from the desmosome junctions formed by multiple cell adhesion molecules (shown simplified in the figure). Exfoliatin toxin acts on the protein filaggrin which is associated with the keratin filaments and the cells split at the desmosomes

Thiol-activated cytolysins

This group of toxins includes cytolysins from 16 different Gram positive bacterial species, including *Streptococcus pneumoniae* pneumolysin, *Bacillus cereus* cereolysin, *Listeria monocytogenes* listeriolysin (involved in intracellular colonisation, see Chapter 8), *Clostridium perfringens* perfringolysin (also known as θ toxin) as well as a number of other clostridial species and *Streptococcus pyogenes* streptolysin O. (Streptolysin S does not belong to this family and is much smaller by comparison, with a molecular mass of only 18 kDa. It must be bound to a carrier molecule such as serum albumin, lipoprotein or RNA to be active.)

These cytolysins are immunologically cross-reactive and have similar biological activity. They contain an internal thiol group which is subject to alterations in the redox potential. When thiol groups on the amino acid cysteine are masked by oxygen the toxins are inactive, but they become active under reducing conditions. If cysteine is replaced by another amino acid, such as alanine, which lacks an -SH group, the full cytolytic activity of the toxin is retained. It therefore seems the thiol group is related to the oxygen sensitivity of the toxin but not its cytolytic action. These cytolysins polymerise to form rings and arc-shaped structures with 25–100 monomeric units on the host cell membrane. For example **streptolysin O** has a monomer subunit of approximately 89 kDa which can form **pores** of up to 30 nm diameter. (These are different from the pores formed by the staphylococcal α toxin which are smaller and homogeneous in size.) There is still some doubt as to the exact lytic mechanism, which may be more subtle than simply the formation of large transmembrane pores. It has been suggested that the concentrations of these toxins present during a natural infection are not sufficient to allow for the formation of these large lytic structures; however, even sublytic concentrations of the toxins are sufficient to interfere with the normal functions of cells such as B-cells and PMNLs. Interestingly, these cytolysins are also cardiotoxic and have an almost instantaneous lethal effect when injected into animals. This suggests that there may be highly specific interactions with host cells and tissues. As cholesterol will block activity of the toxins and membranes lacking cholesterol are not susceptible to their action, it is thought that cholesterol may form the toxin binding site. The protein sequences of some of these toxins have been determined and they show considerable homology. A region containing an 11 amino acid sequence, which includes the cysteine residue, appears to be highly conserved. There is also evidence that pneumolysin shares a region of homology with the acute phase reactant, C-reactive protein. It seems that this homologous region is capable of binding the Fc part of immunoglobulin and it has been suggested that this non-specifically bound immunoglobulin triggers complement activation.

The 'repeats in toxin' family of haemolysins

A number of bacteria, such as *E. coli, Bordetella pertussis, Pasteurella haemolytica* (leukotoxin), *Proteus vulgaris* and *P. mirabilis* produce genetically related toxins. Their activity is dependent on the presence of calcium ions. Characteristically, they have regions of 10 to 47 repeats within the amino acid sequence and are termed the 'repeats in toxin' or RTX gene family. The repeat sequence contains the following nine amino acids; leucine-X-glycine-glycine-X-glycine-asparagine-aspartic acid-X, where X is a variable amino acid. These repeats are required for the haemolytic activity. It is thought that the repeats form a beta-turn structure in the protein and that the aspartic acid binds ionically with calcium ions, which are needed for activity of the haemolysin. A large hydrophobic region of the haemolysin, separate from the repeats, is also essential for activity and may be involved in the interaction with the host cell membrane. Single molecules of the **haemolysin A** of *E. coli* apparently form **pores** of approximately 3 nm diameter on the target cell membrane. This haemolysin has been studied in some detail. It has a molecular mass of 107 kDa and requires the 20 kDa product of another gene, HlyC, before it becomes actively haemolytic. The mode of activation is not yet known, but the following are not involved; proteolytic cleavage of either the amino- or carboxy-terminal end, glycosylation or phosphorylation. Association, either covalently or non-covalently, of phospholipid may be involved in activation of HlyA. In *E. coli*, the operon for the production of the haemolysin contains four genes, *hlyA*, which codes for the structural haemolysin and *hlyC* which is required for activation of the HlyA. The other two genes *hlyB* and *hlyD* are involved in the transport of HlyA to the extracellular environment. The secretion of the haemolysin is unusual in that it is secreted independently of the normal mechanisms for transporting molecules out of Gram negative bacteria. Most proteins to be exported carry an N-terminal signal sequence which 'signals' the export of the molecule across the **cytoplasmic membrane**, the periplasm and then across the outer membrane. Although the exact mechanism of this process is unknown, in some bacteria the C-terminal region of the polypeptide is thought to direct crossing of the **outer membrane**, possibly by forming a pore specific for that protein. A number of additional genes, possibly as many as 13, may be required for the transport of some signal sequence containing proteins across the outer membrane. The signal sequence is normally cleaved from the peptide by a single peptidase enzyme and does not form part of the functional molecule. The HlyA protein lacks a signal sequence and is secreted by an entirely different mechanism, thought to be common to a number of homologous toxins. Examples include, *Pasteurella haemolytica* **leukotoxin** and the *Bordetella pertussis* bi-functional **adenylate cyclase haemolysin**. These toxins have a similar C-terminal sequence and associated genes analagous to those in the *hly* operon. The C-terminal secretion sequence of about 27 amino acids is thought to be the region of the haemolysin which recognises the 'transporter complex' formed by the other gene products within the operon (Figure 5.4). The *hlyB* gene codes for two polypeptides of 66 and 46 kDa and the *hlyD* gene one polypeptide of 53 kDa. These are thought to form a single transporter complex which spans **both** the cytoplasmic and outer membranes, thus bypassing movement through the periplasm. Another gene coding for TolC, a minor outer membrane protein of *E. coli*, is now known to be specifically involved in HlyA secretion. TolC is probably involved in the specific interaction of the HlyB/D transporter with the outer membrane. Sites such as these where the cytoplasmic and outer membranes are joined and which seem to be essential for the transport of molecules into and out of the bacterium are thought to be prime targets for the host's bactericidal molecules such as complement (Chapter 4). A region of the HlyB molecules is similar to regions of other proteins known to be involved in the adenosine triphosphate(ATP)-dependent transport of molecules and is a potential ATP-binding domain. Therefore it may be involved in the coupling of energy to the transportation of the haemolysin. The HlyC activator protein is not involved in the transport, but in the modification of the HlyA protein into an actively haemolytic form: mutants lacking *hlyC* efficiently secrete an inactive polypeptide. This type of transport system may be essential to prevent the lytic toxin from having a detrimental effect on the bacterial membranes. The operon may either be encoded chromosomally or present

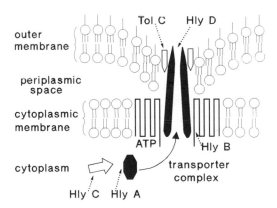

Figure 5.4. Model for the export of haemolysin A. HlyC induces the lytic activity of haemolysin A. The transporter complex is formed by ATP-binding HlyB in the cytoplasmic membrane, HlyD, which spans both the cytoplasmic and the outer membrane, and TolC which is associated with the outer membrane. HlyA may then traverse both the cytoplasmic and outer membranes without entering the periplasmic space. From L. Gray *et al.* 1989. A novel C-terminal signal sequence targets *E. coli* haemolysin directly to the medium. *Journal of Cell Science* Supplement II, pages 45–57. Reproduced by permission of the Company of Biologists Ltd

on a large self-transmissible plasmid. This is therefore another example of a potentially mobile virulence determinant (see Chapter 9).

The **adenylate cyclase/haemolysin** of *Bordetella pertussis* is only active once it has penetrated into the host cell. The adenlyate cyclase activity may be induced by calmodulin, a eukaryotic calcium binding protein. The toxic effects on the cell are thought to be the result of the high intracellular cyclic AMP synthesis. The C-terminal end of the protein has 25% homology with the HlyA of *E. coli* and contains tandem repeats similar to RTX. The *cyaA* gene, thought to encode for the toxin, was cloned into *E. coli*. It produced an enzymatically active, but non-toxic protein. A second gene, *cyaC*, was identified which is thought to confer haemolytic activity on CyaA by post-translational modification. This toxin is therefore bi-functional with both haemolytic and adenylate cyclase activity (this is also under the control of the *bvg* locus: see Chapter 9). There is scant evidence for uptake of the toxin into host cells, but it has been suggested that *B. pertussis* may invade the host cell and release the CyaA protein intracellularly.

Thus bacteria can produce a range of cytotoxic molecules which may allow the bacterium access to essential nutrients and also may be targeted specifically at host cells to avoid the host defence mechanisms.

DEGRADATION OF THE EXTRACELLULAR MATRIX

The macromolecules of the extracellular matrix form an intricate structure with which cells of the tissues are associated. The extracellular matrix can be considered as the glue which holds the tissues together, or the scaffolding which gives the tissues physical structure. It is not, however, an inert component of the body but is thought to be involved in the control of tissue development and, through the activities of associated cytokines, the activation of host cells.

The extracellular matrix is composed of a network of the fibrous proteins collagen, elastin and fibronectin embedded in a hydrated polysaccharide gel of glycosaminoglycans such as hyaluronic acid, chondroitin sulphate and heparin sulphate (Table 5.1). The glycosaminoglycans may be joined to proteins to form proteoglycans, which also contribute to the jelly or ground substance, in which the fibrous proteins are interwoven.

The **collagens** are a family of triple stranded proteins which form a stiff helical structure. They constitute 25% of the total protein of mammals and therefore form one of the major substrates available to the invading pathogen. *Bacteroides* spp. and *Clostridium* spp. are known to have collagenase activity. *Clostridium hystolyticum* expresses two or more enzymes of 72 and 81 kDa with collagenase activity, known as the β toxin. These cause severe tissue damage and are lethal if injected intravenously into animals where they cause pulmonary haemorrhage. The enzymes hydrolyse collagen into peptides of 4–5 amino acids in length. These enzymes may act synergisti-

Table 5.1. Bacteria which degrade components of the extracellular matrix

Extracellular matrix component	Bacterial genus
Collagen	*Clostridium*
	Bacteroides
	Porphyromonas
Elastin	*Bacteroides*
	Pseudomonas
Proteoglycans	*Clostridium*
	Bacteroides
	Streptococcus

cally with other clostridial species in gas gangrene. *Clostridium perfringens* also expresses a collagenase of approximately 80 kDa, called the κ toxin, which is thought to contribute to the softening and pulping of the muscle fibre which occurs in gas gangrene. The degradation of the collagen fibre also removes the supporting reticulum for the capillaries and blood vessels which will cause haemorrhage, while providing the bacterium with a plentiful supply of nitrogen.

Porphyromonas (previously known as *Bacteroides) gingivalis* has a cell-surface associated collagenase enzyme which cleaves the helical domain of types I, II and III collagens. It is also known to secrete a trypsin-like protease which degrades the basement membrane of collagen type IV. Although the precise role of these enzymes in *P. gingivalis* infection is not known, *P. gingivalis* is implicated in periodontal disease and the associated gum destruction.

Elastin as the name implies, is responsible for the elasticity of tissues such as the lungs, blood vessels and skin. It is a glycoprotein molecule of 70 kDa, rich in the amino acids proline and glycine, but has little hydroxyproline and no hydroxylysine. The molecules of elastin form random coils which have physical properties similar to a rubber band. *Pseudomonas aeruginosa* is known to have elastase activity and this is thought to be involved in the damage it causes to lungs and its ability to form corneal ulcers. Degradation of the elastin may indirectly cause haemorrhage. These proteases are not lethal by themselves, as are some of the collagenase enzymes. It is known that the virulence of *Pseudomonas aeruginosa* is also dependent on other factors such as the expression of exotoxin A (see Chapter 6). *Bacteroides* spp. are also reported to produce an elastase enzyme.

The **proteoglycans**, such as hyaluronic acid, chondroitin sulphate and heparin sulphate, which form the jelly-like component of the extracellular matrix, are also subject to bacterial degradation. Proteoglycans differ from glycoproteins in that the major part of the molecule is polysaccharide, rather than protein. A rough guide to the nomenclature of these protein/saccharide molecules is that if 50% or less of molecules is saccharide it is termed a glycoprotein, if more than 50% is polysaccharide it is termed a proteoglycan. The polysaccharide moieties of proteoglycans usually consist of varying numbers of disaccharide repeating units linked in a linear chain called a glycosaminoglycan. The spacing of the polysaccharide chains depends on the nature of the protein backbone to which they are attached, as well as the number of suitable attachment sites. There may be more than one type of polysaccharide chain attached to the same protein. One of the sugars of the repeating disaccharide unit is normally an amino-sugar such as 2-amino-2-deoxy-D-galactose or 2-amino-2-deoxy-D-glucose. These sugars are usually N-acetylated or N-sulphated on the amino group, which counteracts the basicity of the amino group. Uronic acid or O-sulphate groups on the hydroxyl groups make the sugar acidic. The proteoglycans were generally named after the source from which they were first extracted and do not relate to their molecular constituents; for example, chondroitin sulphate from chondros, the Greek for cartilage, heparin from the Greek for liver and hyaluronic acid from hyaloid. The glycosaminoglycan of hyaluronic acid is composed of from 500 to several thousand repeating units of D-glucuronic acid and 2-acetamido-2-deoxy-D-glucose. Chondroitin is composed of D-glucuronic acid and 2-acetamido-2-deoxy galactose in the same linkage as the two sugars of hyaluronic acid. Chondroitin may be present in the host as a sulphated form, where the amino-galactose is sulphated at one of two possible sites. Chondroitin sulphate tends to have a much shorter chain length than hyaluronic acid, with only 10 to 60 repeating units. Thus, the only molecular difference between chondroitin and hyaluronic acid is in the orientation of one hydroxyl group. A number of *Bacteroides* spp. produce hyaluronidase, heparinase and chondroitin sulphatase enzymes and *C. perfringens* μ toxin is a hyaluronidase enzyme. The relevance of these degradative enzymes to the nutrition of these bacteria in vivo is not known; it is not known if the bacteria metabolise the end-products of the degradation and use them as a source of nutrients. *Streptococcus pyogenes* produce a polysaccharide capsule of the same composition as the hyaluronic acid of the host's glycosaminoglycan. They also produce hyaluronidase enzymes which depolymerise their own capsules; however, there is no evidence that the breakdown products are used as a source of nutrient by the bacteria. Bacterial mimicry of mammalian proteoglycans is considered in more detail in Chapter 7.

EFFECTS ON OTHER HOST MOLECULES

It seems likely that the specific degradation of host molecules by bacteria relates to survival mechanisms other than simple nutrition; evasion of the host defences and general interference with the host systems may be involved. With many of these bacterial products, however, the direct link with virulence of the bacterium remains to be proven.

Urea

A number of bacteria produce urease enzymes which degrade urea, notably *Proteus* spp. which causes urinary tract infection. It is not clear, however, if the ammonia released by the enzyme is a suitable nitrogen source for the bacterium, or if the enzyme simply reduces the toxicity of urea. *Helicobacter pylori*, which is associated with gastric ulcers, also produces an abundant and potent urease.

Lipid

Lipid breakdown has already been mentioned in relation to the more specific action of cytolysis (see above). A number of bacteria produce lipases, including *Staphylococcus* spp., *Pseudomonas aeruginosa* and *Legionella pneumophila*. Expression of the lipase produced by *Staphylococcus* spp. is controlled by a lysogenic bacteriophage. The site at which the phage integrates into the chromosome is at the C-terminal end of the protein. Therefore if the phage integrates, a truncated and inactive enzyme is produced, although it may still be detectable with antibodies to the lipase enzyme. The variable expression of the β toxin gene of *S. aureus* may be controlled by a similar mechanism (see above). For a further discussion of phage controlled expression of virulence genes see Chapter 9.

Fibrin–fibrinogen

Monomeric fibrin is an insoluble protein composed of six polypeptide chains, which spontaneously form long fibres. These fibres form the matrix of blood clots and interact with blood platelets. It also forms a type of 'scaffolding' in inflammatory lesions where tissue repair can take place. Fibrin monomer is formed from a soluble precursor molecule fibrinogen by the activity of the proteolytic enzyme, **thrombin**. Thrombin cleaves four short peptides from the six polypeptide chains, resulting in a molecule of much lower solubility. Thrombin itself is synthesised in an inactive form as **prothrombin**. Thrombin contains some sequences similar to the pancreatic serine protease enzymes such as trypsin. The lysis of fibrin clots is controlled by another host molecule, **plasmin**, which is also formed from an inactive form, plasminogen. The activation of plasminogen to form plasmin is normally controlled by a host serine protease enzyme, called **tissue plasminogen activator**, which converts plasminogen into plasmin, resulting in lysis of fibrin clots.

A number of bacterial enzymes can interfere with the clotting/lysis of fibrin (Figure 5.5). The **streptokinase** and **staphylokinase** enzymes of *Streptococcus* spp. and *Staphylococcus* spp., respectively, activate plasminogen to form plasmin. These two bacterial kinases therefore indirectly mediate the lysis of fibrin clots, by mimicking the activity of the host's tissue plasminogen activator. *Yersinia pestis* also produces a plasminogen activator. The genes coding for the staphylokinase enzyme (*sak*) are present on a lysogenic phage and are under the control of the regulatory gene *agr* (see section on staphylococcal cytolysins above). Other than this little is known about the regulation of expression of this gene.

Porphyromonas (Bacteroides) gingivalis, which is thought to be involved in gum disease, expresses surface proteins which specifically bind to and subsequently degrade human fibrinogen. The fibrinogen-binding protein of 150 kDa is a separate molecule from the two fibrinogen proteases of 120 and 150 kDa which degrade **fibrinogen** into two large fragments. *Bacteroides fragilis*, which is a member of the commensal flora of the gut and an opportunistic pathogen frequently isolated from peritoneal infection, also produces **fibrinolysin** enzymes.

Staphylocoagulase, produced by *Staphylococcus* spp., is thought to react with a factor present in prothrombin which causes clot formation, converting fibrinogen to fibrin. Bovine isolates of *Peptococcus indolicus* produce a **peptocoagulase** which has similar activity. The activity of these molecules is not thought to be strictly enzymatic, but they alter the conformation of the prothrombin which make it bind to the active sites on the fibrin molecule.

Bacteria producing molecules such as these will almost certainly interfere with tissue repair mechanisms.

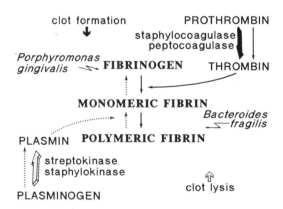

Figure 5.5. Bacterial interference with clot-formation and lysis. Bacteria can cause clot formation (*Staphylococcus* spp., *Peptococcus* spp. coagulases; dark arrows), cause clot lysis (*Staphylococcus* spp., *Streptococcus* spp. kinases; dotted arrows) and degrade fibrinogen (*Porphyromonas gingivalis*) and fibrin (*Bacteroides fragilis*; zigzag arows)

Nucleic acids

Staphylococcus spp. can degrade both deoxyribonucleic acid (DNA) and ribonucleic acid (RNA). The DNase and RNase enzymes hydrolyse the ester bonds between phosphoric acid and carbon in the 5' position of ribose or deoxyribose which results in the formation of 3' phosphate nucleotides. *Streptococcus pyogenes* produce DNase of different activity. This enzyme cleaves the 3' phosphate bond producing 5' DNA fragments of varying lengths. A range of *Bacteroides* spp., including *Bacteroides fragilis* and *Bacteroides ruminicola*, also produce DNase enzymes. Enzymes such as these may supply nutrients required by the bacteria for growth. They may also aid in the spreading of the pathogen as nucleic acid released from lysed host cells will make the immediate environment around the bacterium very viscous.

Oligosaccharides and sialic acids

A number of bacteria, including *Bacteroides fragilis, Vibrio cholerae, Corynebacterium diphtheriae, Streptococcus pneumoniae, Streptococcus agalactiae* and *Clostridium perfringens*, produce enzymes which will remove or destroy the oligosaccharides present on host cell glycoproteins and glycolipids. Included in this group of enzymes are the **neuraminidase** enzymes which specifically remove sialic acids. **Sialic acid** is the general name for a family of sugar molecules which are derivatives of N-acetylated neuraminic acid (see Appendix). By various substitutions and additions to the basic molecule there are 30 different naturally occurring sialic acids. It is now becoming clear that sialic acid residues which are present in the oligosaccharides of the host glycolipids and glycoproteins may play a role in the activities of these molecules, in particular in relation to specific recognition of receptors and cell–cell interactions. One area where sugar residues are known to be important is in the movement or 'trafficking' of lymphocytes around the host (see Chapter 2). Rat T-lymphocytes which were removed from the rat, treated with a sialidase enzyme from *Vibrio cholerae* and then returned to the rat did not migrate as they would normally into the lymph nodes, but migrated into the liver and spleen where they appeared to be re-sialylated. The movement of lymphocytes into and out of lymphoid organs, such as lymph nodes, occurs through specialised high walled capillary venules called high endothelial venules (HEV). The cube-shaped endothelial cells of these venules carry adhesion molecules known as HEV-ligands which are recognised by 'homing' receptors present on lymphocytes. These interactions control organ specific migration of the lymphocytes (see also Chapter 2). Treatment of HEV with sialidase from either *Vibrio cholerae* or *Clostridium perfringens* in vitro prevented the attachment of lymphocytes to the endothelial cells of the HEV. Injection of sialidase intravenously into mice also altered the migration pattern of the lymphocytes. Therefore release of these enzymes by bacterial pathogens could have very subtle effects on cell–cell interactions. Sialic acids are also thought to be important in the adhesion of cells during foetal development. Neural cell adhesion molecules are sialogylcoproteins which contain a polysialic acid. The embryonic forms of these adhesion molecules contain more sialic acid than the adult form. The reduction in sialic acid is thought to relate to an increase in the adhesion between cells.

Some species of *Streptococcus* produce sialidase enzymes. Treatment of human immunoglobulin with the streptococcal enzyme and subsequent injection of the immunoglobulin into rabbits caused acute nephritis. Repeated injections of *Streptococcus agalactiae* (also called Lancefield group B streptococcus) into rats will induce arthritis and rheumatoid factor production. It is possible to speculate that production of neuraminidase by the bacterial pathogen could de-sialate immunoglobulin in vivo and this may in some way relate to glomerulonephritis or arthritis. It is known that the IgG of humans with rheumatoid arthritis have abnormal oligosaccharide chains, in that they lack terminal galactose and sialic acid residues. The lack of these sugar residues decreases the binding of complement to IgG.

Neuraminidase activity in clinical isolates of *Bacteroides fragilis* has been directly correlated with the ability to survive in an animal model of infection, although the underlying mechanism(s) of this is not known.

A number of bacteria produce **endoglycosidase** enzymes which cleave oligosaccharides at different places by hydrolysing the internal sugar linkages. Examples include endo-β-galactosidase produced by *Bacteroides fragilis* and endoglycosidase D and endo-α-acetylgalactosaminidase produced by *Streptococcus pneumoniae*. Whether or not these enzymes play a major role in virulence remains to be determined. It seems likely, however, that as more information becomes available about the role of oligosaccharides and sialic acids in biological interactions the importance of these enzymes in bacterial virulence will become clearer. One area where surface oligosaccharides are known to be important is in host-cell to cell recognition events (see Chapter 2).

Immunoglobulin and complement

The advantage to a pathogenic microbe of degrading the host's immunoglobulin and complement molecules appears to be obvious. *Haemophilus influenzae, Neisseria meningitidis, N. gonorrhoeae, Streptococcus pneumoniae* and a wide range of *Bacteroides* spp. are among the range of bacteria all reported to produce enzymes which specifically degrade human IgA1. *Porphyromonas gingivalis, Bacteroides intermedius, B. assacharolyticus* are capable of degrading IgA1, IgA2, IgG and IgM (see Appendix for Ig structures). The IgA1 proteases of the *Bacteroides* spp. are known to attack the immunoglobulin molecule at a variety of different sites. This may result in complete degradation of the IgA1, degradation of all of the immunoglobulin except for the Fc region, degradation which leaves the Fc and the Fab portion intact, or removal of the oligosaccharide chains of the IgA. The IgA1 proteases which cleave the IgA molecule into the Fav and Fc regions act specifically in a small part of the hinge region of the heavy chain, which is absent in human IgA2, and are therefore specific for IgA1. The IgA1 protease producing bacteria are usually found on mucosal surfaces where secretory IgA is the principal immunoglobulin type present (see Chapter 3). It therefore seems that these enzymes have evolved specifically in relation to the ecological niche in which these bacteria survive, although how much they contribute to the overall virulence of the bacteria is not yet proven.

A number of proteases will non-specifically break down the complement glycoproteins. Included in these is the elastase produced by *P. aeruginosa*. On the other hand some bacteria produce enzymes which specifically degrade complement components. For example, some strains of *Porphyromonas gingivalis* degrade complement factors C3, C4 and C5, and some of the other black-pigmented bacteroides degrade C3, *Streptococcus pyogenes* produces a cell-associated C5a peptidase of 128 kDa which removes a six amino acid sequence from the carboxy-terminus of C5a. This degraded form of the C5a will no longer bind to the surface receptor on human PMNLs and therefore no longer functions as a chemoattractant. *Bacteroides fragilis* isolates contain a protease which cleaves C3b to iC3b. This may be a possible mechanism of resistance to serum killing.

IRON SCAVENGING MECHANISMS

Iron is an essential nutrient for both the host and the pathogen and plays a key role in the growth of bacteria in vivo. To emphasise the point Professor Richard Finkelstein quotes Otto von Bismarck in his speech to the Prussian Diet in 1862, albeit entirely out of context: 'The great questions of the time are not decided by speeches and majority decisions ... but by iron and blood.'

Iron is central to the functioning of a number of biological processes. These include, firstly the cytochrome components of the **electron transport chain**, which by sequential electron donation and acceptance generates cellular energy in the form of adenosine triphosphate (ATP). Secondly, the **reductase enzymes**, which are used for the production of the deoxyribonucleotide subunits of deoxyribonucleic acid (DNA), contain iron. There are also a number of other **iron-sulphur containing proteins** and **enzymes** which require iron to function. In bacteria, the lactobacilli are the exception to this rule of iron requirement; they have incomplete electron transport chains and obtain their energy requirements by fermentation rather than electron transport. Their reductase enzymes contain cobalt, not iron, and are derived from vitamin B12.

The questions to be asked are therefore how do pathogens obtain their iron, what are the sources in the host and how difficult is it for the bacterium to obtain iron? First of all we will consider the availability of iron in the host.

Iron sources in the host

Free iron concentration within the host is estimated to be of the order of 10^{-18}M, clearly insufficient to allow growth of the bacterial pathogen. In serum and body fluids, host iron is complexed or associated with carrier molecules (Table 5.2). These glycoproteins chelate (or sequester) the iron.

The two major serum glycoproteins involved are transferrin and lactoferrin. **Transferrin** is present in serum and lymph and is involved in the transport and transfer of iron to host cells. It has a molecular mass of approximately 70–80 kDa, with a single polypeptide and two iron binding sites. Transferrin receptors are present on host cell membranes and their numbers increase when some cells become activated. After binding to the cell receptor, the iron enters into the intracellular iron pool from where it may either become involved in the metabolic pathways of the cell or be sequestered to **ferritin** in the intracellular iron store.

Lactoferrin is found in human milk, saliva, tears, running noses, granules of polymorphonuclear leukocytes, intestinal fluids, seminal fluids, cervical mucus, respiratory tract mucus and colostrum. Of importance to the pathogen is that lactoferrin can retain iron under the acidic conditions generated at sites of inflammation.

In serum, iron is also found in haem-containing molecules such as **haemoglobin**, which consists of four globin molecules. The haem is carried within a central 'pocket'. Haem is a flat porphyrin ring consisting of four pyrrole groups joined together, with the iron in the centre. In serum haemoglobin is complexed with other proteins such as **haptoglobin**. Small amounts of haemoglobin-free haem may also be present, usually bound to

Table 5.2. Iron sources within the host

Cellular	Body Fluids
Lactoferrin	Lactoferrin
Transferrin	Transferrin
Ferritin	Haem-haemopexin
Haemoglobin	Haemoglobin-haptoglobin
Myoglobin	
Enzymes	

serum albumin or **haemopexin**. Intracellularly iron may either be associated with haemoglobin, transferrin or lactoferrin, or stored in the form of ferritin.

During the course of infection iron availability may be further restricted if a state of hypoferraemia is triggered. This type of defence mechanism of the host is termed nutritional immunity. The induction of hypoferraemia is one of the many host mechanisms which bacterial lipopolysaccharide is thought to induce (see Chapter 2). Iron concentrations are reduced even further by decreasing serum iron while maintaining high levels of transferrin. Polymorphonuclear leukocytes may also release iron-free lactoferrin, apolactoferrin, which will mop up free iron. The lactoferrin containing the iron is then taken up by phagocytic cells.

To the invading pathogen iron is therefore largely inaccessible. As a result of this bacteria have evolved specific adaptive mechanisms to overcome the iron-famine of the host. Despite the evolution of such mechanisms, the effectiveness of the iron restriction as a way of limiting bacterial virulence is clearly illustrated by the wide range of bacteria whose virulence is greatly enhanced if exogenous iron is given to the host (see above).

Bacterial options for obtaining iron

Firstly, bacteria may opt for an **intracellular** existence and take the chance of gaining sufficient iron from the intracellular pool. (For further discussion of intracellular growth and survival of bacteria see Chapter 8.) *Listeria monocytogenes* is one such pathogen. By producing a reductant which reduces Fe^{3+} to Fe^{2+}, iron is released from intracellular chelating glycoproteins. The reducing conditions under which obligate anaerobes grow may also favour release of iron from glycoprotein chelators.

Secondly intracellular iron may be obtained by lysing the host cells with **cytolysins** or haemolysins, providing either free iron, haem or haemoglobin. There is evidence that some bacteria use the haem from epithelial cells which are sloughed off at mucosal surfaces. *Neisseria* spp. *Porphyromonas* and *Prevotella (Bacteroides)* spp. produce specific proteases which degrade transferrin in order to release the iron.

At a more sophisticated level many pathogenic bacteria have evolved specific mechanisms for removing iron from the host's carrier molecules. *Vibrio cholerae* can use haemoglobin as a source of iron by removing the haem group. *Porphyromonas (Bacteroides)* spp. can degrade the other haem-complexing serum glycoproteins, haemopexin and haptoglobin. *Yersinia pestis* will also use haem and *Haemophilus influenzae, Staphylococcus aureus* and *Streptococcus pyogenes* can all use the haemoglobin/haptoglobin complex as a source of iron.

Probably the most widespread mechanism which bacteria have evolved to obtain iron in the host is the production of chelating agents by the bacterium which can compete with the host's; these bacterial products have either an equal or higher affinity for iron (Figure 5.6). The general term for these bacterial derived chelating agents is **siderophore**. Bacteria use their own chelating agents to effectively solubilise iron from inorganic sources or remove it from other chelating agents. They are therefore of general use to the bacterium growing in any low iron environment. (Some of the siderophores which are thought to be important in bacterial virulence and the control of the production of these molecules are considered in detail below.)

In contrast with siderophore production *Neisseria gonorrhoeae* and *N. meningitidis* have taken their level of adaptation a step further. They do not appear to produce their own siderophores but can use the host's lactoferrin and transferrin, which they can bind directly, as sources of iron. It seems that they do this by expressing molecules which mimic the host's receptors for iron chelating glycoproteins (Figure 5.6). Ovotransferrin, from chickens, although a very similar protein to human transferrin, does not support the growth of *Neisseria* spp. Hence, this is an example of a very specific host–pathogen interaction. Growth under iron limitation induces the production of novel outer membrane proteins of approximately 70–100 kDa, which are thought to be the receptors. There is also evidence that *Neisseria gonorrhoeae* expresses haemin-binding proteins under iron-limiting conditions. The various mechanisms by which pathogenic bacteria obtain iron are summarised in Table 5.3.

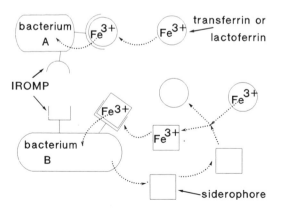

Figure 5.6. Bacterial uptake of iron. Bacterium A expresses an iron repressible outer membrane protein (IROMP) which recognises host iron sequestering glycoproteins such as lactoferrin or transferrin (circle). Bacterium B secretes its own iron sequestering molecule or siderophore (box) which can remove iron from the host's sequestering glycoprotein and expresses an IROMP which recognises the ferric siderophore

Table 5.3. Mechanisms of bacterial iron scavenging

Intracellular bacterial growth
Release of intracellular iron by cytolysis and haemolysis
Degradation of host's iron carriers
Expression of receptors for host's iron carriers
Production of high affinity iron chelators (siderophores)

Siderophores: nature and biosynthesis

Siderophores have a molecular mass of about 600 Da. Although small, they are not small enough to enter the bacterium by diffusion. Therefore they enter into the bacterial cell via specific membrane protein receptors with a high molecular weight (Figure 5.6). Other siderophore specific proteins may be involved in the movement of iron across the periplasmic space and the cytoplasmic membrane in Gram negative bacteria. The production of the siderophores and the proteins involved in their uptake and transfer into the bacterium are all induced by low iron concentrations. Some bacteria express receptors for siderophores, but not the siderophores themselves. It seems that these bacteria effectively commandeer the siderophores produced by other bacteria. This may be very important in polymicrobial infections. As siderophores are effectively obtaining host iron, this could also have a detrimental effect on the cells of the host which also require iron. For example, there is evidence that siderophores may effectively suppress the activities of T-cells. Thus by obtaining iron as a nutrient the bacterium could also be inhibiting the activities of the immune system.

The majority of bacterial siderophores fall into two types, based on their molecular structure; the **hydroxamate-citrate** family and the **phenolate** family (derived from catechol). Table 5.4 lists some bacteria and the siderophores which they are known to produce and Figure 5.7 illustrates the structure of **enterobactin** (catechol family) and **aerobactin** (hydroxamate family).

Aerobactin is an example of the hydroxamate-citrate family of siderophores which is produced by *Escherichia coli*, *Salmonella typhimurium* and *Aerobacter aerogenes* (Figure 5.7). It forms an octahedral complex, with iron chelated by the bidentate hydroxamate arms, central carboxylate and probably the citrate hydroxyl group. Citrate alone is a low affinity chelator. The addition of hydroxamate side chains increases the affinity and stability of the molecule. The three basic constituents of the molecule are hydroxylysine, acetate and citrate. Therefore, it might be anticipated that three genes are required to code for the enzymes necessary for the production of the basic constituents, with probably a fourth gene to code for the membrane receptor for the siderophore. Genetic studies of *E. coli* revealed that aerobactin production required the function of chromosomal genes but was also

Table 5.4. Siderophores produced by bacteria

Siderophore	Bacterium
*Enterobactin	*Escherichia coli*
	Klebsiella pneumoniae
	Salmonella typhimurium
	Shigella dysenteriae
	Shigella sonnei
*Vibriobactin	*Vibrio cholerae*
*Anguibactin	*Vibrio anguillarum*
*Pyochelin	*Pseudomonas aeruginosa*
†Pyoverdin	
†Mycobactin Exochelins	*Mycobacterium* spp.
†Aerobactin	*Escherichia coli*
	Salmonella typhimurium
	Aerobacter aerogenes
	Shigella flexneri
†Desferrioxamine	*Streptomyces* spp.

*Catechol family.
†Hydroxamate family.

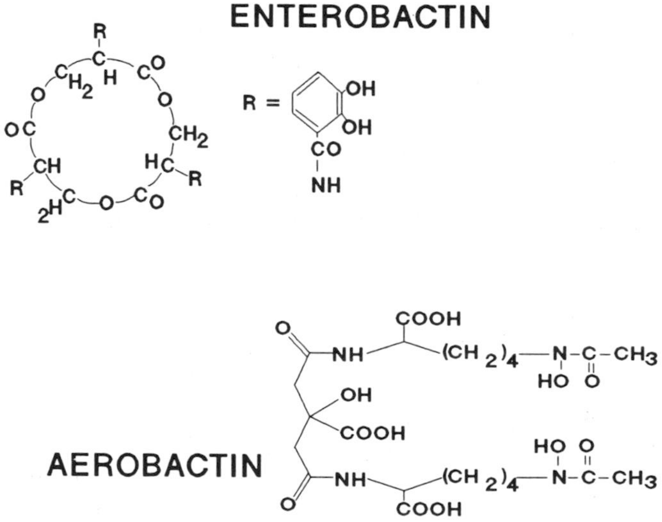

Figure 5.7. Comparison of catechol and hydroxamate siderophores. Enterobactin is a catechol type siderophore derived from phenolates. Aerobactin is a hydroxamate citrate type siderophore derived from citrate with two bidentate hydroxamate arms. These can both be produced by *Escherichia coli*

linked with the presence of a plasmid, known as pColV. This plasmid was known to code for the gene for the bacteriocin, colicin. (Bacteriocins are bacterial products which kill bacteria of a different species.) Removal of the gene for colicin production from the plasmid did not interfere with aerobactin production. This indicated that aerobactin formation was a separate function of the plasmid. The problem was then to identify which part of the plasmid **was** involved in aerobactin production. To do this use was made of the sensitivity of *E. coli* to the bacteriocin, cloacin, which is produced by *Enterobacter cloacae*. It is common for siderophore receptors to be also receptors for bacteriocins; in this case the aerobactin receptor is also a receptor for cloacin. Different parts of the colicin plasmid were put or inserted into another plasmid, carrying an ampicillin resistance marker. Bacteria containing the 'hybrid' plasmids were then screened for both ampicillin resistance, to make sure that they contained the plasmid, and sensitivity to cloacin, to see if the aerobactin genes were present (Figure 5.8). By doing this, genes for aerobactin production were narrowed down to a 7–8 kilobase (kb) region of the plasmid which coded for five gene products. These were defined as polypeptides of 62, 63, 33, 53 and 74 kDa. The 74 kDa polypeptide was identified as the aerobactin **membrane recep-**

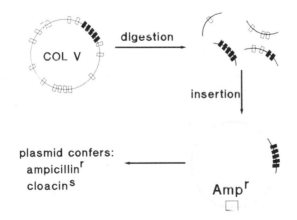

Figure 5.8. Cloning of the aerobactin biosynthesis genes. Segments of the colicin V (COL V) plasmid (pColV), which is known to carry the genes for both aerobactin biosynthesis and the aerobactin receptor, are cloned into another plasmid which carries an ampicillin resistance gene. Plasmids are then transferred into a bacterium which does not produce aerobactin and is ampicillin sensitive. After the plasmid transfer, bacteria are then selected which are ampicillin resistant and are sensitive to the bacteriocin cloacin, as the aerobactin receptor is coincidentally a receptor for cloacin. (The cloacin selection is done by replica plating). These bacteria will therefore contain a plasmid which is carrying the gene for the aerobactin receptor and probably the genes associated with biosynthesis. Further investigation of the plasmid aerobactin operon has shown that it contains five genes, four for biosynthesis and one for the receptor

tor and the gene was given the name *iron uptake transport (iut) A*. It was discovered that the other four polypeptides were all required for aerobactin biosynthesis. Therefore four gene products are necessary for aerobactin synthesis, not three as initially anticipated. The genes were designated *iron uptake chelate (iuc) A, B, C* and *D*. The synthesis of aerobactin and the enzymes involved is represented in Figure 5.9. The IucA and the IucC enzymes are unusual as they catalyse the synthesis of non-peptide amide bonds. The *iucD* gene product is also interesting as it is a **hydroxylysine monooxygenase**. The reaction which it catalyses, the direct oxidation of a primary amine to a hydroxyamine, is a reaction which does not normally occur in animal tissue. This is therefore an example of an enzyme which catalyses the first step in the production of an important virulence determinant, and which appears not to occur in the host. This is therefore a potential target for chemotherapeutic agents designed to block aerobactin synthesis in vivo, as a potent inhibitor of the enzyme is not likely to be toxic to the host.

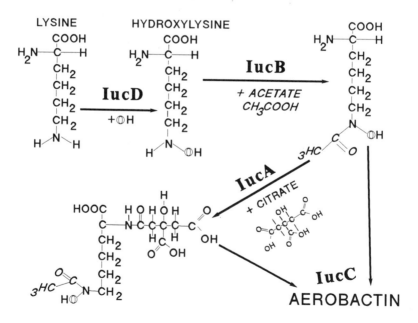

Figure 5.9. Aerobactin biosynthesis. Lysine is converted to hydroxylysine by a monooxygenase enzyme (IucD) and then acetyl hydroxylysine by an acetylase enzyme (IucB). The addition of one acetyl hydroxylysine to citrate is catalysed by IucA to form one of the arms of aerobactin (see Figure 5.7). The addition of a second acetyl hydroxylysine is catalysed by IucC

Siderophores: genetic control of production

Although the genes for aerobactin production in *E. coli* were found on the colicin V plasmid (pColV), *Salmonella* spp. and some strains of *E. coli* are known to produce aerobactin, although lacking a plasmid. Mapping of the aerobactin operon revealed insertion sequence (IS) 1 about 4–5 kilobases (kb) upstream of the promoter region and an inverted copy of IS1, immediately downstream of *iutA* gene, which is the last gene in the operon. Therefore the aerobactin operon forms a potential **transposable element** which can move from the plasmid to the chromosome and back (see Chapter 9). This ability to mobilise a set of genes coding for virulence *en bloc* must confer a tremendous selective advantage to the population of pathogenic bacteria.

The **induction** of the iron uptake operon occurs at the transcriptional level. The promoter is of the 'strong' variety, which results in a high yield of mRNA transcript. It has been postulated that the control is similar to that of the *lac* operon, with negative control of transcription (Figure 5.10). The repressor requires iron to bind to the promoter and this prevents transcription. Without iron the repressor no longer binds and transcription occurs. There is also some evidence for control at the translational level. A possible ribosome binding sequence 7 base pairs (bp) upstream of the ATG start codon has also been identified and mRNA-ribosome binding may be controlled in some way by iron concentration.

Much of this work was done with *lacZ* fusions, whereby the *lacZ* gene was placed in the aerobactin operon. Therefore expression of the *lacZ*-fusion was used as an indication of aerobactin production. Mutants were obtained

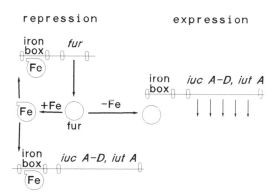

Figure 5.10. Iron mediated repression of the aerobactin operon. In the presence of iron, the ferric uptake regulation (*Fur*) gene product, multimeric Fur (circle), binds to a palindromic DNA sequence called the iron box, upstream of the aerobactin operon and also upstream of *fur*. The genes for aerobactin biosynthesis (*iuc A–D*) and uptake (*iutA*) are repressed. In the absence of iron, Fur does not bind to the iron box and the aerobactin genes are expressed

which were de-repressed, that is they still expressed aerobactin even at high iron concentrations, and the mutation was mapped to a region of chromosome which encoded for a polypeptide of 148 amino acids. The gene was termed *ferric uptake regulation (fur)* gene. Addition of the exogenous *fur* gene product in the presence of high iron stopped aerobactin production in mutants.

Interestingly, the *fur* gene also interacted with manganese (II), cobalt (II) and cadmium (II) ions, but not aluminium (III) ions. It therefore seems that the *fur* gene regulates the uptake of a number of different ionic nutrients, which all activate the *fur* gene product to repress operon activity.

The region of DNA to which the *fur* gene product binds has been identified and a common sequence has been found upstream of the iron sensing genes on both the *E. coli* chromosome and plasmids. This is a palindromic sequence — GATAATGATAATCATTATC—and has been termed the 'iron box'. A region with some homology for the iron box has also been detected **upstream** of the *fur* gene, which suggests that there is also some autologous regulation (Figure 5.10). The genes which are controlled by the *fur* gene product include those necessary for transport of iron within the periplasmic space, cytplasmic proteins and outer membrane protein receptors and may be either chromosomally or plasmid encoded. Some of the regulated genes are listed in Table 5.5. This use of one gene product to control a number of different operons is termed **pleiotropic** gene regulation. Aspects of regulation of gene expression are discussed in detail in Chapter 9.

As well as the iron sensing *fur* gene, there is also apparently a separate temperature regulation of siderophore synthesis in *E. coli*. Synthesis decreases with a rise of temperature from 31 to 37 °C and is not detectable at 41 °C. This strongly suggests that the use of siderophores as a mechanism for nutrient scavenging initially evolved in such bacteria outside the host and may have been subsequently adapted to survival within the host.

Table 5.5. Iron regulated genes in *Escherichia coli*

Gene	Function
fur	Ferric uptake regulator (repressor)
iucA, B, C, D	Aerobactin biosynthesis
iutA	Aerobactin outer membrane receptor
fhuB, C, D	Hydroxamate siderophore transport
entA, B, C, D, E, F, G,	Enterobactin biosynthesis
fepA	Enterobactin outer membrane receptor
fes	Ferric enterobactin esterase for release of iron from enterobactin
fepB, C, D, E, F	Ferric enterobactin transport
slt	Shiga-like toxin

Enteric bacteria in particular can survive in natural environments outside of the host, for example in fresh waters which may be nutrient poor (termed oligotrophic). Thus an efficient nutrient scavenging mechanism at lower temperatures may also be important for the survival of pathogenic bacteria between hosts. The reduction in bacterial siderophore synthesis with increase in body temperature indicates that the febrile response may limit bacterial growth.

CONCLUSION

The human host therefore provides the bacterium with a wide range of readily degradable substrates, which the pathogen makes full use of. The host does, however, restrict access of the bacterium to certain essential nutrients, thereby successfully limiting growth and consequently the evolutionary success of the pathogen.

FURTHER READING

General

Alberts B., Bray D., Lewis J., Raff M., Roberts K., Watson J. D. 1994. Molecular biology of the cell (3rd Edn). Garland Publishing, New York, USA.
Holder I. A. (Ed). 1985. Bacterial enzymes and virulence. CRC Press, Boca Raton, Florida, USA.
Stephen S., Pietrowski R. A. 1986. Bacterial toxins. (2nd Edn). Chapman and Hall, London.

Cytolysins

Boulnois G. J., Mitchell T., Saunders K., Mendez X., Andrew P. 1991. Structure, function and role in disease of pneumolysin, the thiol-activated toxin of *Streptococcus pneumoniae*. In: Microbial surface components and toxins in relation to pathogenesis (Eds E. Z. Ron, S. Rottem). Plenum Press, New York, USA.
Braun V., Focareta T. 1991. Pore-forming bacterial protein haemolysins (cytolysins). Critical Reviews in Microbiology 18, 115–158.
Geoffroy C., Mengaud J., Alouf J. E., Cossart P. 1990. Alveolysin, the thiol-activated toxin of *Bacillus alvei*, is homologous to listeriolysin O, perfringolysin O, pneumolysin and streptolysin O and contains a single cysteine. Journal of Bacteriology 172, 7301–7305.
Gray L., Baker K., Kenny B. 1989. A novel C-terminal signal sequence targets *Escherichia coli* haemolysin directly to the medium. Journal of Cell Science Supplement 11, 45–57.

Host molecules

Corrigan J. J. 1986. Clotting and fibrinolysis during bacterial infection. Medical Microbiology 5, 265–278. Academic Press, London.

Lantz M. S., Allen R. D., Vail T. A., Switalski L. M., Hook M. 1991. Specific cell components of *Bacteroides gingivalis* mediate binding and degradation of human fibrinogen. Journal of Bacteriology 173, 495–504.
Lottenberg R., Minning-Wenz D., Boyle D. P. 1994. Capturing host plasmin(ogen): a common mechanism for invasive pathogens? Trends in Microbiology 2, 20–24.
O'Connor S. P., Darip D., Fraley K. *et al.* 1991. The human antibody response to streptococcal C5a peptidase. Journal of Infectious Diseases 163, 109–116.

Oligosaccharides

Faillard H. 1989. The early history of the sialic acids. Trends in Biochemical Science 14, 237–241.
Moncla B. I., Braham P., Hillier S. L. 1990. Sialidase (neuraminidase) activity among Gram-negative anaerobic and capnophilic bacteria. Journal of Clinical Microbiology 28, 422–425.
Raedmacher T. W., Dwek R. A. 1989. The role of oligosaccharides in modifying protein function. In: Carbohydrate recognition in cellular function. Ciba foundation symposium 145, 241–256. J Wiley, Chichester.
Rosen S. D., Chi S., True D. D., Singer M. S., Yednock T. A. 1989. Intravenously injected sialidase inactivates attachment sites for lymphocytes on high endothelial venules. Journal of Immunology 142, 1895–1902.
True D. D., Singer M. S., Lasky L. A., Rosen S. D. 1990. Requirement for sialic acid on the endothelial ligand of a lymphocyte homing receptor. Journal of Cell Biology 111, 2757–2764.

Iron uptake

Autenrieth I., Hantke K., Heesmann J. 1991. Immunosuppression of the host and delivery of iron to the pathogen: a possible dual role of siderophores in the pathogenesis of microbial infections? Medical Microbiology and Immunology 180, 135–141.
Bullen J. J., E. Griffiths (Eds). 1987. Iron and infection. J Wiley, Chichester.
Finkelstein R. A., Sciortino C. V., McIntosh M. A. 1983. Role of iron in microbe-host interactions. Reviews of Infectious Diseases 5, Supplement 4 S759–S777.
Lee B. C. 1992. Isolation of haemin-binding proteins of *Neisseria gonorrhoeae*. Journal of Medical Microbiology 36, 121–127.
Neilands J. B. 1990. Molecular biology and regulation of iron acquisition by *Escherichia coli* K12. In: Molecular basis of bacterial pathogenesis (Eds B. H. Iglewski, V. L. Clark). Academic Press, London. Chapter 10.
Otto B. R., Verweij-van Vught A. M. J. J., MacLaren D. M. 1992. Transferrin and heme-compounds as iron sources for pathogenic bacteria. Critical Reviews in Microbiology 18, 217–233.
Payne S. M., Lawlor K. M. 1990. Molecular studies on iron acquisition by non-*Escherichia coli* species. In: Molecular basis of bacterial pathogenesis (Eds B. H. Iglewski, V. L. Clark). Academic Press, London. Chapter 11.
Williams P., Morton D. J., Towner K. J., Stevenson P., Griffiths E. 1990. Utilization of enterobactin and other exogenous iron sources by *Haemophilus influenzae, H. parainfluenzae, H. paraphrophilus*. Journal of General Microbiology 136, 2343–2350.

6 Bacterial Exotoxins Which Act Inside Host Cells

INTRODUCTION

Historically the term 'toxin', in relation to bacteria, has been used for any part of the bacterium which has noticeably toxic effects on the host. As a clearer understanding of the inter-relationships of these bacterial molecules with the systems of the host has been gained, many of these molecules can be re-grouped and considered under different headings, such as immuno-modulation and nutrition.

It is now abundantly clear that many of the toxic effects associated with these molecules are due to systems of the host being pushed out of control. The toxicity is therefore the result of excess or uncontrolled host molecules. Where the bacterial products interfere with regulation of the immune system they can be considered as immunomodulators (Chapter 2). A prime example is lipopolysaccharide, which is classically referred to as endotoxin. The bacterial superantigens can also be included in this category. Whether the effects of the bacterial molecules on the host constitute immune recognition of the foreign molecules or bacterial virulence in the form of interference with the immune system remains a complex and largely unanswered question. For example, there is a subtle, but important distinction between a host cell which releases particular cytokines in response to a bacterial molecule (recognition) and a host cell which is subverted from its **normal** activities and responses within the host by the bacterial molecule (interference). It may be that both aspects are involved and have become inextricably interwoven during evolutionary time. It is, however, important that we attempt to unravel the tangle not only to gain a better understanding of the immune system but also if future therapies are to involve the administration of host molecules.

The bacterial toxins which can degrade host molecules and lyse host cells have the potential to provide nutrition for the bacterium in vivo (Chapter 5). Cytolytic toxins are sometimes categorised as membrane damaging toxins, to distinguish them from toxins which act intracellularly but whose effects ultimately result in cell lysis. Where lytic toxins are specifically targeted towards cells of the host immune system, they may also have a gross immunomodulatory effect. In such cases there is a fine line between cytolysins which may have a primarily nutritional role and those which can be considered primarily as virulence determinants.

This chapter will deal with some of the better characterised bacterial protein exotoxins, most of which interfere with the normal function of intracellular molecules of the host cells. (Toxins which are essentially immunomodulators are considered in Chapter 2 and those which may aid bacterial nutrition in Chapter 5.) Many of these bacterial extoxins, do not appear to have a functional relationship with bacterial cell growth; many have characteristics typical of bacterial secondary metabolites. In general they are synthesised for short periods by bacteria which have recently ceased multiplication and just entered into the stationary phase of growth. Therefore the selective pressures in favour of their production are unclear. If the damage caused by the toxins results in sufficient nutrient release to allow the population to re-enter into exponential growth, they may represent a last ditch attempt at survival of the bacterial population. Their toxic effects on the host may be purely coincidental. Interestingly many of the antibiotics derived from bacteria, such as *Streptomyces* spp., are secondary metabolites. As a result of commercial production of these antibiotics, the precise details of the environmental conditions (e.g. temperature, redox potential, nutrient concentration) under which they are produced are known. Perhaps if food and medical microbiologists put a similar amount of effort into studying the physiological conditions under which this type of toxin is produced, such knowledge could be used to **prevent** their formation. These toxins are generally termed exotoxins as they are secreted from the bacterium. This term was initially used to differentiate them from the 'endotoxin' of the Gram negative bacterial envelope; however, it should be noted that the outer membrane of Gram negative bacteria is also excreted from the bacterial cell in the form of outer membrane vesicles (Chapter 2).

A common feature of many exotoxins is that they have **two components**, a B component which mediates **binding** to specific host cell receptors and an A component which is the **active** part of the molecule. The site of action of many of these toxins is intracellular. Therefore the active part of the toxin must be able to enter into the cell. As it is unlikely that the host cells carry 'suicide' receptors which have evolved specifically for the uptake of bacterial toxins, the toxin has to hijack the normal mechanisms by which molecules enter into the host cells. This aspect of the use of normal host cell uptake mechanisms is also relevant to the uptake of whole bacteria which grow intracellularly (see Chapter 8). Molecules enter cells by three separate mechanisms. Firstly, the internalisation may occur by the process of **receptor mediated endocytosis**. This is the pathway by which the host cell internalises cytokines and hormones such as insulin and epidermal growth factor. Receptor mediated endocytosis can be followed by the clustering of a number of ligand–receptor complexes and the entry of the molecules, usually still associated with the receptor, into the host cell inside endocytic vesicles known as **clathrin coated pits**. These vesicles migrate through the cytoplasm and reach the Golgi endoplasmic reticulum lysosome system in about 15–20 min, finally fusing with primary lysosomes after about 30–60 min. Receptor mediated endocytosis can also occur in **uncoated vesicles** when the clustered ligand–receptors interact with myosin and actin containing fibres in the cytoplasm. Molecules enter cells in a less specific manner by **pinocytosis** which is pinching off or folding of the cell membrane to form vesicles containing the surrounding fluid phase. Pinocytosis could be thought of as the cell drinking the surrounding fluid. Direct transfer across the membrane, perhaps in a manner similar to that associated with proteins which carry signal sequences, is another possible mechanism for entry into host cells. Although there are several potential mechanisms by which toxins can enter cells, the efficiency of their toxicity on the host cell may be determined by the route of entry. The bulk uptake of toxin via pinocytosis may be largely non-productive in terms of toxicity to the cell, that is the toxin which enters the cell by this mechanism is essentially non-toxic to the cell. On the other hand specific uptake of the same toxin by receptor mediated endocytosis may help to target the activity of the toxin, rendering it more toxic to the cell. It seems that for some toxins productive toxicity is reliant on receptor mediated endocytosis. A recurrent difficulty in determining the route of productive toxin uptake is that where a very few, or even a single, toxin molecule is required to kill the host cell, as is the case for diphtheria toxin, minor routes of productive uptake may be overlooked within the experimental system.

Another characteristic common to many of the bacterial protein toxins is the necessity for post-translational modification to convert the toxin from a proenzyme into an active form. This point will be considered in more detail in relation to specific toxins.

Many of the bacterial protein toxins have a common biochemical activity in that they act as **ADP-ribosylating enzymes** and these toxins will be considered as a group. Despite concerted effort by a number of workers the precise molecular detail of the activity of toxins, such as tetanus toxin, botulinum toxin and *Clostridium difficile* toxins, remains to be determined.

THE ADP-RIBOSYLATING ENZYMES

This family of bacterial toxins catalyses the removal of an **ADP-ribose** moiety from **NAD⁺** and its subsequent transfer to specific target proteins within mammalian cells. Hence they have dual enzymic activity and are both **NAD glycohydrolases** and **ADP-ribosyl transferases** (Figure 6.1). As the target host cells and proteins within the cells differ from one toxin to another, although the mechanism of action is common, the effect on the host is different. Examples of these bacterial toxins are listed in Table 6.1. It should be noted that this is a virulence characteristic common to a range

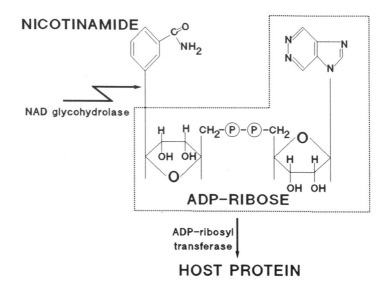

Figure 6.1. Enzymic activity of ADP-ribosylating toxins. These toxins catalyse two processes: the cleavage of nicotinamide from the substrate NAD$^+$ (glycohydrolase) and the transfer of the ADP-ribose moiety to the host target protein (ADP-ribosyl transferase)

of taxonomically divergent bacteria. These toxins will be considered below in relation to the effect they have on the host cell.

Effects on protein synthesis

Diphtheria toxin which is encoded by a lysogenic phage of *Corynebacterium diphtheriae*, was the first bacterial toxin in which ADP-ribosylating activity was identified. Productive uptake of the toxin probably occurs by receptor mediated endocytosis. The pro-enzyme is converted into the active form by proteolytic cleavage at two sites and the reduction of disulphide bonds. This can occur in the supernatant of cultured *C. diphtheriae* from the activity of bacterial products; in the host it is thought that these modification steps occur within the host cell vesicle. Diphtheria toxin effectively halts protein synthesis within the cell by catalysing the transfer of ADP-ribose to **elongation factor-2** (Ef-2) which is a transfer RNA (tRNA) translocase, mediating the movement of tRNA to the nascent polypeptide at the ribosome. EF-2 is one of a family of host **guanine nucleotide binding proteins** (GNBP) with intrinsic GTPase activity; when GDP is bound they are inactive and

Table 6.1. The ADP-ribosylating toxins

Bacterium	Toxin	Molecule to which ADP-ribose is added	Effect on host cell
Pseudomonas aeruginosa	Exotoxin A	Elongation factor-2	Peptide chain elongation blocked, inhibits protein synthesis
Corynebacterium diphtheriae	Diphtheria toxin		
Vibrio cholerae	Cholera toxin	Signal transducing stimulatory G protein	Adenylate cyclase activation
Escherichia coli	Heat-labile toxin		
Bordetella pertussis	Pertussis toxin	Signal transducing inhibitory G protein	Adenylate cyclase activation
Clostridium botulinum	C3	Small GTP-binding proteins	Effects on cytoskeleton
P. aeruginosa	Exoenzyme S	ras gene superfamily proteins	Disruption of intracellular vesicular traffic and secretion of granules?
		Vimentin (cytoskeletal intermediate filament)	Effects on cytoskeleton
Clostridium botulinum	C2	Actin	Breakdown of intracellular microfilament network
C. perfringens	iota		
C. difficile			
C. spiroforme			

when GTP is bound they are active. The intrinsic GTPase activity allows 'self-controlled' decay of activity. Other members of this family include the G proteins, which are involved in signal transduction. It is these GNBPs on which most of the ADP-ribosylating enzymes act.

With respect to EF-2, active EF-2 binds aminoacetylated tRNA and translocates it to the ribosome. Stimulation by the ribosome results in increased GTPase activity of EF-2 and generation of EF-2-GDP. The EF-2 therefore becomes inactive and dissociates from the tRNA which is left behind to allow formation of the peptide. Thus EF-2 regulates protein synthesis by controlling the unidirectional movement of tRNA to the ribosome. The catalytic activity of diphtheria toxin results in the covalent binding of ADP-ribose to an unusual amino acid in EF-2. This amino acid is a histidine residue which has been post-translationally modified to produce 2-(3-carb-oxyamido-3(trimethylammonio)propyl)histidine, which has been named **diphthamide**. The successful catalytic activity of diphtheria toxin is not only reliant on the presence of a diphthamide residue but also other structural features of the EF-2.

The **exotoxin** A of *Pseudomonas aeruginosa* has been shown to have not only identical catalytic activity, but the same target molecule within the host cell. These two toxins bind ADP-ribose to the diphthamide residue of EF-2 in a stereochemically identical manner. Despite this, these two bacteria are pathogenically very different. Detailed comparison of the two toxins indicates that, amongst other things, the toxins have different host cell receptor specificities, are internalised by different routes within the host cell and show little immunological cross-reactivity. The two toxins are compared in Table 6.2.

The gene for exotoxin A has been cloned and the function of different regions of the molecule determined by deletion mutagenesis. The various activities of different regions of the molecule are summarised in Figure 6.2. Exotoxin A is synthesised as a 638 amino acid precursor polypeptide, which is processed to a 613 amino acid pro-enzyme. The pro-enzyme then has to undergo conformational change before it becomes toxic. Four regions of the molecule have been defined with different biological function. The bac-

Table 6.2. Comparison of diphtheria toxin and *Pseudomonas* exotoxin A: toxins with the same substrate but different characteristics

	Diphtheria toxin	Exotoxin A
Molecular mass	60 kDa (B subunit 39 kDa, A subunit 21 kDa)	66 kDa (A and B regions in one molecule)
Active toxin generated by	Proteolytic cleavage and disulphide bond reduction	Conformational change or limited proteolytic cleavage
Sensitivity of tissue culture cell lines:		
Vero cells	Sensitive	Resistant
L-929	Resistant	Sensitive
Uptake mechanism	RME, but not into clathrin coated pits	RME into clathrin coated pits
Site of enzymic activity	Towards N-terminus	Towards C-terminus

A, active; B, binding; RME, receptor mediated endocytosis.

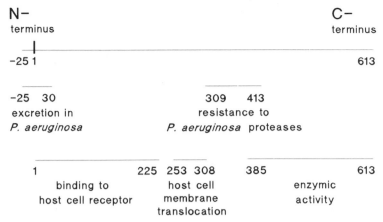

Figure 6.2. Summary map of *Pseudomonas aeruginosa* exotoxin A. *P. aeruginosa* exotoxin A is produced as a single mature polypeptide of 613 amino acids (a.a.). Amino acids −25 to 1 form a leader peptide and this region, along with a.a. 1 to 30, is required for secretion of the toxin from the bacterium. The other major functional domains are related to: resistance to *P. aeruginosa* protease activity (a.a. 309 to 413); binding to the host cell receptor (a.a. 1 to 225); translocation across the host cell membrane (a.a. 253 to 308); NAD glycohydrolase and transfer of ADP-ribose to elongation factor 2 (a.a. 385 to 613)

terium has an N-terminal signal sequence which is necessary for secretion from the bacterium, the binding region which binds the toxin to an as yet unidentified eukaryotic receptor, a region involved in the translocation and internalisation of the toxin into the host cell and finally the region with ADP-ribosylating enzymic activity. A limited amount of information is known about the control of expression of exotoxin A. The *regA* gene which codes for a 29 kDa cytoplasmic membrane protein but with no DNA binding activity, is known to be involved. The *regA* gene is itself controlled by two promoters, one of which is positively regulated by low iron concentration. The mRNA for exotoxin A is not constitutively expressed and optimal production of the toxin is obtained in media with low iron concentration. Interestingly, the production of diphtheria toxin is also regulated by iron concentration.

Comparison of diphtheria toxin and exoenzyme A has revealed DNA homology in the enzymic domains of the protein. There is a requirement for the presence of glutamic acid residues in this region for activity. This strongly suggests that both these enzymic domains diverged from a common ancestral protein and that there is a common evolutionary origin of all ADP-ribosylating enzyme toxins.

The exoenzyme S of *Pseudomonas aeruginosa* also has ADP-ribosylating activity but its site of action is entirely different (see below).

Effects on adenylate cyclase

Cholera toxin which is produced by *Vibrio cholerae*, is another ADP-ribosyl-ating enzyme; however, although the enzymic activity in terms of NAD glycohydrolysis and ADP-ribosyl transfer to a host protein (Figure 6.1) is the same as in diphtheria and exotoxin A, this is essentially the only simi-larity.

Cholera toxin is composed of five binding subunits which form a circular structure, with the active subunit in the centre of the ring (Figure 6.3). A single B subunit binds to the oligosaccharide residues of the **monosialyl ganglioside** GM_1 (galactosyl-N-acetylgalactosaminyl-(N-acetylneuraminyl) galactosylglucosylceramide) on intestinal epithelial cells. The other five B subunits eventually also bind to individual GM_1 molecules, as a result of lateral diffusion in the plane of the host cell membrane. A similar lateral diffusion is then thought to occur to bring the cholera toxin into contact with the cAMP cyclase enzyme/regulatory complex, which is the target of the ADP-ribosylating activity. The A subunit consists of two disulphide bonded parts, A1 and A2. A2 is thought to be involved in the internalisation of A1, which possesses the enzymic activity. The target for this enzymic activity is another GNBP, a member of the **G protein** family involved in transmembrane signalling. These G proteins are coupled to receptors for host cell messengers such as cytokines, hormones and neurotransmitters and physical signals such as light. When the receptor receives the message (usually by attachment of the extracellular messenger molecule) the G pro-

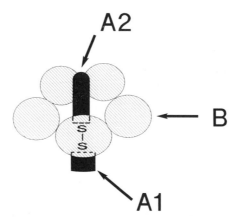

Figure 6.3. Diagram of cholera toxin. The five subunits (B) of cholera toxin which mediate binding to the host cell receptor, ganglioside GM_1, form a doughnut shape, with the enzymically active subunit (A) in the centre of the ring. The A subunit is composed of two parts, A1 and A2, which are bonded together by a disulphide bond. When the toxin interacts with the host cell the disulphide bond is reduced (see Figure 6.4)

tein, located on the cytoplasmic side of the host cell membrane, becomes associated with the receptor. The G protein then passes on the 'message' to the effector molecules within the cell such as adenylate cyclase, phospholipases and phosphodiesterases. These G proteins are heterotrimers with α, β and γ subunits. (The small GTP-binding proteins, which are also G proteins involved in intracellular signals, are discussed below).

In the case of cholera toxin, the target G protein is a stimulatory protein designated G_s. It is the α subunit of the G protein which has intrinsic GTPase activity. In a normally functioning cell, in response to specific stimulation of the transmembrane receptor, the α-GDP is converted to a α-GTP. The β-γ subunit has lower affinity for α-GTP than α-GDP, therefore the α unit dissociates from the heterotrimer. The α subunit, now in its active form, binds to and activates adenylate cyclase. This results in the generation of several thousand cAMP molecules from ATP. The intrinsic hydrolysis of the GTP to GDP produces the inactive α unit which reassociates with the β and γ. Only the β-γ-α-GDP complex can bind to the membrane sensor. Thus the formation of cAMP has an in-built braking system (Figure 6.4) which could be thought of as a wind-up timer switch. The A1 unit of cholera toxin catalyses the linkage of ADP-ribose to the α subunit of G_s, effectively blocking the internal hydrolysis of GTP to GDP, and removing the brakes from the production of cAMP, effectively leaving the switch in the on position. Host cell derived ADP-ribosylation factors (ARFs) are probably involved in the initial activation of the ribosylating activity of cholera toxin. cAMP activates protein kinases which modulate protein activities within cells by phosphorylating them. Phosphorylation may activate or inactivate proteins. It is the over-production of cAMP which is thought to be ultimately responsible for the disruption of normal ion fluxes in the intestinal epithelium, namely the increase in chloride secretion and inhibition of sodium absorption. This generates the watery diarrhoea and dehydration associated with cholera. The details of the events between cAMP production and the associated fluid loss from the intestine are the subject of current study. It is now clear that the trimeric G proteins are also involved in the regulation of vesicle formation from the Golgi network. Therefore as cholera toxin prevents the deactivation of the G α stimulatory subunit, vesicle production is continuously stimulated. The small GTP-binding proteins are also involved in the regulation of intracellular vesicle movement (see below).

Cholera toxin also has **immunomodulatory activity** and will act as a potent adjuvant. If it is given orally, along with an unrelated antigen, it enhances the production of mucosal IgA and serum IgG antibody specific for the antigen. In an experimental system, cholera toxin promotes production of IgG1 in B-cells, causing them to switch from production of membrane-IgM. Cholera toxin will act synergistically with IL4, the host cytokine which promotes class switching in B-cells from membrane-IgM to IgG1.

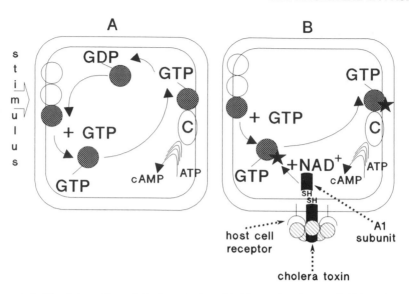

Figure 6.4. The interaction of cholera toxin with Gs, a stimulatory GTP-binding protein. In the normal microvillus cell (Cell A), an external signal (stimulus) is passed into the cell via the addition of GTP to the α subunit of the Gs protein (cross-hatched circle). The α-GTP then dissociates from the β-γ subunit (open circles) and binds to and activates adenylate cyclase (C). This generates cAMP from ATP. The intrinsic GTPase activity of the α subunit results in the decay of GTP to GDP and the consequent inactivation of the α subunit, which reassociates with the β-γ subunit. The A1 subunit of cholera toxin (cell B) catalyses the cleavage of ADP-ribose (star) from NAD^+ and its transfer to the α-GTP subunit of the Gs protein. This blocks the intrinsic hydrolysis of the GTP and therefore the decay of the signal. cAMP is therefore produced in excess

The A subunit and the associated ADP-ribosylating activity are not essential for this induction of B-cell Ig isotype switching, although the complete cholera toxin is more efficient that the B subunit alone. How this activity relates to the pathogenesis of cholera is unclear, but this adjuvant effect could be useful in the production of oral vaccines. Binding of the B subunit alone to GM_1 causes lymphocyte activation and the initiation of DNA synthesis in resting B-cells, possibly in a manner analogous to the mitogenic action of staphylococcal protein A. Some of these immunomodulatory activities are shared by the pertussis toxin of *Bordetella pertussis*.

Molecular genetic studies of the expression of the cholera toxin gene have shed some light on the differential control necessary for the production of different quantities of five B subunits for every individual A subunit. The genes coding for the A and B subunits of cholera toxin, *ctxA* and *ctxB*; have been mapped to a single operon. Within this operon they are tightly linked and the two open reading frames overlap. The termination codon of the A subunit gene shares two nucleotides with the B subunit initiation codon.

As five copies of B are required for every one of A, and there is therefore no room for a separate promoter, this presents the bacterium with a regulatory problem. It appears that the two genes are not translationally coupled as upstream of each of the open reading frames is a Shine-Dalgarno ribosomal binding site. It is thought that differential translation of the messages for A and B is dependent on the efficiency of their respective ribosomal binding sites.

Fusion of the *ctxB* gene to the *ctxA* transcriptional and translational signals resulted in production of about nine times less B protein. In other words if the *ctxB* message is coupled to the *ctxA* ribosomal binding site fewer copies of B are produced. In most *V. cholerae* strains the *ctx* genes have been duplicated and are present in multiple copies. This therefore allows for the amplification of cholera toxin production. The duplication is probably mediated by *recA* homologous recombination events (see Chapter 9) as *ctx* genes are flanked at either end by direct repeats of the 2.7 kb sequence termed RS1.

Attempts are being made to produce a *V. cholerae* strain lacking in all the copies of the *ctxA* gene and which only expresses the immunogenic B subunit. Such strains would be potential live oral vaccines.

Two genes have been identified which are involved in the transcriptional activation of the cholera toxin operon, the *toxR* (regulatory) and *toxS* (sensory) genes. It is likely that the two component, **sensory/regulatory mechanism** of environmental modulation of cholera toxin production is similar to that observed in a number of other bacterial types (see Chapter 9). The *toxR* gene codes for a 32.5 kDa protein which has a 16 residue hydrophobic domain and a transmembrane helix; *toxS* is present in the same operon as *toxR* and encodes a 19 kDa protein. The precise mechanism for environmental modulation of expression of cholera toxin is not clear, but taking into account that the agent which mediates environmental signal transduction for regulation of toxin genes is also known to have DNA-binding acitivity, the following model has been proposed. Prior to the environmental signal, ToxR and ToxS are present in the cytoplasmic membrane in an inactive state. Environmental signals then cause ToxR to become an activator of transcription of the *ctxA* and *ctxB* genes by binding to the DNA upstream of these genes. The dimerisation of the ToxR may be involved in the process (Figure 6.5). Superimposed on this is regulation of gene activity by DNA supercoiling, which is considered in Chapter 9.

The **heat labile toxin** (LT) of the enterotoxigenic *E. coli* is very similar to cholera toxin. Not only does it ADP-ribosylate the same target molecule, but it also binds to GM_1. The difference in the pathogenesis of the diseases caused by these two bacteria may by due, in part, to the efficient transport system for export of toxin by *V. cholerae*, which is apparently lacking in *E. coli*. The LT of *E. coli* remains associated with the bacterial cell. Comparison of the genes for the A and B subunits shows a 75% identity with the LTA

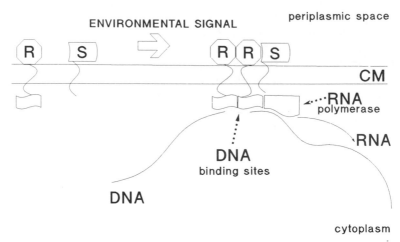

Figure 6.5. Model of environmental control of cholera toxin gene transcription. The membrane proteins ToxR and ToxS associate in response to an environmental signal. ToxR activates transcription of the *ctxA* and *ctxB* genes by binding to the DNA upstream of these genes

gene and 77% identity with the LTB gene. The LT genes are carried on plasmids in *E. coli* and a comparison of the G+C ratio of the plasmid and chromosomal DNA and the frequency of usage of particular codons specifying amino acids indicates marked differences between the plasmid DNA and the chromosomal DNA. It seems that the LT genes of *E. coli* are foreign genes which were acquired in the more recent evolutionary past. On the other hand, there is evidence which points to an ancient association of the cholera toxin genes with the *V. cholerae* genome and the suggestion that they were present before the appearance of humans on the planet. A number of other bacteria are also known to produce cholera related toxins. They include *Aeromonas hydrophila* and *Campylobacter jejuni*. It remains to be seen if they also obtained their genes from an ancestral *V. cholerae*.

The **pertussis toxin** of *Bordetella pertussis* (also known as pertussigen, lymphocytosis promoting factor, histamine-sensitising factor and islet-activating protein) is another bacterial toxin with ADP-ribosylating activity. The binding unit of pertussis toxin is composed of two sets of dimers, S2–4 and S3–4, and a connector molecule, S5 (Figure 6.6). Similarly to cholera toxin there is a single active subunit with enzymic activity. By comparison with the cholera and cholera related toxins, the outcome of the activity of the pertussis toxin is similar, vis-à-vis the over-production of cAMP within the target host cell. The mechanism by which this is brought about, however, is essentially the opposite to that of cholera toxin. Again the target molecule is a G protein, but in this instance the α subunit of an **inhibitory G protein**, G_i, which in response to extracellular signals, shuts down mem-

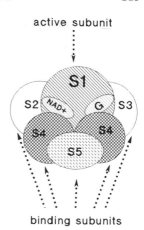

active subunit

binding subunits

Figure 6.6. Diagram of pertussis toxin. Subunits S2 to S5 (dimers S2–4 and S3–4 and the connecting subunit S5) mediate the binding of pertussis toxin to the host cell receptor. The enzymically active subunit S1 has an internal disulphide bond and binding sites for NAD^+ and the host cell target protein (G). From Grershik P. 1992 *Current Topics in Immunology*, Volume 175, page 72. Reproduced by permission of Edward Arnold

brane associated adenylate cyclase activity. Thus pertussis toxin stimulates over-production of cAMP by interfering with inhibition of adenylate cyclase rather than by enhancing stimulation of adenylate cyclase. This elevation of cAMP can persist for weeks. As with cholera toxin, the formation of vesicles in the Golgi network is also affected. Alpha subunits of inhibitory G proteins negatively regulate vesicle formation. ADP-ribosylation of the α subunit removes this inhibitory control, leading to over-production of vesicles from the Golgi network. Bacterial cell associated pertussis toxin can also act as an adhesin, which along with filamentous haemagglutinin, mediates adherence of the bacteria to ciliated human respiratory cells. The cAMP activity of the host cell is further increased by the production of bacterial derived adenylate cyclase. *B. pertussis* produces a number of other toxins which are considered below, although it is thought that pertussis toxin is largely responsible for the symptoms of the disease. The genetic basis of the environmental modulation and antigenic variation of many of the virulence determinants of *B. pertussis* is dealt with in Chapter 9.

As with cholera toxin, pertussis toxin is mitogenic for B-cells and also acts as a potent adjuvant. The effects which both of these molecules have on B-cells are probably related to the multimeric nature of the binding molecules of the toxin which effectively cross-link surface receptors.

Effects on small GTP-binding proteins

Another family of intracellular GTP-binding proteins which are targets for bacterial toxins are exemplified by the products of the *ras* gene family. These small cellular GTP-binding proteins, of molecular mass in the region of 20–26 kDa, include the Ras proteins, H-Ras, K-Ras, N-Ras (sometimes called p21[ras]), and the related proteins Rap, Rab, Ral and Rho. These proteins are inactive when GDP is bound and active when GTP is bound. They are involved in triggering effector molecules within the cell and some of them could be considered to form a class of monomeric G proteins. Although they are known to be involved in controlling a wide range of intracellular processes, the precise function of many of these molecules remains to be elucidated. Indeed the activities of the bacterial toxins which ADP-ribosylate these molecules have been used as a tool in determining the normal cellular function of the small GPT-binding proteins.

The **C3 toxin** of *Clostridium botulinum*, which is phage encoded, ADP-ribosylates Rho at an asparagine residue. Rho protein (not to be confused with *rho factor* which is involved in the termination of mRNA synthesis in *Escherichia coli*) is involved in some aspect of the regulation of the cytoskeletal architecture. C3 toxin is known to destroy the microfilament network, but leave the microtubule network intact. This causes visible morphological changes in the cell.

Pseudomonas aeruginosa **exoenzyme S** was originally considered to catalyse the transfer of ADP-ribose to many different proteins, but it is now clear that the preferred substrates of the enzyme are the *H-ras* and *K-ras* gene products, which are p21 proteins. These G proteins are located on the inner side of the plasma membrane and are involved in some way in the control of cell growth and division. The genes encoding these proteins were initially characterised because some viruses code for mutated *ras* genes. If the viral genome is integrated into the host chromosome and mutated Ras proteins expressed, the cells proliferate in an uncontrolled manner resulting in tumour formation. The viral mutated genes are termed oncogenes and the normal host cell genes, proto-oncogenes. How this relates to the activities of the bacterial toxins is unclear.

One of the normal functions of some of these small GTP-binding proteins is the control of the movement of vesicles through the exocytic and endocytic pathways. It is thought that the small GTP-binding protein, with attached GDP, binds to a receptor on an intracellular membrane. This triggers the assembly of a coated pit or vesicle. The binding site remains on the donor membrane, but the GTP-binding protein, now with GTP attached, moves with the vesicle through the cytosol to another membrane site. One of the effects of the toxin could therefore be to alter the secretion of granules from phagocytic cells, thus limiting the effectiveness of phagocytic killing (see Chapter 4). The microfilament protein **vimentin** is also a target for exoenzyme S. Therefore the cellular cytoskeleton may be disrupted. Interestingly, exoenzyme S has higher enzymic activity at 25°C than at 37°C, which suggests that it primarily evolved in *Pseudomonas* spp. to attack eukaryotic microorganisms in soil and water habitats. Many questions remain to be answered with respect to the relationship of these bacterial toxins with virulence.

Effects on actin

Actin is a major component of the cell cytoskeleton and is involved in all aspects of cell movement from muscle contraction to the migration of leukocytes. It is not a GTP-binding protein but binds ATP and can be present either as a monomer (monomeric G-actin) or in a polymerised form (F-actin). A number of bacterial ADP-ribosylating enzymes can transfer ADP-ribose to actin, thus modifying its activity. These toxins include *Clostridium botulinum* C2 toxin, *C. perfringens* ι toxin, *C. spiroforme* toxin and a toxin of *C. difficile*. Interestingly, these toxins have independent A and B moieties which are not linked and are therefore termed **binary toxins**. The C2 toxin of *C. botulinum*, unlike the C3 toxin (see above), is not phage encoded. Production of C2 toxin is linked with the sporulation phase of *C. botulinum*. The two constituents of the binary C2 toxin are CI, which has ADP-ribosylating activity (the A unit), and CII, which binds to the host cell (the B unit). CII is released from the bacterium as an inactive pro-form of molecular mass of about 95–105 kDa. This is then cleaved by proteolysis to form a 74 kDa unit which has haemolytic and haemagglutinating activity. Binding of 74 kDa CII to the cell surface creates a binding site for CI, which probably enters the cell via receptor mediated endocytosis. CI will add ADP-ribose to monomeric G-actin, but not polymeric F-actin. This inhibits the ability of G-actin to polymerise. It appears that the bound ADP-ribose blocks the intrinsic ATP-ase activity of actin. A proposed model of the effect of C2 toxin is illustrated in Figure 6.7. The actin-ADP ribosylating enzymes may have different substrate specificities. For example, C2 is active against non-muscle and γ-smooth muscle actin, whereas the ι toxin of *C. perfringens* is active against all mammalian actins.

OTHER BACTERIAL EXOTOXINS

This section covers the activities of toxins other than those known to have ADP-ribosylating activity. As yet the precise mechanisms of activity of some of these toxins remains to be determined. It is not impossible that some of these may also have ADP-ribosylating activity.

The heat stable (ST) toxins of *Escherichia coli*

The heat stable group of toxins (ST) of enterotoxigenic *E. coli* are low molecular weight peptides in the order of 2 kDa. These toxins stimulate cyclic-GMP synthesis in the intestinal brush border. Although less fluid is secreted than would be associated with cholera toxin and LT, the overall effect of fluid loss and lack of fluid absorption is similar. This toxin is very tissue specific and receptors for it are apparently only present in the intestine. The ST toxins can be divided into two groups, STI and STII. The genes

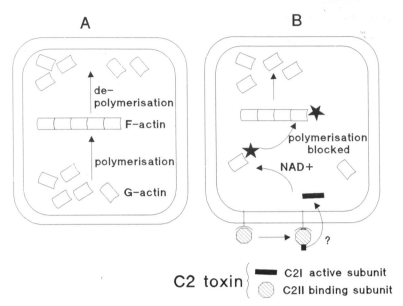

Figure 6.7. The interaction of *Clostridium botulinum* C2 toxin with actin. In normal cells (cell A) actin monomers (G-actin) reversibly polymerise to form F-actin in the dynamic equilibrium of the microfilament network in response to the need for cell movement. C2 is a binary toxin with two unlinked units, CII the binding unit and CI the enzymically active unit. CII binds to the host cell surface, thereby allowing CI to bind. Once inside the cell CI catalyses the cleavage of ADP-ribose (star) from NAD$^+$ and its subsequent transfer to F-actin monomer. ADP-ribose-actin binds to the fast-growing end of the actin filament, termed capping. The normal equilibrium between polymerisation and depolymerisation is upset; capping prevents further polymerisation and depolymerisation occurs at the other end of the actin filament. The outcome is the breakdown of the microfilament network

coding for these toxins (*estA* and *estB*) are generally found on plasmids and it is now clear that they are located within composite transposons which are mobile. *EstA* is flanked at either end by inverted repeats of insertion sequence 1 (IS1); it is therefore capable of independent movement and indeed these genes have been located on plasmids, bacteriophage and the chromosome. (See Chapter 9.) Comparison of the G+C ratio indicates that, as with the genes for LT, it is unlikely that these genes evolved in *E. coli*, but were probably obtained from another bacterial source, on at least two separate occasions. This is a prime example of genetic plasticity allowing for acquisition of virulence determinants and the subsequent rapid evolution of a pathogen. Other bacteria, including *Yersinia enterocolitica* and *Klebsiella pneumoniae*, produce similar toxins.

The Shiga toxin family

Shiga toxin of *Shigella dysenteriae* and the Shiga-like toxins of *Escherichia coli* are a family of related toxins which have similar amino acid sequences and biological activity. Infection with bacteria producing these toxins characteristically results in bloody diarrhoea and has more recently been shown to be associated with haemolytic uraemic syndrome, often caused by *E. coli* of serotype O157, in which bloody diarrhoea is following by acute renal failure. *E. coli* which produce Shiga-like toxins may also be responsible for oedema disease of pigs. Some of the Shiga-like toxins of *E. coli* were called verotoxins because of their toxicity to Vero tissue culture cells. As in the ADP-ribosylating toxins, the Shiga and Shiga-like toxins have both binding and active subunits. The A subunit of Shiga toxin has a molecular mass of 31 kDa which is thought to associate with five of the 7 kDa B subunits. The A subunit is proteolytically cleaved into A1 and A2, and it is the A1 fragment which is biologically active. The host cell receptor for Shiga toxin is the glycolipid Gal(α1-4)Gal(β1-4)GlcCeramide (globotriosylceramide; Gb3) and for Shiga-like toxin I (SLTI) and SLTII of *E. coli* is Gal(α1-4)GalCeramide (galabiosylceramide). The binding specifity is dependent on both the sugar residues and the lipid moiety. After binding to the glycolipids there is evidence that Shiga toxin is taken up by receptor mediated endocytosis into clathrin coated pits. It then appears that the toxin is transported to the Golgi, before translocation into the cytosol. Its gross effect on the cell is to inhibit protein synthesis. It is now known that Shiga toxin is an RNA N-glycosidase enzyme whose site of action is the 60S ribosomal subunit. Specifically, the Shiga toxins remove an adenine base from one particular position (4324) on the aminoacyl-transfer RNA (A) binding site of 28S ribosomal RNA, but leave the phosphoribose backbone of the RNA intact. By removing the adenine from the A site, elongation factor 1 dependent binding of aminoacyl-transfer RNA is prevented, and peptide chain elongation is stopped (Figure 6.8). Although the enzymic mechanism is different, the effect on protein synthesis is similar to that of diphtheria toxin and *Pseudomonas aeruginosa* exotoxin A.

The SLTI and II toxins of *E. coli* are encoded by lysogenic phage, but although there are regions of the *S. dysenteriae* chromosome which are homologous with the *E. coli* bacteriophage DNA as yet it has not been possible to induce production of phage. The Shiga-like toxin of *E. coli* is one of the many products whose expression is controlled by iron concentration in the growth medium, by way of the *fur* gene and the 'iron box' repressor protein binding site (see Chapter 5). The relationship of toxin production to the virulence of *Shigella* spp. is interesting, as *Shigella* spp. are facultatively intracellular bacteria, which can invade and grow inside host cells. Human volunteers given large doses of toxin-producing but non-invasive *S. dysenteriae* were not affected. Volunteers given non-toxigenic but invasive

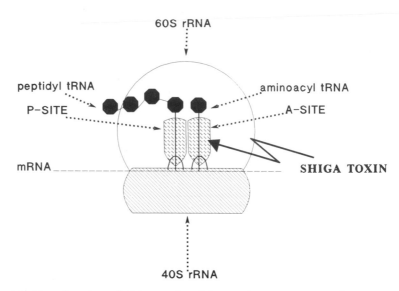

Figure 6.8. Site of action of Shiga toxin. Shiga toxin removes an adenine residue from the aminoacyl-transfer RNA (tRNA) binding site (A-site) on the 60S (larger) ribosomal RNA subunit. Thus new amino acids (hexagons) are not added to the nascent peptide and synthesis is halted

mutants had a less severe disease, although they did have loose, mucoid stools. It seems that the toxin causes microvascular damage, resulting in bloody stools, but is not involved in the intracellular survival of the bacterium.

Interestingly, the enzymatically active subunit of the Shiga-like toxin of *E. coli* has amino acid homology with ricin, the castor bean derived toxin, and the activity of ricin is identical to that of the Shiga toxin family. This could represent convergent evolution, alternatively the evolutionary origin of these molecules could pre-date the separation of prokaryotes and eukaryotes.

Anthrax toxin

Anthrax toxin, produced by *Bacillus anthracis*, has three separate components which are called protective antigen, oedema factor and lethal factor. These combine to form an 88 kDa toxin. It appears that the protective antigen is the B component of the toxin with the A component either the oedema or lethal factor. There is evidence that the oedema factor is an adenylate cyclase enzyme which elevates levels of cAMP within the target cell. As with the adenylate cyclase of *Bordetella pertussis* host cell calmodulin acts as a cofactor for the adenylate cyclase activity.

The neurotoxins, tetanus and botulinum

Tetanus toxin (TeTx) produced by *Clostridium tetani* and botulinum toxin (BoTx) produced by *Clostridium botulinum* are both neurotoxin polypeptides with active (A) and binding (B) domains. By blocking exocytosis of neuro-transmitter-containing small synaptic vesicles from neurones at neuro-muscular junctions, the normal contraction and relaxation of the muscles is indirectly halted. In the case of TeTx, it is **inhibitory** spinal cord interneu-rones which are affected. The release of inhibitory neurotransmitters is pre-vented and the muscles continuously contract against each other resulting in a **spastic** paralysis. BoTx acts on spinal cord **motor** neurones thus having the opposite effect; a lack of muscle contraction and a **flaccid** paralysis.

Despite many years of study, there is still no clear understanding of the mechanism of tetanus and botulinum toxin action at a molecular level. The amino acid sequence of TeTx does not show homology with the ADP-ribo-sylating toxins and no ADP-ribosylating enzymic activity has been detected. (ADP-ribosylating activity has, however, been detected in the *C. tetani* C3 toxin.) There is some evidence that both toxins are metalloprote-ases which require Zn^{2+} for activity. How the protease activity blocks the release of vesicle contents from neurones is as yet unclear, but it may be that modification of proteins in the vesicular membrane results in the vesicle remaining stuck to the cytoskeleton, thus preventing fusion with the plasma membrane. It therefore seems that this is another instance of different toxins having similar enzymic activity, the specificity being apparently dependent on the ganglioside receptor molecules of the target cells.

Clostridium difficile toxins

The obligate anaerobe *Clostridium difficile* is a minor member of the com-mensal gut flora of a small proportion of adults and a larger proportion of neonates. It is normally considered to be kept at low numbers by compe-tition from the other normal flora. Its importance as a pathogen has only come to light with the use of antibiotic therapy. Problems occur during antibiotic therapy with for example ampicillin, clindamycin, tetracyclines, chloramphenicol, which kill other members of the gut commensal flora which appear to keep the *C. difficile* in check. Antibiotic associated diarrhoea is common, but may develop into the more serious **pseudomembranous colitis** as a result of the over-growth of *C. difficile*. The mixture of fibrin, mucus and leukocytes, which is the host's response to the infection, form patches on the mucosa, the pseudomembranes observed by histology. If untreated, mortality may be as high as 10%; however, treatment with van-comycin or metronidazole, which act on the *C. difficile*, is effective. The virulence of *C. difficile* is associated with the production of two toxins A and B, neither of which appears to have ADP-ribosylating activity. Toxin

A is a tissue-damaging enterotoxin which causes the production of viscous fluid in the gut. The receptor of toxin A is thought to contain the trisaccharide, di-galactose, N-acetyl glucosamine. Toxin B may have similar activity to toxin A, but does not bind to the same receptor. Toxin B alone is not active in the intestine, but only becomes lethal when given with sublethal doses of A. This suggests that initial tissue damage by A allows for activity of B on other cell types.

CONCLUSION

Although the gross effects of these toxins on the host have been known for a long time, it is only now apparent that these enzymes are in fact tinkering with normal cellular function in an extremely complex way. As a result of this, studies of the activities of these toxins have not only shed light on the virulence of bacteria but have also been useful in unravelling the intricacies of intracellular communication. It is clear that many of these toxins have a devastatingly destructive effect on the host even though their role in the successful colonisation of the host by the bacterium is obscure. As these toxins affect **fundamental** functions of the host cells their potential to cause rapid death within the human population is immense. Perhaps it is not surprising that some of the bacteria which produce these toxins, notably anthrax, have been the subject of biological warfare studies. The knowledge that at least some of these genes are on moveable genetic elements points to the possibility of the evolution of a wider range of virulent bacteria carrying these determinants. If the human host had to rely solely on genetic evolution, survival could require mutation of the molecules central to normal cellular activity. Thankfully, our social evolution has allowed us to attain a level of civilisation sufficient to enable vaccine design and production.

On the more positive side, many of these toxins are being investigated as possible tools in the treatment of cancer. It is hoped that the toxic activity can be targeted specifically to tumours. By cloning the genes for antibody specific for host-cell surface molecules along with the genes for the enzymic activity of bacterial toxins it is possible to produce chimaeric molecules. It is therefore essential to be able to identify which part of the bacterial toxin genes are responsible for toxicity and separate them from those involved in binding. Antibody–toxin fusion proteins composed of single chain antibodies (sFv) fused to bacterial ADP-ribosylating toxins have already been genetically engineered. Where the antibody is specific for a molecule unique to the surface of transformed cells, the 'immunotoxin' should selectively kill the tumour cells.

FURTHER READING

Bourne H. R., Sanders D. A., McCormick F. 1991. The GTPase superfamily: conserved structure and molecular mechanism. Nature 349, 117–127.

Burton J. L. 1990. The shiga toxin family: molecular nature and possible role in disease. In: Molecular basis of bacterial pathogenesis (Eds Iglewski B.H, Clark V.L). Academic Press, London. Chapter 18.

Dugas B., Paul-Eugene N., Genot E. *et al.* 1991. Effect of bacterial toxins on human B cell activation II Mitogenic activity of the B subunit of cholera toxin. European Journal of Immunology 21, 495–500.

Field M., Rao M. C., Chang E. 1989. Intestinal electrolyte transport and diarrheal disease. New England Journal of Medicine 321, 879–883.

Finkelstein R. A. 1988. Cholera, the cholera enterotoxins and the cholera enterotoxin-related enterotoxin family. In: Immunochemical and molecular genetic analysis of bacterial pathogens (Eds Owen P., Foster T.J.). Elsevier Science, NL. pp 85–103.

Frank D. W., West S. E. H., Iglewski B. H. 1990. Molecular studies of *Pseudomonas aeruginosa* exotoxin A. In: Molecular basis of bacterial pathogenesis (Eds Iglewski B. H., Clark V. L.). Academic Press, London. Chapter 20.

Goldschmidt-Clermont P. J., Mendelsohn M. E., Gibbs J. B., 1992. Cytoskeleton: Rac and Rho in control. Current Biology 2, 669–671.

Hall A. 1990, The cellular functions of small GTP-binding proteins. Science 249, 635–640.

Halperin S. A., Issekutz T. B., Kasina A. 1991. Modulation of *Bordetella pertussis* infection with monoclonal antibodies to pertussis toxin. Journal of Infectious Diseases 163, 355–361.

Melancon P. 1993. Vesicle traffic. Current Biology 3, 230–233.

Middlebrook J. L., Dorland R. B. 1984. Bacterial toxins: cellular mechanisms of action. Microbiological Reviews 48, 199–221.

Parker C. D. 1986. Monoclonal antibodies to *Bordetella pertussis*. In: Monoclonal antibodies against bacteria. Vol III. Academic Press, London. pp 165–179.

Pozzam T. 1992. Bacterial toxins. Current Biology 2, 621–623.

Schmid S. L. 1993. Coated-vesicle formation in vitro: conflicting results using different assays. Trends in Cell Biology 3, 145–148.

Spangler B. D. 1992. Structure and function of cholera-toxin and the related *Escherichia coli* heat-labile enterotoxin. Microbiological Reviews 56, 622–647.

van Heyningen S. 1992. Tetanus toxin. Reviews in Medical Microbiology 3, 145–150.

Wren B. 1992. Molecular characterisation of *Clostridium difficile* toxins A and B. Reviews in Medical Microbiology 3, 21–27.

7 Bacterial Surface Molecules and Virulence

INTRODUCTION

The bacterial cell surface is perhaps the most obvious site of interaction between the pathogen and the host. It is important in many aspects of virulence.

In the initial stages of colonisation surface appendages allow the bacterium to gain a foothold on host cells and structures in body environments where host secretions would otherwise wash them away. In the case of intracellular parasites cell surface interactions are the first stage in gaining access to the intracellular environment. For pathogenic bacteria which remain extracellular, attachment to host cells may work against them at other points in infection where they need to avoid attaching to phagocytic cells which are endeavouring to ingest and kill them. Avoidance of the attachment to the opsonising host complement and immunoglobulin molecules is advantageous in avoiding phagocytosis. For the Gram negative bacterium it is also important for avoiding the lethal effects of the other stages of the complement cascade. From the point of view of the bacterium, interactions with the host's defence molecules can be considered to be unwanted attachment of host molecules; from the point of view of the host it can be seen as recognition and potential destruction of non-self. For the bacterium to be virulent and therefore survive within the host it must have evolved suitable mechanisms for avoiding this 'host recognition'. Therefore one of the major selective pressures governing the nature of the surface molecules of pathogenic bacteria is undoubtedly the host. This is most obvious in bacteria which colonise only one host such as *Neisseria gonorrohoeae* which is an **obligately** human pathogen, without any free-living stage. In cases such as this very subtle interactions between particular host and bacterial molecules have evolved. In many other instances it seems that, to cope with the host's defences, bateria have adapted surface molecules which are integral to the survival of the bacterium in environments outside the host.

The general role of cell envelope components in immunomodulation is considered in Chapter 2. This is partly because it is not clear if the interactions which we now consider in general terms as immunomodulation form part of the host's defence and recognition of the bacterium, or part of the virulence of the bacterium. In the evolutionary past these interactions may have been strictly one or the other, but whether the distinction is less clear because of our lack of detailed understanding of the molecules and mechanisms involved, or because of the co-evolution of the host/bacterium resulting in the two becoming inextricably interwoven remains to be determined. This difficult question should not be ignored as it underlines the complexity of the possible interactions between the host cells and the bacterium. If future therapies to counteract disease are to involve not only drugs aimed at the invading bacterium, but also the manipulation of the host's immune response by the administration of manufactured host components, such as cytokines or agents which block cytokine activity, it is particularly important that this potential complexity is taken into account. In this chapter we will consider the interactions of the bacterial surface molecules which seem to clearly enhance the virulence of the bacterium. Details of the surface structures and molecules of the Gram positive and Gran negative bacterial cell envelope can be found in the Appendix.

ATTACHMENT TO HOST CELLS AND STRUCTURES

Attachment to host cells and the extracellular matrix is a necessity for bacteria colonising sites such as mucosal surfaces and the urinary tract which are constantly being washed by host secretions. Bacterial ligand mediated attachment is also a prerequisite for entry into host cells which are not normally phagocytic, but in which phagocytosis can be induced. (These cells are sometimes termed non-professional phagocytes.) This is a major route of entry of bacteria across for example the gastrointestinal tract in the case of *Salmonella typhi* or the urethral mucosa in the case of *Neisseria gonorrhoeae*. Attachment may also be advantageous for the bacterium which obtains nutrients by lysing the host cells: host cell contact followed by lysis ensures that the release nutrients are directly accessible to the bacterium. The same can be said for bacteria which attach to the extracellular matrix and subsequently degrade these molecules to obtain nutrients. The first major barrier to attachment is charge, as both the bacterial surface molecules and the surface glycoproteins of the host cell confer a net-negative surface charge. Once this is overcome very specific interactions occur between the bacterial and host molecules. Bacteria also attach to surfaces artificially introduced into the host, such as prosthetic devices. The concentration of nutrients on solid substrates in fluid environments is a general phenomenon and is an obvious advantage to the bacterium which can attach to the surface. A general term for bacterial structures involved in attachment is **adhesin**.

Historically many studies on the ability of bacteria to attach to host cells have centred on their ability to agglutinate erythrocytes, not perhaps because this activity was considered to be central to bacterial virulence, but because such experiments are easy to perform, giving by and large a clear-

cut answer. If the bacteria agglutinate erythrocytes the aggregates are clearly visible by eye, thus providing a very simple assay system which may
be indicative of the general ability of the bacterium to attach to host cell
surface glycoproteins and glycolipids. Structures involved in host cell
attachment include fimbriae/pili, outer membrane proteins, lipoteichoic
acids, lipopolysaccharide and extracellular polysaccharides. It therefore
seems likely that any exposed bacterial surface molecule may have been
adapted to allow the bacterium to attach. Conversely, these same structures
may also have evolved to **avoid** attachment to host phagocytic cells, as is
discussed in relation to evasion of the host defences (see below). Some of
these structures exhibit phase and antigenic variation (see Chapter 9), which
may enable the bacteria to evade the specific host defence and probably
also colonise different tissues within the host.

Fimbriae/pili

Fimbriae are long protrusions, built up from protein subunits in the molecular mass range of 15–30 kDa, and which extend from the bacterial cell
surface (Figure 7.1). There may be as many as 500 of these structures on
an individual cell and they allow bacteria to attach to not only mammalian

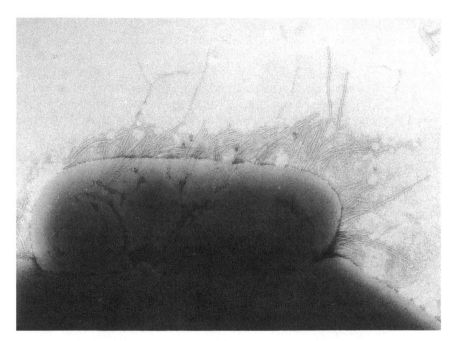

Figure 7.1. Fimbriae of *Escherichia coli*. Electron micrograph of negatively stained
whole bacterium

cells but also non-living surfaces. Thus the attachment process may be due to a specific interaction with receptor molecules or one which allows the bacterium to overcome repulsive charge or hydrophobic/philic effects of different surfaces. The specific host cell receptors are known for a few bacteria and the examination of the binding of bacteria to well characterised mammalian glycoproteins is the subject of much current research. Fimbrial expression is a common feature of Gram negative bacteria as most genera can be demonstrated to express fimbriae when cultured under the correct conditions. Fimbriae have been described in fewer of the Gram positive bacteria, examples being *Corynebacterium* spp. and *Actinomyces* spp.; however, they may be very different from those of Gram negative bacteria. The term 'fimbria(e)' was introduced in 1955 by Duguid and co-authors from the Latin for thread or fibre. In 1959 Brinton used the term 'pilus(i)' from the Latin for hair-like for the same type of structure. It has been suggested that the term pilus should only be used for the filamentous structures encoded by conjugative plasmids and involved in conjugation (i.e. the movement of DNA from one bacterium to another); however, in practice in the literature the two terms are still used for the same type of structure. Neither is there any consensus for the nomenclature of fimbriae from different bacteria, the names of some of which are listed in Table 7.1. Throughout the text fimbria(e) will be used as the general term for these structures and pilus(i) where this is the term normally used in the literature for a particular bacterial species (e.g. *Neisseria* spp.).

Fimbriae can be grouped by their morphology when viewed with an electron microscope after negative staining of whole bacteria (for example, see Figure 7.1). They can be divided into three categories: firstly, **rigid filaments** of 5–10 nm in diameter; the *E. coli* Type 1 fimbriae fall into the category of rigid filaments, in which the subunits form a right-handed helix with an axial hole of approximately 2 nm; secondly, the **N- methylphenylalanine fimbriae** which form flexible filaments of about 6 nm in which the subunits are arranged in a helix with a central pore of about 1 nm and mediate twitching motility of bacteria; and thirdly, very thin wiry **flexible filaments** of about 4 nm or less (e.g. K88, K99, CS3) which have an open helical structure which lacks an axial hole. Some fimbriae cannot be neatly classified on the basis of morphology as they have both rigid and flexible parts (e.g. *E. coli* Pap). The adhesive sites may be located either at the end of the fimbriae furthermost from the bacterial surface or located along the length of the fimbriae. The host cell receptors for a number of fimbriae are listed in Table 7.2.

A number of fimbriae undergo phase and antigenic variation. Phase variation is when a given structure is either produced or not produced and antigenic variation is when different antigenic types of the same structure are produced. In both instances the underlying mechanism for variation involves DNA rearrangement (see Chapter 9 for detailed discussion). The

Table 7.1. Some examples of bacterial fimbriae

Bacterium	Fimbrial name	Approx. molecular mass of fimbrial subunit (Da $\times 10^3$)
Escherichia coli	Type 1	18
	Pap	18
	CFA I	14
	CFA II CS1	16
	CFA II CS2	15
	CFA II CS3	15
	K88	27
	K99	18
	S	17
Salmonella typhimurium	Type 1	21
Klebsiella pneumoniae	Type 1	18
Bordetella pertussis	ST2	22
	ST3	22
Actinomyces viscosus	Type 2	59
Neisseria gonorrhoeae*	α and β	19.5 and 20.5
Pseudomonas aeruginosa*	PAO	18
	PAK	15
Bacteroides nodosus*	91B	18
Moraxella bovis*	α and β	18 and 16
Vibrio cholerae*	TCP	20

*The first amino acid at the N-terminus of these fimbrial subunit proteins is N-methylphenylalanine (NMePhe). They are also sometimes called Type IV and have a common mechanism of biogenesis.

ability to express fimbriae when necessary for attachment to host cells, and then reversibly switch to non-expression, may be of great advantage to a pathogen where it colonises different parts of the body during the course of infection. For example in a model of ascending pyelonephritis in rats, fimbrial expression by the bacterium *Proteus mirabilis* is thought to prevent the bacterium from being washed away as it ascends from the bladder to the kidney. Once in the kidney, however, the fimbriae enhance the attachment of the bacteria to phagocytic cells (probably because of lectinophagocytosis); therefore a population expressing an anti-phagocytic capsule is selected for and fimbrial expression selected against. Fimbrial expression is also affected by environmental factors such as nutrients, temperature and liquid or solid culture. The details of the factors controlling this environmental modulation of fimbrial expression, as distinct from phase and antigenic variation (see above), are by and large unknown.

One type of bacterium may be capable of producing more than one type

Table 7.2. Examples of host cell receptors for adhesins

Bacterium	Receptor
Escherichia coli *Klebsiella pneumoniae* *Salmonella* spp.	
Type 1	D-Mannose
E. coli	
K99	NeuGc(α2–3)Gal(β1–4)Glcβ1)ceramide
Pap	Gal(α1–4)Galβ (on P blood group antigen)
S	NeuAc(α2–3)Gal(β1–3)GalNAc
Neisseria gonorrhoeae *Pseudomonas aeruginosa*	GalNAc(β1–4)Gal
Streptococcus pneumoniae	Gal(β1–4)GlcNAc(β1–3)Gal(β1–4)Glc
Vibrio cholerae	L-Fucose
Helicobacter pylori *Bordetella bronchiseptica*	NeuAc(α2–3)Galβ
Actinomyces viscosus	Gal(β1–3)GalNAc

of fimbria and there may be more than one type of fimbria present on the surface of a single bacterial cell at the same time. This suggests that different fimbriae may have different functions and that a detailed understanding of the protein molecules of the fimbriae and of the host molecules with which they interact is important for the understanding of their role in virulence. The host molecules which act as receptors for the bacterial ligands are now known for some bacteria and from this, together with detailed genetic studies of the bacteria, we are beginning to unravel the underlying molecules and mechanisms responsible for the initial observation of bacterial haemagglutination.

The **P pilus** of *E. coli* (also called pap or Gal-Gal pili) is a good example of a system which is now known in detail at the level of both the molecules which make up the fimbriae and the genes coding for the constituents. *E. coli* is known to produce a range of different types of fimbriae which differ in the cell surface receptor to which they adhere (Table 7.2). The genes encoding the proteins involved in both the structure and assembly of these fimbriae have been located on the chromosome in some instances and on plasmids in others. One gene cluster which has been studied in detail is the one which encodes for the P pili which are commonly expressed by *E. coli* associated with acute pyelonephritis in children. The host cell receptor for the pili is the Gal(α1–4)Gal moiety of the P blood group antigen, hence the name 'P pilus'. A number of proteins are encoded by the P pilus or *pap* operon and the functions of most of these have been determined. The gene cluster has been located at several different sites on the chromosome of clinical isolates of E. coli and is often linked to the genes for other virulence determinants such as the K1 capsular polysaccharide and haemolysin. The *pap* gene cluster is bordered by conserved sequences, which indicates that it may have been acquired initially by transposition events during the course of evolution; however, transposition to plasmids has not been demonstrated, which suggests that the transposing ability is now degenerate.

Although there is considerable between-strain variation in the antigenicity of the pilin proteins, there are regions of amino acid homology at both the amino and carboxy termini. These are probably the regions involved in the joining of one subunit to another, while the antigenically varied central regions are not involved structurally and are exposed on the fimbrial surface. It is likely that this type of organisation of the fimbrial subunits is common to the majority of fimbriae.

The major structural protein of the P pilus is a 16.5 kDa protein known as PapA, encoded by the gene *papA*. Each individual pilus is composed of approximately 1000 monomers of this pilin subunit which are thought to be arranged in a right-handed helix which forms a rigid rod-shaped structure of about 10 nm in diameter.

Two other pilin subunits are required for the adhesive properties of the P pili and are located at the tip of the P pilus; namely the PapG, which contains the binding site for the $Gal(\alpha 1-4)Gal$ residues, and the PapF, which is thought to interact in some unknown way with PapG to enable it to bind. A third protein, PapE, is also located at the tip of the pilus and is the major structural protein of the flexible fibrillar tip which is attached to the rigid rod. The PapE forms an open helix approximately 3 nm in diameter and varying in length from 26 to 58 nm. The PapG adhesin protein is thought to be at the distal tip of the fibrillum. Another protein, PapK, is also associated with the fibrillar tip but as yet its precise position and function are now known (Figure 7.2). Two other proteins encoded within the *pap* operon are involved in the assembly of the fimbriae; the PapD protein is a member of the chaperone family of proteins and 'chaperones' each of the subunit proteins within the periplasm. The PapC is embedded in the outer membrane and is thought to form a channel through the outer membrane and a location for polymerisation of the pilus. The PapH protein is the final subunit incorporated into the pilus and effectively anchors the pilus to the outer membrane. It also appears to govern the length of the pilus, as mutants which over-produce PapH produced shortened pili.

The organisation of the genes involved in P pilus formation is summarised in Figure 7.3. Two genes which positively control the transcription of the operon have been mapped upstream of *papA*: *papB* and *papI*. The PapB protein is a specific DNA binding protein which binds to the *pap* DNA. Catabolite repressor protein with attached cAMP also positively regulates

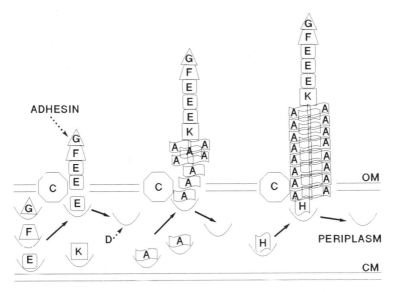

Figure 7.2. Schematic diagram of model of assembly of *Escherichia coli* P pilus. After the pilus subunits are secreted across the cytoplasmic membrane (CM) they associate with the chaperone PapD in the periplasm. The pilus is assembled at the outer membrane (OM) in association with the 'molecular usher' PapC. When the subunits join onto the assembling pilus, they disassociate from PapD. The adhesin (PapG) is linked to the tip fibrillum polymer of PapE by PapF. PapK forms the link between the tip fibrillum and the polymerising pilus rod of PapA. Attachment of PapH terminates polymerisation of PapA and anchors the pilus to the OM. From Jacob-Dubuisson F. *et al.* 1993. A novel secretion apparatus for the assembly of adhesive bacterial pili. *Trends in Microbiology*, Volume 1, pages 50–54. Reproduced by permission of Elsevier Trends Journals

the *pap* operon. This is no doubt related to the decrease in pilus expression at high glucose concentration. This decrease in fimbrial expression at high glucose concentration, or catabolite repression, has also been observed for Type 1 and K99 fimbriae. Two promoters have been mapped to the region between *papI* and *papB*, one which acts as a promoter for all the genes in the operon downstream of *papB* and the other which acts divergently for *papI* (see Chapter 9).

Differential expression of these genes is thought to occur at both the transcriptional and translational level. The majority, but not all, of mRNA transcripts, starting at the promoter (P) terminate between the *papA* and *papH* genes, where a terminating stem-loop structure is thought to form in the DNA. Therefore PapA is produced in quantity and the other pilin proteins at reduced levels from the few transcripts which extend the whole length of the operon. Further control of the expression of PapA is obtained by processing of the mRNA and differential stability of the transcripts. For example, the mRNA transcribed immediately downstream of the promoter

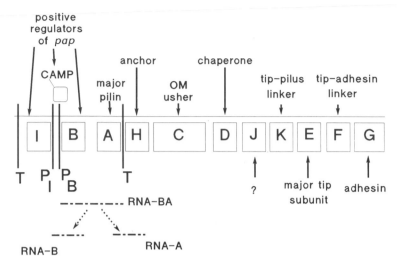

Figure 7.3. Diagram of the *Escherichia coli* P pilus gene cluster. Promoter P_I acts on the regulatory gene *papI* and promoter P_B acts on all the genes in the cluster. *papI* and *papB* code for transcription activators of the *pap* genes. The catabolite repressor protein also positively regulates the gene cluster when cAMP is bound. The transcriptional terminator (T) between *papA* and *papH* is thought to terminate most, but not all, of the mRNA transcripts. Thus more copies of PapA are produced than the other Pap proteins. Gene expression may also be controlled by the stability of the mRNA transcripts. RNA encoding both PapB and PapA (RNA-BA) is processed into two separate messages (RNA-B and RNA-A). RNA-B is rapidly degraded; however, RNA-A has an unusually long half-life, possibly because the terminator sequence (T) also acts as a stabilising element

contains RNA coding for PapA and PapB. PapB is a cytoplasmic regulatory protein. The RNA-BA is cleaved into RNA-A and RNA-B. RNA-A has a long half-life, whereas RNA-B is more rapidly degraded.

There is evidence that many of the fimbriae of *E. coli* are heteropolymeric in nature and have a similar gene cluster organisation, although in some instances the clusters are located on plasmids (e.g. K88, K99) and in others chromosomally (e.g. P). Examples include the *fim* (or *pil*) genes of the Type 1 fimbriae, *fan* genes of K99, *fae* genes of K88, the *afa* genes AFA-1 and the *sfa* genes of the S pili. Common features include the formation of the outer membrane channel through which the fimbriae are extruded. In spite of these similarities the structures of these fimbriae may be very different. The fimbriae may be either the rigid filamentous structures of, for example, the P, type 1, S pili, or the loose helix of the K88 and K99 fimbriae where the major pilin is also the adhesin. It is therefore likely that the P pilus has evolved as a combination of these two different types with a rigid filament bearing the distal flexible adhesive tip. This combination may increase the accessibility of the host cell receptor and suggests that it may be possible for the rigid filament to carry more than one type of adhesin. It is likely that as the fine detail of the structure of fimbriae is better understood common themes and relationships will emerge.

The P pili and Type 1 fimbriae of *E. coli* are known to undergo phase variation whereby within a population a genotypic switch from production to non-production of the fimbriae occurs. Type 1 fimbrial expression varies at a rate of about 10^{-3} to 10^{-4} per cell per generation. The region of the DNA involved in the switch is adjacent to the *fim* genes and is a 314 base pair region with 9 bp inverted repeats which is just upstream of the *fimA* structural gene. More details of this and other genetic mechanisms controlling phase and antigenic variation can be found in Chapter 9. The genes coding for colonisation factor antigen (CFA) I and CFA II are found on plasmids which may also carry the genes for heat stable and heat labile enterotoxin (ST and LT respectively). The genes for CS1, 2 and 3 are usually all present, but some form of controlling mechanism results in the expression of only one or two of these at one time. The details of this remain to be worked out.

Another well characterised group of fimbriae are the **N-methylphenyl-alanine** pili, which are included in the category of flexible fimbriae of intermediate size (5–6 nm). These fimbriae are generally polar and confer a twitching motility to the bacteria. They derive their name from the methylated phenylalanine residue which is present at the N-terminus of the pilin subunits. The subunits are in the order of 15–18 kDa. An extensive region of amino acid homology at the N-terminal end is common to a wide range of bacterial genera including *Pseudomonas aeruginosa*, *Neisseria gonorrhoeae*, *N. meningitidis*, *Moraxella bovis* and *Bacteroides nodosus*. This N-terminal region is highly hydrophobic, which is in contrast to the fimbriae of the Enterobacteriaceae which either have a hydrophobic region at the C-terminal end or lack a hydrophobic region altogether. In general the pilin genes are encoded chromosomally. In *N. gonorrhoeae* and *meningitidis* intergenic recombination events and slipped stranded mispairing of DNA are known to generate tremendous within-strain antigenic variation of the pilin proteins. In *Moraxella bovis* a DNA inversion event within the pilin gene generates two antigenic types, α and β (see Chapter 9). Different serogroups and serotypes of the other species are known and it has been generally assumed that these do not exhibit within-strain phase and antigenic variation to the extent observed in *N. gonorrhoeae*. Some antigenic variation has been observed in *P. aeruginosa* which relates to differences in molecular mass of the pilin subunits. Only a single copy of the gene is found; therefore the genetic variation must be the result of recombination events within the single gene, as occurs with the streptococcal M protein, rather than recombination events between multiple gene copies, as is the case for *Neisseria gonorrhoeae* pili (see Chapter 9). In *Bacteroides nodosus*, the pilus contains two proteins, the subunit of 17 kDa and an 80 kDa minor protein associated with a structure at the base of the pilus. It may be that *B. nodosus* also exhibits a limited amount of antigenic variation in these proteins as again differences in molecular mass relating to different serotypes have been observed. A comparison of the pathogenesis of *B. nodosus* and *N. gonorrhoeae* perhaps explains why the tremendous antigenic variation of *N. gonorrhoeae* is of little or no advantage to *B. nodosus*. *N. gonorrhoeae* colonises the genital epithelial surface where it is subject to the onslaught of the specific mucosal immune response with the generation of specific blocking IgA. In contrast *B. nodosus* colonises the epidermal tissue of the interdigital skin and the hoof of sheep in foot-rot, which results in lameness and the eventual separation of the hoof from the soft tissues. The twitching motility conferred by the fimbriae is thought to help in the penetration of the tissues. Even after severe foot-rot only minimal immune protection is gained against future infection. This is thought to be because the disease is superficial and restricted to the avascular epidermis, thus there is little stimulation of the specific immune response. Therefore, by inhabiting a very different ecological niche within the host, *B. nodosus* and *N. gonorrhoeae* are subject to different selective pressures. It is likely that the high concentrations of IgA present in the mucosal secretions favour antigenic variation of surface structures in *N. gonorrhoeae*. This selective pressure will be absent in *B. nodosus* infections where there is little stimulation of the specific immune response. Interestingly, inoculation of a vaccine containing fimbriae has proved to be very successful in protecting sheep from foot-rot. This indicates that although antigen movement from the site of a natural infection is not sufficient to generate a strong immune response, the bacterial components are immunogenic and the host's defences can reach the site of infection. Immunity is apparently mediated by agglutination of the bacteria by antibodies specific for the fimbriae. It will be interesting to see if continued use of the vaccine exerts enough selective pressure to result in the evolution of greater antigenic variation in the fimbriae of *B. nodosus* in the future.

Comparison of the amino acid sequences of the pilin subunits has allowed the mapping of regions of homology and variation. This has allowed the identification of those regions of the protein which have a common function. The amino acids at the N-terminus form a hydrophobic region which is thought to be involved in subunit–subunit interaction and also possibly in assembly of the fimbriae. It is also thought that this region forms a β-sheet during synthesis of the subunit and transport to the membrane, then taking on an α-helical shape in the assembled fimbriae. By X-ray crystallography, it has been shown that the subunits of *P. aeruginosa* pili are arranged in a helix with an internal central pore or channel of 1.2 nm and an overall diameter of 5.2 nm. The major antigenic sites can vary with different genera. For example, the major antigenically hypervariable region of *N. gonorrhoeae* is in a C-terminal loop formed by disulphide bonding between cysteine residues whereas in *P. aeruginosa* the most strongly immunogenic region is in the central part of the peptide between amino acids 70 and 81. The regions of the *P. aeruginosa* and *N. gonorrhoeae* fimbriae are compared in Figure 7.4.

Non-fimbrial adhesins

Although, technically, any other component of the bacterial cell surface which mediates attachment to host cells could be called a 'non-fimbrial adhesin', the term is generally reserved for bacterial components which are thought to be related to fimbriae. In some instances these may be constructed from the adhesive subunits of the fimbriae, without the non-adhesive structural components. The gene organisation of one of these non-

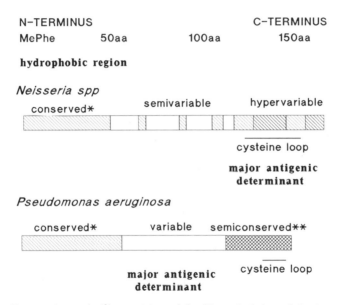

Figure 7.4. Comparison of pilin proteins of the N-methylphenylalanine pili of *Neisseria* spp. and *Pseudomonas aeruginosa*. The pilin subunits have a homologous conserved region at the N-terminal end and both have a cysteine loop towards the C-terminus. In *Neisseria* the region with the cysteine loop forms the major antigenic determinant of the pilin and is also the region which undergoes **within**-strain antigenic variation (see Chapter 9). Both the semivariable and the hypervariable region may be involved in attachment to host cells. In contrast, in *P. aeruginosa* the central region contains the major antigenic determinant and is variable **between** strains. The region containing the cysteine loop is relatively less variable between strains. The central and C-terminal regions of both of these proteins are the exposed regions of the molecule and the constant region is probably involved in holding the subunits together to form the intact pilus. *Conserved, region conserved between species; ** semiconserved, region conserved between strains. aa, amino acid

fimbrial adhesins of *E. coli*, AFA-1 (for *afimbrial adhesin*), is similar to that
of the P pilus. These adhesins are composed of non-covalently linked subunits of apparent molecular mass of about 15–30 kDa. After stabilisation with
specific antibody, electron microscopy shows that the adhesin NFA-1 (for
non-fimbrial adhesin) of *E. coli* forms an extensive encapsulating structure
outside the outer membrane of the bacterium. Co-expression of a polysaccharide capsule and an encapsulating non-fimbrial adhesin has been observed
by electron microscopy of *E. coli*. The polysaccharide capsule, K98, was
associated intimately with the bacterial surface and the adhesin, NFA-4,
seemed to be on the outer surface.

Outer membrane proteins

Attachment to host cells is one of the many diverse functions of the outer
membrane proteins of Gram negative bacteria. A number of these are
involved in the initial attachment stage, which occurs prior to entry into
the host cells of bacteria which either grow intracellulary or transiently pass
through the host cells, as a means of gaining access to other sites within
the body (Chapter 8). Some of the best studied outer membrane proteins
are those of *Neisseria gonorrhoeae* (also termed OP for opacity proteins due
to the appearance of colonies of bacteria which express these proteins). The
PII (or Opq) protein (27–32 kDa) is known to mediate attachment to epithelial cells, along with the fimbriae. It is likely that it is the PII which
mediates specific attachment to glycoprotein receptors on human fallopian
tube and uterine epithelial cells. As with the pili, PII undergoes extensive
antigenic variation, although the underlying genetic mechanism is different
(see Chapter 9). The PI protein also attaches the *Neisseria* to the host epithelial cells, but in a manner which is thought to trigger the uptake of the
bacterium into the cell. The PI is an anion selective porin which does not
undergo antigenic variation. It appears to insert into the host target cell
membrane in the opposite orientation to that of the bacterium (see Figure
8.2). This insertion of an ionophoric channel in the host cell could alter the
ionic and nutrient balance of the host cell and the membrane potential and
may trigger the endocytosis of the bacterium, thus enabling it to invade.
There is a direct correlation between expression of the PII protein and virulence of *Neisseria gonorrhoeae*. Other bacterial outer membrane proteins
associated with attachment and invasion of host cells include the Yad (also
called YopA or P1) and Inv of *Yersinia* spp. These and other outer membrane proteins associated with host cell invasion are discussed in detail in
Chapter 8. The outer membrane proteins of Gram negative bacteria have a
diverse range of functions and it is likely that many of the proteins which
are involved in attachment remain to be characterised.

Proteins of the Gram positive cell envelope

This diverse group of proteins will doubtless yield many examples of bacterial molecules involved in attachment to host cells and molecules as more detailed studies are undertaken, but at present the precise molecular interactions are known for only a few. Included in these are cell envelope proteins of *Streptococcus mutans*, which is associated with caries formation in teeth. The host receptors for the bacterial proteins are salivary glycoproteins, adsorbed onto the tooth enamel. This therefore enables the bacteria to stick to the tooth surface. One of these proteins, of 150 kDa, binds to salivary amylase.

Lipoteichoic acids

Lipoteichoic acids (LTA) may be involved in the adhesion of a number of different Gram positive bacteria to a range of host cell molecules, although few of these interactions have been characterised in detail.

One exception is the polyglycerol phosphate of the lipoteichoic acid of *Streptococcus pyogenes* which links to lysine residues on the streptococcal M protein to form a cross-linked network at the bacterial cell surface. The exposed fatty acid moieties of the LTA can then attach to fibronectin on the epithelial cell surface (Figure 7.5). Thus the LTA mediates attachment to a component of the extracellular matrix, rather than a specific host cell receptor. Adhesion of *S. agalactiae* (group B) may also be mediated by lipid moieties of the LTA.

Lipopolysaccharide and polysaccharides

In general terms more detailed molecular information is available on the involvement of extracellular polysaccharides in avoiding attachment to cells in their antiphagocytic capacity rather than in mediating attachment; however, where bacteria form colonies within a glycocalyx or biofilms, particularly on prostheses and teeth, then they become very important in attachment in general terms. The identification of specific ligands and receptors is the subject of future study. Lack of information again is perhaps not a reflection of a lack of importance, but rather a lack of investigation.

Haemagglutination can be inhibited by the treatment of some bacteria with reagents such as periodate and neuraminidase which will destroy or remove sugar residues from the cell surface. A good example of this is provided by the obligate anaerobe *Bacteroides fragilis*. In most instances specific ligands and receptors remain to be defined.

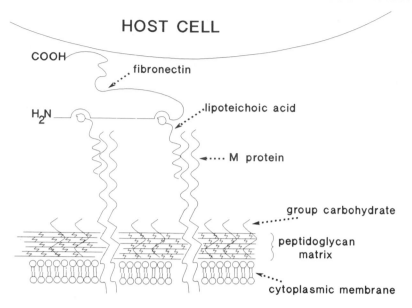

Figure 7.5. Adhesion of *Streptococcus pyogenes* to host cells: the role of M protein and lipoteichoic acid. M protein, anchored in the cytoplasmic membrane, extends through the peptidoglycan–teichoic acid matrix of the Gram positive cell envelope and out from the bacterial cell surface. The poly-glycerol phosphate region of the lipoteichoic acid (LTA) binds to the M protein. The exposed lipid moiety binds to fibronectin, a component of the extracellular matrix of the host. Fibronectin has a binding site for host epithelial cell receptors and forms a bridge between the bacterium and the host cell

Host cell receptors

An increase in our understanding of the structure of mammalian cell surface glycoproteins has helped considerably in defining the molecules of the host to which the bacteria bind. Oligosaccharides of mammalian cell surfaces may be bound to either proteins, by N- or O- linkage, or to lipids, to form glycoproteins and glycolipids respectively (see Appendix). In the N-linked glycoproteins, the oligosaccharides are linked to an asparagine residue in the peptide, and in the O-linked to serine, threonine or hydroxylysine. N-linked oligosaccharides come in three major types. The **high mannose-type** are composed of branched mannose antennae and are joined by a stalk of 2 N-acetyl glucosamines to the lipid or protein. The **complex-type** of N-linked oligosaccharides are produced from a precursor with a di-N-acetyl glucosamine stalk and antennae containing nine mannose and three glucose residues in the endoplasmic reticulum. This is then processed in the Golgi by removal of the glucose and six of the nine mannose residues. These may then be replaced with a range of sugars such as galactose, N-acetyl neuraminic acid and glucose. The **hybrid-type** of N-linked oligosaccharide has features of both the high-mannose and complex types. Examples of N-linked and O-linked oligosaccharides are illustrated in the Appendix. The significance of the sugar sequences of these oligosaccharides in the normal cell–cell interactions is only just beginning to be understood and is discussed in Chapter 2. One important point is that the same oligosaccharide unit may be attached to different proteins or lipids, and in general the oligosaccharides present at the mammalian cell surface are characteristic of the cell type. For example the blood group antigens A, B and O are oligosaccharides which may be attached to either proteins or lipids. A well documented example of this phenomenon is the Thy-1 glycoprotein, which is a member of the immunoglobulin superfamily of molecules and present on thymocytes and brain cells. Although it has an identical polypeptide component, the sugars of N-linked oligosaccharide moieties differ depending on whether the Thy-1 is derived from thymus or brain. These variants of the glycoprotein are referred to as 'glycoforms'. As the majority of cell surface receptors for bacterial fimbriae (and probably other adhesins) are oligosaccharide moieties, knowledge of the sugar constituents of the oligosaccharides involved is of prime importance in understanding the cell types to which the bacteria can bind. To date most of the information about the host molecules to which the bacteria bind is limited.

The Type 1 fimbriae of *E. coli* are thought to bind to three adjacent mannose residues whereas the binding site of Type 1 fimbriae of *Salmonella* spp. is thought to be smaller and may accommodate fewer mannose residues. Thus, although both of these fimbriae probably mediate attachment by binding to high-mannose containing oligosaccharides, they differ in their sugar specificity.

A number of fimbriae require sialic acids in the oligosaccharides to which they bind. As this family of sugars is now thought to be important in the normal functioning of mammalian systems, the binding of bacteria to these residues may possibly have effects on the host which are at present unknown (Chapter 2 and 5). The K99 fimbriae of *E. coli* are known to bind to N-glycolyl neuraminic acid present, along with galactose and glucose, on a glycolipid of erythrocytes. In contrast, S fimbriae of *E. coli* bind to N-acetyl neuraminic acid, galactose and N-acetyl galactosamine containing oligosaccharides of glycophorin A, one of the major constituents of the erythrocyte membrane. The *E. coli* CFA I and II fimbriae also bind to sialic acid containing N-linked oligosaccharides of the complex type. *Vibrio cholerae* produces an adhesin which can be inhibited by L-fucose. L-Fucose is usually a constituent of the di-galactosamine stalk of the oligosaccharide antennae. Where these oligosaccharides are also present on phagocytic cells, bacterial attachment may no longer be advantageous to the bacterium and phase variation may play a very important role. The S fimbriae of *E. coli* may be involved in the specific adhesion of *E. coli* associated with meningitis. The host receptor has been identified as the terminal Neu-Ac(α2–3)Gal disaccharide unit of oligosaccharides which is present in neonatal mice on vascular endothelium and the lining of the choroid plexus and brain ventricles. It has been suggested that the S fimbriae are therefore responsible for the neurotropism of *E. coli* with the capsular antigen K1 which causes neonatal meningitis (see below in relation to capsular polysaccharides and evasion of the host defence). The sugar components of host cell receptors for a number of fimbriae are listed in Table 7.2.

EVASION OF THE HOST DEFENCES

The two major areas of bacterial evasion of host defence which can be related to the surface molecules of the bacterium are the avoidance of phagocytic uptake and killing and resistance to complement mediated cell lysis (Chapter 4), termed serum resistance. Central to these is the deposition of complement and Ig molecules on the bacterial cell surface. These either act as, (a) **opsonins** if C3b, iC3b, C4b and Ig are recognised by the CR1, 3, 4 or Ig receptors respectively on phagocytic cells or (b) initiators of bacterial lysis by either the **alternative** or **classical complement pathways**. Bacteria avoid phagocytosis and the activities of complement, in broad terms, by either physical–mechanical means, for example where complement is activated but is ineffectual, or by subtle interaction dependent on highly specific molecular interactions. Antigenic variation of bacterial surface molecules and a lack of immunogenicity are both strategies used by bacteria to avoid specific recognition by immunoglobulin. (See Chapter 9 for a discussion of the genetic basis of bacterial antigenic variation.) The enzymatic degradation of host molecules such as Ig and complement glycoproteins, as well as the targeted lysis of leukocytes, are both potential mechanisms for avoiding the immune system. As such activities may be closer, in evolutionary terms, to nutrient scavenging by bacteria and may indeed still play some role in this aspect of bacterial colonisation of the host, they are dealt with in Chapter 5.

Physical/mechanical mechanisms

The thick three-dimensional matrix of peptidoglycan and teichoic acids of Gram positive bacteria protects the cytoplasmic membrane from complement mediated lysis, thus rendering Gram positive bacteria serum resistant. Complement is activated on the bacterial surface, but the membrane attack complex is physically at a distance from the membrane and therefore not effective. Complement and Ig deposited on the surface may still have opsonic activities and products of the complement cascade act as chemoattractants for leukocytes. Gram negative bacteria are more vulnerable as the outer membrane is relatively more exposed; however, where the bacteria produce very long O-antigens, this affords a similar protection to that of the Gram positive envelope (Figure 7.6). Some very elegant experiments have been done using *Salmonella* spp. in which both the length and distribution of O-antigen on the cell surface could be related to serum sensitivity. The experiments were done with a strain of *S. montevideo* which lacked the ability to convert glucose to galactose, or break down galactose into glucose as it was mutated in the gene encoding for uridine diphosphate galactose 4 epimerase. It was also mutated in the gene coding for mannose-6-phosphate isomerase. This strain, when fed exogenous galactose, incorporated it only into the core region of the lipopolysaccharide (LPS) molecule. Exogenous mannose was only incorporated into the O-antigen. By feeding the bacterium tritiated mannose and carbon-14 labelled galactose and then comparing the ratio of 3H to 14C, a measure of both the length of O-antigen and the density of O-antigen over the surface of the bacterium was estimated. At low concentrations of mannose the bacterium continued to produce long chains of O-antigen, but in fewer numbers over the cell surface. The sensitivity to the killing action of complement was directly related to the density of the long chain LPS molecules on the bacterial surface. The conclusion is that the long chains of O-antigen **sterically hinder** the access of the membrane attack complex (MAC) to the outer membrane, the C3 is deposited towards the end of the LPS furthest from the cell surace and the MAC is formed too far from the membrane to be effective. Where there are fewer long side chains distributed on the bacterial surface, the steric hindrance is less effective and serum killing can occur (Figure 7.6). Antibody and C3b have been observed beneath the capsule in some bacteria, which will sterically hinder the opsonic activities of these molecules. They may also hinder the lytic activities of complement.

Bacteria can also limit the effects of complement and opsonisation by **shedding** some of their surface molecules which do activate complement, thus reducing the quantity of complement available for reaction with the bacterial cell surface. Capsular polysaccharide is excreted as cell free slime by a number of bacteria. *Pseudomonas aeruginosa*, which infects the lungs of people with cystic fibrosis, is a good example. The shed polysaccharide binds C3 which is then cleaved by factor B. *Staphylococcus aureus* sheds soluble teichoic acid which also has de-complementary activity. The budding of vesicles of outer membrane is well documented in pathogens such as *Haemophilus influenzae*, *Bacteroides* spp. and *Neisseria* spp. (See Figure 2.4). Deposition of opsonin and complement activation on such shed 'decoys' diverts the host's immune system away from the bacterial cell, while the bacterium laughs up its metaphorical sleeve.

The TraT outer membrane lipoprotein is associated with resistance to serum killing in *E. coli*. Although the exact mechanism of its action is not yet known, it is included in this section as complement is activated and MAC deposited at the bacterial cell surface, but for some unknown reason, possibly because the MAC is not assembled correctly, it does not kill the

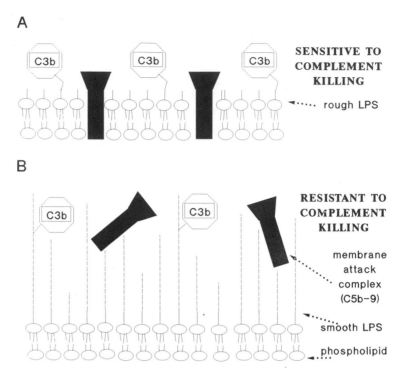

Figure 7.6. The role of O-antigen in resistance to complement mediated killing. A. Complement, activated at the bacterial surface by the deposition of C3b, results in the insertion of the membrane attack complex and lysis of bacteria which lack O-antigen (rough LPS). B. In bacteria with O-antigen (smooth LPS), complement is activated too far from the outer membrane surface for the membrane attack complex to be effective

bacterium. TraT is lipoprotein which maintains a non-covalent association with peptidoglycan. It has a molecular mass of approximately 25 kDa and bacteria are known to express 3000 to 20 000 molecules per cell. TraT is plasmid encoded and many bacteria which are not pathogenic are known to express TraT. Its presence on the bacterium prevents the formation of stable mating aggregates between bacteria, thus preventing the entry of a second F-plasmid into the bacterium. In a way it confers 'maleness' to the bacterium. The phenomenon is known as surface exclusion. This is therefore a molecule which has not evolved as an adaptive mechanism for the pathogen, but for a different purpose and is only coincidentally linked with virulence.

Purely physical characteristics of the bacterial surface, in relation to that of the phagocytic cell, play some role in the avoidance of phagocytosis by bacteria, in the absence of opsonin. The **surface charge** and **relative wettability** or affinity of a cell surface for water relates to phagocytosis. The more hydrophilic the bacterial cell surface is in relation to the hydrophobicity of the phagocytic cell, the more likely it is that the bacterium will resist phagocytosis (Table 7.3). During the course of an infection, opsonins will no doubt be present and have an over-riding effect on the phagocytic process. These physicochemical interactions may reflect, in evolutionary terms, an earlier adaptation in bacteria, which enabled them to avoid phagocytosis by single celled eukaryotes in aquatic environments. Capsular structures may also impede phagocytosis where opsonins are bound at the bacterial cell surface, but beneath the capsule. For example there is evidence that C3b can bind beneath the capsules of *Streptococcus pneumoniae* and *Staphylococcus aureus*. The capsule therefore acts as a physical barrier to the recognition of the opsonin by phagocytes.

Molecular interactions

An understanding of the subtlety of bacterial–host molecular interactions is still in an early stage of development. This section is concerned with how bacteria subvert the activities of complement and thus have the potential to avoid both complement mediated lysis and phagocytosis. Many structures,

Table 7.3. The hydrophobicity/hydrophilicity of bacterial surfaces in relation to those of phagocytic cells

	Bacterium	Contact angle*	
Hydrophilic; resistant to phagocytosis by human PMNL	*Staphylococcus aureus* Smith strain	16.5°	
	Salmonella typhimurium	17.0°	
	Streptococcus pneumoniae	17.0°	
	Escherichia coli 0111	17.2°	resistant to phagocytosis by guinea pig macrophages
	Haemophilus influenzae group B	17.6°	
	Human PMNL	18.0°	
	Shigella flexneri	18.1°	
	H. influenzae (rough)	18.6°	
	Salmonella typhimurium (rough)	20.0°	
	Streptococcus pyogenes	21.3°	
	Guinea pig macrophages	21.3°	
	E. coli 07	23.0°	
	Staphylococcus aureus Smith strain (decapsulated)	26.0°	
	Listeria monocytogenes (rough)	26.5°	
	Neisseria gonorrhoeae	26.7°	
Hydrophobic	*Brucella abortus*	27.0°	

*Contact angle: this is determined by placing a sessile standard drop of saline on a flat monolayer of air-dried cells (bacteria or phagocytes); the curvature of the drop (measured as the angle of the tangent to the drop, the contact angle) relates to the hydrophobicity/hydrophilicity of the cells forming the monolayer. The bigger the angle, the more hydrophobic the cells.
Rough, rough lipopolysaccharide.
PMNL, polymorphonuclear leukocyte.

originally identified as anti-phagocytic, are in fact interfering with complement activation and reducing opsonisation. Some bacteria avoid the specific immune response by expressing surface structures which mimic molecules present within the host. Finally bacteria can also avoid the specific immune response by varying the antigenicity of their surface molecules in a genetically reversible manner (see Chapter 9).

Biological molecules have long been divided into complement activating and non-activating. It is now known that **all** molecules which contain $-NH_2$ and $-COOH$ groups are potential activators of the complement cascade (see Chapter 4). Host cells avoid the activities of complement by patrolling their cell surfaces with molecules such as decay accelerating factor (DAF) which down-regulate the complement cascade. Therefore for a bacterium to have non-activating molecules this must involve very subtle interactions with the host at the molecular level. The presence of a layer which forms a physical barrier between the site of MAC deposition and the membrane, thus preventing the killing mechanism of complement without preventing the deposition of opsonin, is discussed above. A number of bacteria produce enzymes which degrade components of the complement cascade (see Chapter 5) which may also afford protection; however, many bacteria possess very highly evolved mechanisms for interfering with complement activity. Much of our current knowledge is based on studies of the surface molecules present in bacteria known to be resistant to complement and a comparison of these with similar bacteria which are sensitive. In the case of saccharide molecules, patterns are beginning to emerge and particular moieties, or even substitutions of moieties, are being identified as important. For the most part, however, how these particular moieties interact with host molecules is a subject for the future and very much dependent on our understanding of molecular immunology.

Figure 7.7 summarises the complement cascade and details the points at which the host controlling molecules act and also where bacteria are known to interfere with the normal complement cascade. These aspects will now be considered in relation to the different molecular components of the bacterial cell envelope.

Extracellular polysaccharide

Capsular polysaccharides (Figure 7.8) can be considered as perhaps the classical virulence determinant of bacteria, in that the elegant experiments on *Streptococcus pneumoniae* indicated a clear-cut relationship between the presence of the capsule and virulence. The importance of the capsule as a structure which prevents phagocytosis is perhaps one of the most widely known 'facts' in bacterial pathogenesis. As discussed above, some capsules do provide a physical barrier to phagocytosis in the absence of opsonin; however, with our current understanding of the complex interactions of

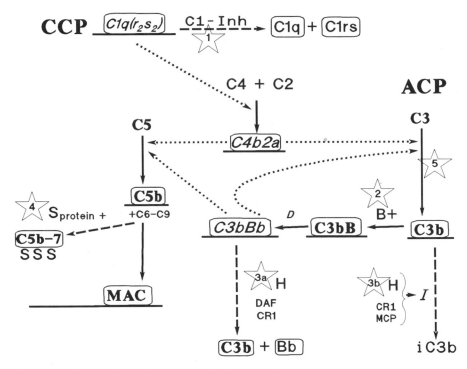

Figure 7.7. Bacterial interference with the complement cascade. The regulation of the complement cascade by the host (dashed line) is used by some bacteria to mediate resistance to complement killing (star). 1. Sugars in the outer core region of bacterial LPS prevent direct binding of C1 to sugars in the inner core, possibly by binding C1 esterase inhibitor (C1-Inh) which down regulates C1 activation; 2. Some bacterial polysaccharides decrease the affinity of factor B for C3b and therefore prevent up-regulation; 3. Streptococcal M protein binds factor H and N-acetyl neuraminic acid in bacterial polysaccharides is thought to enhance the binding of factor H to membrane bound C3b. Factor H down-regulates the activity of C3 convertase enzyme at two points (3a) by accelerating its decay and (3b) by acting as a cofactor for the serine protease factor I which cleaves C3b; 4. *Neisseria gonorrhoeae* binds S protein which binds to C5b-7 and therefore inhibits the deposition of MAC; 5. Poly-ribose phosphate of *Haemophilus influenzae* is resistant to binding of C3b. Other host molecules which regulate complement are decay acceleration factor (DAF), membrane cofactor protein (MCP) and complement receptor type 1 (CR1). (See also Chapter 4, Figure 4.1.)

the bacterial capsule with host molecules it is perhaps naive to consider the capsule as being simply 'anti-phagocytic'.

Capsules and extracellular polysaccharides are produced by a wide range of bacteria, pathogen and non-pathogen alike. They therefore play a role in the survival of bacteria in a wide range of different environments far removed from the mammalian immune system. The question is, therefore,

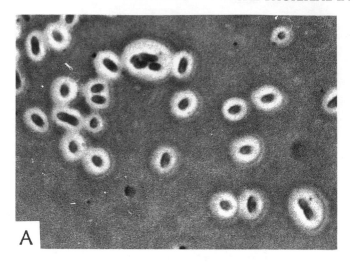

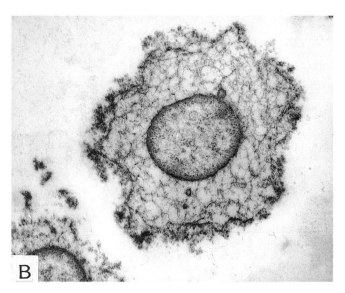

Figure 7.8. Capsules of the Gram negative bacterium *Bacteroides fragilis*. A. Light micrograph of bacteria negatively stained with carbol fuchsin and eosin; the large white areas around the bacteria are the capsules. B. Electron micrograph of an ultra-thin section of an equivalent population to A. The large fibrous network corresponds with the white area in the light micrograph

'what is unusual or special about the capsular polysaccharides associated with virulence?' To answer this question the possible strategies adopted by the bacterium to avoid the host defence must be considered: namely, prevention or inhibition of the activation of the alternative complement pathway (ACP) and the generation of opsonin on the bacterial cell surface; and the avoidance of the specific immune response by antigenic variation and/or mimicry of host molecules. Extracellular polysaccharides of bacteria are biochemically diverse, with those of *E. coli* among the most studied. Therefore the composition of the capsular or K (from Kapselantigene) antigens of *E. coli* will be considered in detail.

The **K antigens** were initially assigned different numbers according to their antigenic cross-reactivity, but with more detailed knowledge of the biochemical composition of the polysaccharides it is now clear that although some of them are not antigenically cross-reactive, the differences in the sugar residues may be very slight. Indeed in some instances strains of one particular antigenic type have turned out to be mixtures of more than one type, which appear to be undergoing within-strain antigenic variation. Examples of K antigens which are antigenically different, but biochemically identical except for the presence or absence of an acetyl group, are detailed in Table 7.4.

The **K18** and **K22** antigens are both polymers of ribose and ribitol phosphate. They are therefore structurally similar to the teichuronic acids of the Gram positive cell envelope, being polymers of sugar phosphates. They are also related to the **K100** and the *Haemophilus influenzae* type B polysaccharide as discussed below. The only difference between the K18 and K22 is in

Table 7.4. Capsular antigens of *Escherichia coli* in which the sugars are the same but the antigenicity is altered by O-acetylation

Sugars in polymer	Antigenic type	
	(O-acetylated sugars)	(no O-acetylated group on sugars)
Galactose-glycerol	K2ab*	K2a
Ribose-ketodeoxyoctonate (KDO)	K13 (KDO acetylated) K20 (ribose-acetylated)	K23
N-Acetyl neuraminic acid	K1+[†]	K1−
Ribose-ribitol phosphate	K18[‡]	K22

*Originally designated K62.
[†]Population a mixture of K1+ and K1−.
[‡]Population a mixture of K18 and K22.

the presence of an O-acetyl group at the C3 position of the ribose (Figure 7.9). Closer examination of individual cells within the strains identified as K18 showed that only a proportion of the population had the acetylated form of the polymer and it was effectively a mixture of the K18 and K22 serotypes. Separated populations do not retain one antigenic type, but revert to a mixture of K18 and K22.

The **K1** antigen, a polymer of N-acetyl neuraminic acid, undergoes a similar type of within-strain antigenic variation, whereby within an individual population, some of the bacteria have O-acetylated N-acetyl neuraminic acid, termed K1+, and some lack the O-acetyl group, termed K1−. It is likely that the variation is controlled by altering the expression of a transacetylase enzyme. The significance of O-acetylation in relation to virulence is discussed below. In strains of *E. coli* identified as K22, either the gene for the transacetylase enzyme is no longer functional or the on-off switch controlling the antigenic variation is stuck in the 'off-position'.

Within-strain antigenic variation of capsule antigens may be common to a number of bacterial types. Among these is the obligate anaerobe *Bacteroides fragilis*, which like *E. coli* is commensal in the gut, but may cause disease of faeces or the contents of the lower intestine contaminate other sites in the body. An example is peritonitis after rupture of the appendix. As yet, the components of the polysaccharides responsible for the antigenic variation in *B. fragilis* are not known, but examination of the pattern of labelling with monoclonal antibodies clearly illustrates antigenic heterogeneity of

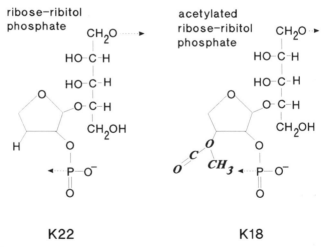

Figure 7.9. Comparison of *Escherichia coli* K18 and K22 capsular antigens. The K22 and K18 serotypes are composed of a polymer of ribose and ribitol phosphate. In the K18 serotype a proportion of the bacteria have an acetyl group added to the ribose. The K18 serotype is therefore a mixture of bacteria with capsules composed of either poly ribose-ribitol phosphate or poly-acetylated ribose-ribitol phosphate. The dotted arrows represent the position of linkage to another sugar residue

structurally similar bacteria (Figure 7.10). It is likely that this phenomenon of within-strain variation in surface polysaccharides will be identified in many bacterial types when the labelling patterns of monoclonal antibodies are examined by immunofluorescence and immunoelectron microscopy. Other examples of K antigens where O-acetylation causes a lack of antigenic cross-reactivity include the **K2** and **K62** antigens, which have been renamed K2a and K2ab respectively. K2ab(K62) is essentially an O-acetylated K2b(K2). **K13**, **K20** and **K23** differ only in either the position of the O-acetyl group (K13 and K20) or a lack of O-acetyl group (K23). Whether there is the potential for within-strain variation in these polysaccharides is not clear. These examples illustrate that in some cases serotyping of bacterial strains has masked the underlying subtlety of the variation in bacterial surface molecules. Another example of this is in serotyping of the streptococcal M protein (see below).

Sialic acids, and the structurally related keto-deoxyoctonate (see Figure 7.11), are common constituents of polysaccharides present on virulent bacteria. As sialic acids are common constituents of host molecules and their importance in the regulation and communication within the host is becoming more apparent (see Chapter 5 for discussion in relation to neuraminidase production by bacteria), host molecule mimicry by bacteria may enable

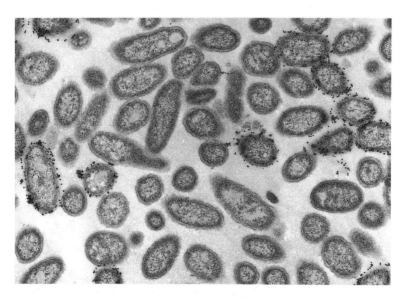

Figure 7.10. Within-strain antigenic variation illustrated by immunolabelling with a monoclonal antibody. Electron micrograph of ultrathin section of *Bacteroides fragilis* labelled with a mouse monoclonal antibody specific for a surface polysaccharide and anti-mouse antiserum conjugated to particles of gold (black dots). Note that not all of the bacteria in the population are labelled

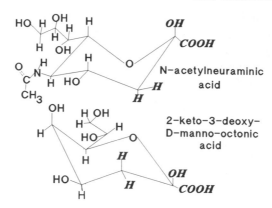

Figure 7.11. Comparison of N-acetyl neuraminic acid (NANA) and 2-keto-3-deoxy-D-manno-octonic acid (KDO). These two structurally related sugars (bold) are frequently found as components of the polysaccharides of virulent bacteria. KDO is also a constituent of the core of lipopolysaccharide

the bacterium to interfere with host functions in ways which remain to be discovered. It is known that this mimicry is related to poor specific immune recognition (see below) and with interference with complement activity.

The polysaccharide capsules of *E. coli* K1- and *Neisseria meningitidis* type b are identical polymers of α-2,8 linked N-acetyl neuraminic acid (NANA) and associated with poor activation of the ACP as is the type III capsule of group B streptococci which also contains NANA, but not as the sole constituent. Other bacteria with α-2,8 linked NANA in their capsular polysaccharides include *Pasteurella haemolytica*, which causes pasteurellosis in pre-weaned lambs, and *Moraxella liquefaciens*. The mechanism of down-regulation of the ACP is probably related to enhancement of the binding of factor H to C3b. Sialic acids on erythrocyte surface oligosaccharides are known to enhance the binding of factor H to membrane bound C3b, thus enhancing the decay of membrane bound C3bBb convertase (Figure 7.7). If the sialic acids are removed complement is activated on the erythrocyte membrane. One possible explanation of this phenomenon could be that sialic acid-containing host molecules are involved in complement regulation. The bacteria may therefore be mimicking a host mechansim for the regulation of complement activity. Although there is as yet no evidence for the direct minicry of host complement regulators in bacteria, the protozoan parasite, *Trypanosoma cruzi*, expresses a surface structure which mimics decay acceleration factor. Other pathogens which contain sialic acids exposed on the surface, such as viruses, may have adopted mechanisms similar to those observed in bacteria to avoid complement activity.

E. coli K92 and *N. meningitidis* group c polysaccharides are also NANA polymers, although relatively less virulent than K1 and *N. meningitidis* group b. In the K1 and group b polymers the linkage is between the second and eighth carbon atom of NANA ((α2–8) NeuAc) In *N. meningitidis* group c the linkage is between the second and the ninth carbons ((α2–9) NeuAc; Figure 7.12). The K92 polymer alternates between 2–8 and 2–9 linkages ((α2–9) NeuAc(α2–8) NeuAc). The *Haemophilus influenzae* type b and *E. coli* K18/22 and K100 polysaccharides are all polymers of ribose and ribitol phosphate, which again differ in the linkage position of the sugars. Computer aided modelling reveals that this is sufficient to considerably alter the three dimensional structure of the polymers. That a structural change such as this is apparently sufficient to alter the virulence of the bacteria again points to the importance of subtle molecular recognition events in host–bacterial interactions. These undoubtedly involve the three dimensional position of the relevant moieties of both the host and bacterial molecules.

Streptococcus pneumoniae capsules which do not contain sialic acids (e.g. type 7 and 12) down-regulate complement by decreasing the affinity of factor B for bound C3b, thus preventing up-regulation. In contrast, the type b polyribose-ribitol phosphate capsule of *Haemophilus influenzae* binds very little C3, thus interfering with initial deposition of complement (Figure 7.7).

In many cases there is an apparent relationship between virulence and a lack of complement activation. *Haemophilus influenzae* type b are highly virulent in neonates whose maternal antibody levels are low and before adult levels and subclasses of immunoglobulin have been attained. In this

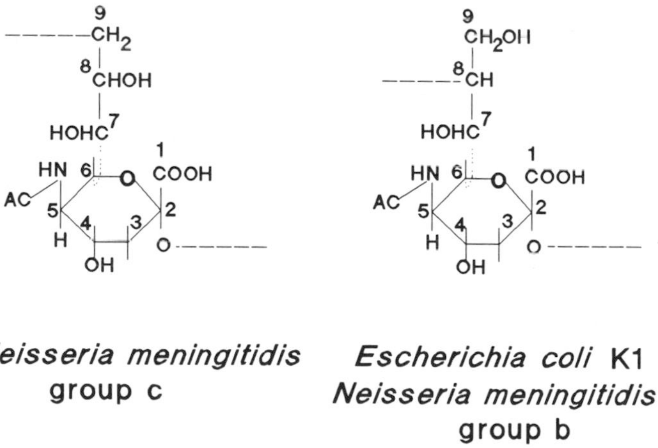

**Neisseria meningitidis
group c**

**Escherichia coli K1
Neisseria meningitidis
group b**

Figure 7.12. Linkage to polymers of N-acetyl neuraminic acid in bacterial capsules. In *Escherichia coli* K1 and *Neisseria meningitidis* group b capsules the 2nd carbon atom of the sugar is linked to the 8th carbon atom of the next sugar (dashed lines). In *N. meningitidis* group c, which is less virulent, the 2nd carbon atom is linked to the 9th carbon of the next sugar. (*E. coli* K92 capsule has alternating α2–8, 2–9 linkage and is also of low virulence.)

age group the ACP is one of the major defence mechanisms, and as a result of bypassing this the bacteria can survive in the blood in large numbers. It is thought that this sustained bacteraemia leads to seeding of the bacteria in the meninges. The bacteria colonise the subarachnoid space and the ensuing inflammatory response can result in disruption of the blood–brain barrier. *E. coli* K1 and *N. meningitidis* group b, probably also rely heavily on down-regulation of complement for virulence, although they are successful pathogens in individuals from a wider age range. This may in part relate to a lack of specific immune recognition of their polysaccharides (see below). Therefore a single molecule may play more than one role in virulence.

A number of bacterial polysaccharides resemble or are identical to components of host cell oligosaccharides and components of the extracellular matrix (Table 7.5). This is thought to relate directly to the poor or non-existent specific immune response to these polysaccharides; the bacterial capsule is regarded by the host as a self-antigen and protective hyper-immune antibody is not generated. Neither is there the potential for the memory-dependent rapid production of specific antibody if the host encounters the bacterium on a second occasion.

Examples of bacterial polysaccharides which mimic host structures include the K1− capsule of *E. coli* and the *N. meningitidis* group b. These two identical polymers are antigenically cross reactive with the oligosaccharides on host gangliosides and cell surface glycoproteins. They share the same NANA linkage pattern as the terminal sialic acids on the embryonic form of the oligosaccharide on a neural cell adhesion molecule (N-CAM). As the brain develops, there is a reduction in the number of sialic acid residues and in the adult the terminal residues are absent (Figure 7.13). The lack of immune recognition of the bacterial polysaccharides in adults is therefore a result of an immunological memory of self. Interestingly, the NANA of the K1+ capsule is O-acetylated and slightly more immunogenic.

For a number of years the **K5** polysaccharide remained undetected due to its lack of antigenic reactivity. The structure of the K5 polymer is identical to the first polymeric intermediate produced during the biosynthesis of heparin. In broth culture the **K4** polysaccharide is similar to chondroitin,

Table 7.5. Bacterial polysaccharides which mimic host components

Bacterium	Host component
Escherichia coli K1	Oligosaccharides of cell surface
Neisseria meningitidis group b	glycoproteins and gangliosides
E. coli K5	Heparin biosynthetic intermediate
E. coli K4	Chondroitin
Streptococcus pyogenes	Hyaluronic acid

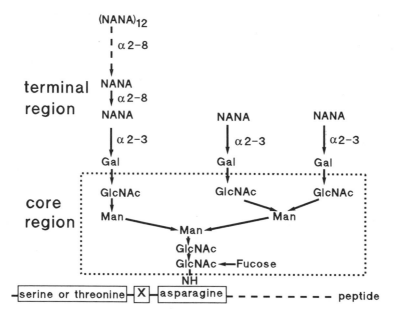

Figure 7.13. Diagram of the oligosaccharide on neural cell adhesion molecule which cross-reacts with *Escherichia coli* K1 and *Neisseria meningitidis* group b polysaccharides. The oligosaccharide is N-linked to an asparagine residue on the peptide. The oligosaccharide is of the complex tri-antennary type. The cross-reactivity is thought to be due to the chain of 12 or more ($\alpha2-8$) linked N-acetyl neuraminic acid (NANA) residues. In adults the length of the NANA polymer is reduced. Man: mannose; GlcNAc: N-acetyl glucosamine; Gal: galactose; X: any amino acid

but with fructose residues which form part of an immunodominant epitope. When the K4 expressing bacteria are grown at pH4, however, the fructose linkage is labile and the bacterial molecule is converted to non-immunogenic chondroitin. It is likely that the bacterium will encounter low pH during the course of an infection due to the release of components from phagocytic cells at sites of inflammation. This is another example where it is important to consider the growth of the bacterium in vivo to obtain a clear understanding of virulence. *Streptococcus pyogenes* can express a capsule with identical structure to hyaluronic acid. These three bacterial polysaccharides, the K4, K5 and *S. pyogenes* hyaluronic acid, are mimicking the proteoglycans which form the gel in which the proteinaceous components of the extracellular matrix are embedded. Therefore by mimicking these major host components the bacterium can remain 'unseen' by the specific arm of the immune system. Bearing in mind that many of these polysaccharides are also protected from recognition by the ACP, it is not surprising the bacteria expressing them are associated with invasive disease.

Mimicry of host regulatory molecules increases the complexity of the possible interactions of the bacterium with the host from simply an avoid-ance of the specific immune response. This was discussed above in the context of the ACP. Direct mimicry of cytokines by polysaccharides is another possible mechanism for interfering with the immune response. The polysaccharide of *Haemophilus actinomycetemcomitans*, which is associated with periodontal disease, is reported to mimic many of the activities of IL1. The mimicry of cytokines by other bacterial molecules is considered in the context of immunomodulation in Chapter 2.

An area in which it is essential to have a clear understanding of the composition of the bacterial capsule in relation to host molecules is in the development of vaccines. If the bacterial structure is altered so that host tolerance is broken, there is always the possibility that the antibodies gener-ated to the modified bacterial molecule will cross-react with the host, thus generating an autoimmune response. This is particularly important for bab-ies and children who are usually at most risk from these pathogens and therefore prime candidates for vaccination. In this age group the immune system is still developing and we do not as yet have a complete understand-ing of the complexities of this developmental process, particularly in relation to immune recognition of polysaccharides. The introduction of new polysaccharide vaccines is therefore treated with extreme caution.

Lipopolysaccharide

Lipopolysaccharide (LPS) has already been considered in detail in Chapter 2 in relation to its role as a biological response modifier and in endotoxic shock (see Appendix for structure). The activity of the O-antigen as a physi-cal barrier to MAC deposition is considered above. It is now clear, however, that the sugar components of LPS are also important in its interactions with complement.

In general the classical complement pathway (CCP) requires bound Ig for activation. *Escherichia coli* LPS both with and without O-antigen (i.e. rough and smooth) can, however, bind the first component of the CCP, C1, directly, although the whole cascade sequence is not normally triggered. The key to the lack of complete activation of the CCP is the host's own control molecule C1 esterase inhibitor (C1-Inh). The function of C1-Inh is to bind to activated C1r and C1s and remove them from the C1 complex (Figure 7.7). In serum depleted of C1-Inh, complement is directly activated by the rough LPS, but not smooth LPS. It seems that in *E. coli* and *N. gonorrhoeae* LPS core sugars near the lipid A bind the C1. LPS core sugars further from the bacterial surface, such as keto-deoxyoctonate and D-man-noheptose, are involved in the inhibition of direct activation, possibly by enhancing C1-Inh binding, or blocking binding of C1 at a second site. These core sugars therefore convert LPS from a classical pathway activator to an alternative pathway activator. The relevance of this to bacterial–host evolution is open to speculation, but perhaps some of the outer sugar constituents of the LPS have been selected for as a result of this direct activation of the CCP.

The ability of *Salmonella* spp. to cause systemic disease is thought to relate, in part, to the structure of the O-antigen (for intracellular survival of *Salmonella* spp. see Chapter 8). The greater virulence of *S. typhimurium* in mice, when compared with *S. enteritidis*, is thought to be related directly to complement activation. The sugar constituents of the O-antigen have been examined in relation to their ability to avoid complement deposition. The amount and degradation of C3b to iC3b and the binding of factor H were the same for both types of O-antigen. In this instance, therefore, it appears that it is the binding of factor B to C3b to form the C3bBb convertase which is influenced by the fine structure of the bacterial O-antigen. The only apparent biochemical difference between the LPSs is that an abequose sugar residue in the *S. typhimurium* is replaced by a tyvulose in *S. enteritidis*. The two sugars are epimers which only differ in the position of an -OH group, yet it seems that this is sufficient to alter the activity of the C3bBb convertase enzyme.

In *N. gonorrhoeae*, both outer membrane proteins (see below) and the lipooligosaccharide (LOS; essentially the same type of molecule as LPS, but lacking long polysaccharide chains) are involved in resistance to complement. The involvement of LOS is intriguing, as this form of resistance is only apparent if the bacteria are grown in vivo, or in the presence of serum. The complement resistance is therefore induced by host factors. The essential host component is the sialic acid, N-acetyl neuraminic acid (NANA) attached to the nucleotide carrier, cytosine monophosphate (CMP). The bacterial sialyl transferase enzymes use the host CMP-NANA to add NANA residues to the LOS. By electron microscopy a thickened layer can then be seen at the bacterial cell surface. This underlines the importance of examining bacteria which have grown in vivo when trying to identify virulence determinants. In this instance, the mechanism by which the addition of NANA interferes with complement activity is not known, but evidence from studies of capsular polysaccharides (see above) indicates that sialic acids are key components in complement resistance.

Neisseria gonorrhoeae also evades complement by binding S protein, serum spreading factor (also called vitronectin). S protein is a fluid phase inhibitor of MAC formation and binds to the host integrin molecules via the sequence of three amino acids RGD (arginine, glycine, aspartic acid); however, the component of *N. gonorrhoeae* which binds S protein has not yet been identified (Figure 7.7)

Streptococcus pyogenes M protein

The streptococcal M protein is classically described as anti-phagocytic, in much the same way as capsular polysaccharides (see above). It is now clear that although the net negative charge of the N-terminal region of the M protein, which is furthest removed from the bacterial cell surface (Figure 7.14), may be responsible for some physico-chemical repulsion of phagocytes, the molecular basis of the anti-phagocytic activity is due to the affinity of the M protein for the factor H regulator of complement. This seems to be slightly different from the polysaccharide interference with the activities of H in that the M protein binds factor H, thus increasing the concentration of H at the bacterial cell surface. The factor H then both accelerates the decay of the C3bBb convertase enzyme and in association with factor I enhances the cleavage of C3b to inactive (i)C3b which cannot associate with B. As a result the amplification loop, and therefore the deposition of opsonising C3b, is limited (Figure 7.7). Evidence for this mechanism of protection from the ACP includes experiments in which M+ and M− variants were compared in serum which was depleted of factor H. Under these conditions the M+ bacteria bound similar amounts of C3b to the M−. The M protein is also subject to a high degree of antigenic variation, probably as a result of intra-genomic recombination events between regions of repeated DNA within the *emm* gene (see Chapter 9). Interestingly, the distal

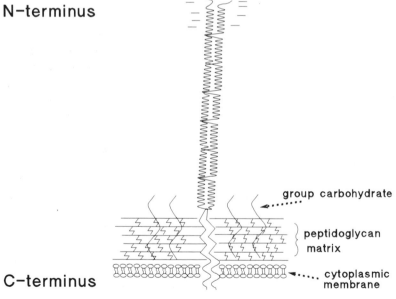

Figure 7.14. M protein of *Streptococcus pyogenes*. The M protein is a dimer which is anchored to the cytoplasmic membrane. A small coiled region at the C-terminus is associated with the cytoplasmic membrane, a β sheet region is associated with the peptidoglycan/teichoic acid matrix and the extended α helices of the dimer form a coiled coil which extends from the cell surface. The region towards the N-terminus is negatively charged (−)

portion of the M protein is a relatively conserved region. This is thought to be the region involved in H factor binding. Obviously too much variation in this region could result in a loss of the ability to bind H; therefore variation is constrained by function.

Immunoglobulin-binding proteins

Both Gram positive and Gram negative bacteria produce a number of surface proteins which bind immunoglobulins of a variety of different isotypes and from a variety of different species (Table 7.6). These proteins bind to immunoglobulin molecules in regions other than the antigen-binding region, for example in the Fc region. By doing this they potentially impede both the activation of the CCP by immunoglobulin and the direct recognition of the Ig by receptors on phagocytic cells. Much of the work concerning these molecules relates to their potential as research and clinical tools in the identification, purification and removal of antibodies of different types. For example there is the possibility of their use for the extra-corporeal removal of immune complexes from patients with autoimmune disease. Their precise relationship with virulence remains to be proven, although one of the strongest arguments in favour of their role in virulence is that molecules of similar function have evolved independently in a wide range of different bacterial types. If the DNA and amino acid sequences of, for example, the staphylococcal A protein, streptococcal G protein and the H protein of *Streptococcus pyogenes* are compared, there is no obvious relationship. The *S. pyogenes* M protein (see above), streptococcal H and Arp protein do, however, have regions of homology. This is most striking in the regions of the molecule which anchor the protein to the cytoplasmic membrane and are associated with other components of the envelope. There is also considerable homology with the internal repeats in the genes. The implications of this are that these proteins with diverse function arose as a result of gene duplication in the evolutionary past. Indeed the genes for protein M and H have been mapped next to each other on the *S. pyogenes* chromosome. The expression of immunoglobulin-binding proteins by virulent Gram negative bacteria adds weight to the argument that there is a strong selective pressure in favour of this trait for success as a pathogen. The *hpd* gene which codes for the D protein of *Haemophilus influenzae* has been sequenced and shows no homology with the Ig-binding proteins of the Gram postive bacteria. It lacks any internal repeat sequences. In contrast to the Gram postive Ig-binding proteins, it is the N-terminal end of the protein which is associated with the bacterial cell surface and the C-terminus which is involved in Ig-binding. This protein binds to human IgD, which is only detectable in trace amounts in serum and is generally present as a surface immunoglobulin on B-cells. IgD is, however, secreted in both the nasopharynx and middle ear cavity. It is therefore likely to be important

Table 7.6. Bacterial immunoglobulin-binding proteins

Bacterium	Protein	Specificity
Gram positive *Staphylococcus aureus*	A (Type I)	Range of mammalian IgG Fc
Lancefield Group A *Streptococcus pyogenes*	H (Type II)	Human IgG1, IgG4; rabbit IgG Fc
	52 kDa	Human IgG1, IgG2, IgG4; rabbit IgG; pig IgG Fc
	38 kDa	Human IgG3 Fc
	Arp	IgA
Lancefield Group C *Streptococcus equisimilis* *S. dysgalactiae*	G (Type III)	All human IgG subclasses, range of mammalian IgG Fc
Lancefield Group G *Streptococcus anginosus* Bovine isolates	(Type III) (Type IV)	All human IgG subclasses, range of mammalian IgG Fc Human IgG1, IgG4, rabbit, pig, equine IgG Fc
Lancefield Group C *S. zooepidemicus*	(Type V) (Type VI)	Range of mammalian IgG Range of mammalian IgG, greater reactivity with rat IgG than Type V
Lancefield Group B *Streptococcus agalactiae*	β	Human IgA Fc
Peptococcus magnus	L	IgG, IgM, IgG, IgA, IgD, IgE light chain
Clostridium perfringens	P	Human IgM Fab
Gram negative *Haemophilus influenzae*	D	Human IgD Fc
Haemophilus somnus		Bovine IgG, IgM, IgA Fc
Brucella abortus		Bovine IgM Fc
Branhamella catarrhalis		Human IgD Fc
Taylorella equigenitalis		Equine IgG Fc

in immunity in the primary site of colonisation by *H. influenzae*, the upper respiratory tract. In this instance there does appear to be a relationship between the production of an Ig-binding protein and virulence.

Investigations of streptococcal protein G, which binds to human IgG, present a slightly more confusing picture. Protein G binds to not only IgG, but also human serum albumin and two major plasma protein protease inhibitors, α-2-macroglobulin and kininogen (staphylococcal protein A also binds to these plasma proteins). Both IgG and α-2-macroglobulin bind at the same site on the protein G. Binding of protein G to α-2-macroglobulin does not affect the inhibition of protease activity by the α-2-macroglobulin, which suggests that protein G is not a protease. It is not immediately clear that the expression of protein G will be advantageous to the pathogen. If α-2-macroglobulin is bound to protein G at the bacterial cell surface it could inactivate bacterial cell surface proteases and therefore inhibit bacterial growth. α-2-macroglobulin may also act as an opsonin, if attached to the bacterial cell surface; α-2-macroglobulin–protease complexes are cleared from circulation by macrophages which carry receptors for α-2-macroglobulin. Protein G can, however, also allow the bacterium to **avoid** opsonisation by binding Ig the wrong way round (Figure 7.15). This example perhaps illustrates the difficulties in relating molecules to virulence and the need for studies with models of infection and isogenic bacterial mutants. On balance, Ig-binding proteins probably have evolved as virulence determinants, given the wide range of divergent bacteria which produce them. The affinity of these bacterial molecules for other host proteins may represent an area where evolution of host molecules has 'muddied the water' to an extent where it is impossible to distinguish between a bacterial viru-

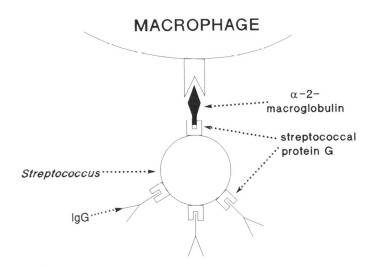

Figure 7.15. Binding of streptococcal protein G. Streptococcal protein G (SPG) can bind to both immunoglobulin G (IgG) and the plasma protease inhibitor α-2-macroglobulin via the same binding site. Expression of SPG at the bacterial cell surface can therefore potentially either inhibit phagocytosis by binding IgG the wrong way round, thus masking the Fc region which binds to the Fc receptor on the phagocytic cell, or enhance phagocytosis as α-2-macroglobulin also binds to macrophage

lence determinant and a host defence strategy. On the other hand the interactions of Ig-binding proteins with other host proteins may be purely
coincidental.

Outer membrane proteins

This diverse group of molecules is involved in many aspects of bacterial
virulence. Outer membrane proteins (OMP) involved in Ig-binding are considered above. One other area in which OMPs play a direct role in escaping
the host defence is in avoiding the activities of specific antibody. Antigenic
variation of OMPs has been described in *Borrelia* spp., which are responsible
for a classical relapsing fever, where repeated cycles of illness are associated
with altered antigenicity of the variable membrane protein of the *Borrelia*
spp. Similarly the PII OMP of *Neisseria gonorrhoeae* undergoes within-strain
antigenic variation, such that different PII variants can be isolated from
different sites of infection within an individual host. In both of these
instances it is thought that the generation of specific antibody to the OMP
drives the selection of new bacterial variants produced as a result of genetically controlled antigenic variation. Details of the genetic mechanisms
involved in the generation of within-strain variation of these and other bacterial surface molecules are described in Chapter 9.

The PIII OMP of *N. gonorrhoeae* does not undergo antigenic variation and
although specific antibody is generated to PIII, any MAC generated following binding of anti-PIII antibodies is not lethal to the bacterium. The PIII
and the specific antibody block the lethal deposition of MAC. The antibody
generated by PIII is therefore termed 'blocking antibody'. This is turn protects unrelated epitopes on PI and the LPS from specific recognition.

The *Yersinia* outer proteins (Yops) are secreted proteins, rather than
strictly outer membrane proteins, with antiphagocytic activity. One theory
is that some of the Yop proteins effectively paralyse phagocytes by depoly-
merising the actin within the phagocytic cell. These proteins are discussed
in more detail in Chapter 8.

Some OMPs mimic host proteins. Whether or not this is a bacterial strategy to avoid host immune recognition is not clear, but the end-result may
be detrimental to the host as a result of the generation of cross-reacting
antibodies, rather than from a successful bacterial infection. After infection
with a number of bacteria, including species of *Shigella, Salmonella, Yersinia,
Campylobacter* and *Chlamydia*, reactive arthritis, a chronic aseptic arthritis,
develops in some individuals several weeks later. This is generally associated with individuals who carry the HLA B27 cell surface glycoprotein. In
the enterobacteria there is evidence that the cross-reacting antigen is OmpA.
The precise mechanism by which the reactive arthritis is included is not
clear. Again a clearer understanding of host-bacterial evolutionary relation-

ships may help in our understanding of how and why such interactions have arisen.

As studies of bacterial OMP progress it is likely that many more will be characterised and found to play a role in the evasion of the host defences.

CHEMOTAXIS AND MOTILITY

Bacterial movement is generated by either twitching of fimbriae or the rotation of flagella. Flagella extend out from the cell surface (Figure 7.16) or, in the case of spirochaetes, are enveloped at the cell surface below the outer membrane in the form of periplasmic flagella or endoflagella. Motility without chemotaxis is probably of little use to the bacterium; however, little is known about the chemoattractants of pathogenic bacteria. At least 60 genes are involved in generating bacterial motility. It can therefore be argued that with such a high genetic commitment there must be very strong selective pressures acting in favour of motility. Motility and chemotaxis are thought to increase the efficiency with which bacteria contact the host mucosal surfaces and possibly also provide sufficient propulsive force for

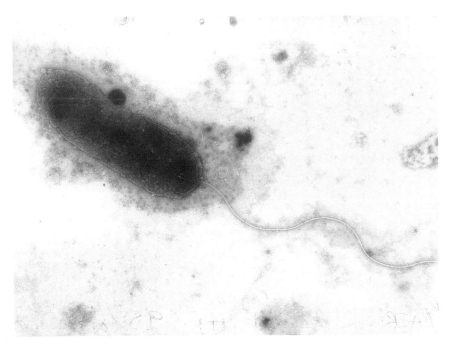

Figure 7.16. *Pseudomonas aeruginosa* flagellum. Electron micrograph of negatively stained whole bacterium illustrating the rigid flagellum extending from the cell surface

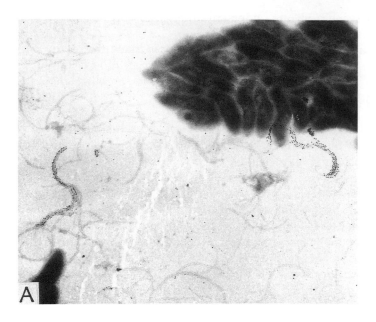

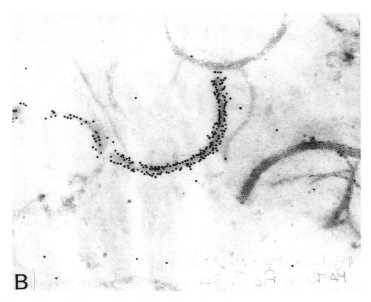

Figure 7.17. *Campylobacter jejuni* flagella. The whole bacterial cells have been labelled with a mouse monoclonal antibody specific for the flagella and anti-mouse antiserum conjugated to particles of gold (black dots) and then negatively stained (A). Detail of labelled flagella at higher magnification (B). Note that not all of the flagella are labelled by the monoclonal antibody which suggests that there is antigenic variation

the movement of the bacteria through the mucous layer to the epithelial cell surface. This may be important for the initial colonisation by enteric pathogens such as *Salmonella* spp. and *Vibrio cholerae*. Studies with mutants indicate that non-motile variants are less adept at colonising mucosal surfaces. They did not penetrate as deeply between the villi of the intestinal epithelium as motile cells, nor did they colonise at as many sites. Non-chemotactic mutants were less able to penetrate the mucus layer. In a mouse model of infection with *Campylobacter jejuni* polyclonal anti-flagellar antiserum, which inhibited motility, protected against infection. Interestingly, monoclonal antibodies specific for the flagella did not. This could have been due to within-strain antigenic variation of the flagella (Figure 7.17) or, as the authors suggest, to inactivation of the MAb in the gut. In a similar way, motility of *E. coli* which cause urinary tract infections may enhance bacterial colonisation of the host by enabling the bacterium to move upwards through the urinary tract towards the kidney, against the urine flow.

Motile *Pseudomonas aeruginosa* are more virulent in infections of burns and inoculation with purified flagellar protein is protective in a model of infection. This indicates a direct relationship between flagella and virulence. In contrast, *P. aeruginosa* isolated from the chronically infected lungs of cystic fibrosis patients lack flagella or are poorly chemotactic. It therefore seems that the selective pressures favouring chemotaxis and motility are absent in the lungs of these patients. Detailed comparison of these two sites of infection may increase our understanding of the role of flagella in virulence. It would also be interesting to determine the genetic basis of the phase variation from flagellate to non-flagellate.

The endoflagella of spirochaetes almost certainly are involved in colonisation of the host, where it is thought that the corkscrew motility of the whole bacterial cell enables the bacterium to bore through host tissues. In *Treponema pallidum*, the bacteria may invade and spread by penetrating at the junctions between cells of the epithelium and endothelium (see Chapter 8).

Antigenic variation of the *Salmonella typhimurium* flagella is one of the classical examples of reversible genetic switching. Although the genetic basis of the switch is known in detail (see Chapter 9), the relationship of flagellar variation with virulence remains to be proven.

Investigations of the host molecules which act as chemoattractants and studies of the genetic basis of motility and chemotaxis of virulent bacteria are areas ripe for study.

FURTHER READING

General

Doyle R. J., Sonnenfeld E. M. 1989. Properties of the cell surfaces of pathogenic bacteria. International Review of Cytology 118, 33–92.
Hormaeche C. E., Penn C. W., Smyth C. J. (Eds). 1992. Molecular biology of bacterial infection; Current status and future perspectives. Symposia of the Society for General Microbiology 49. Cambridge University Press, Cambridge, U.K.
Iglewski B. H., Clark V. L. (Eds). 1990. Molecular basis of bacterial pathogenesis. Academic Press, London.
Owen P., Foster T. J. (Eds). 1988. Immunochemical and molecular genetic analysis of bacterial pathogens. Elsevier, NL.
Ron E. Z., Rottem S. 1991. Microbial surface components and toxins in relation to pathogenesis. Plenum Press, New York, USA.
Roth J. A. (Ed). 1988. Virulence mechanisms of bacterial pathogens. American Society for Microbiology, Washington DC, USA.

Attachment

Costerton J. W., Cheng K-J., Geesey G. G. et al. 1987. Bacterial biofilms in nature and disease. Annual Review of Microbiology 41, 435–464.
Denyer S. P., Gorman S. P., Sussman M (Eds). 1993. Microbial biofilms: formation and control. Society for Applied Bacteriology Technical Series 30. Blackwell Scientific Publications, Oxford.
Elleman T. C. 1988. Pilins of Bacteroides nodosus: Molecular basis of serotypic variation and relationships to other bacterial pilins. Microbiological Reviews 52, 233–247.
Evans D. J., Evans D. G. 1990. Colonization factor antigens of human pathogens. Current Topics in Microbiology and Immunology 151, 129–145.
Hoepelman A. I. M. Tuomanen E. I. 1992. Consequences of Microbial attachment: Directing host cell functions with adhesins. Infection and Immunity 60, 1729–1733.
Jacob-Dubuisson F., Kuehn M., Hultgren S. J. 1993. A novel secretion apparatus for the assembly of adhesive bacterial pili. Trends in Microbiology 1, 50–54.
Jann K., Hoschutzky H. 1990. Nature and organization of adhesins. Current Topics in Microbiology and Immunology 151, 55–70.
Krogfelt K. A. 1991. Bacterial adhesion: Genetics, biogenesis and role in pathogenesis of fimbrial adhesins of Escherichia coli. Reviews of Infectious Diseases 13, 721–735.
Kuehn M. J., Heuser J. Normark S. Hultgren S. J. 1992. P pili in uropathogenic E. coli are composite fibres with distinct fibrillar adhesive tips. Nature 356, 252–255.
Ofek I., Sharon N. 1990. Adhesins as lectins: specificity and role in infection. Current Topics in Microbiology and Immunology 151, 91–113.
Paranchych W., Frost L. S. 1988. The physiology and biochemistry of pili. Advances in Microbial Physiology 29, 53–114.
Read R. 1989. Bacteria with a sticky touch. New Scientist, 28 October, 38–41.
Rosenstein I. J., Mizuochi T., Hounsell E. F. et al. 1988. New type of adhesive specificity revealed by oligosaccharide probes in Escherichia coli from patients with urinary tract infection. Lancet, December 10, 1327–1330.
Tennent J. M., Hultgren S., Marklund B.-I. 1990. Genetics of adhesin expression in

Escherichia coli. In: Molecular basis of bacterial pathogenesis. (Eds Igleswki B. H., Clark V. I.) Academic Press, London. Chapter 5.
Wick M. J., Madara J. L., Fields B. N., Normark S. J. 1991. Molecular cross talk between epithelial cells and pathogenic microorganisms. Cell 67, 651–659.

Evasion of host defence

Bacterial immunoglobulin-binding proteins Volumes 1 and 2. 1990. Academic Press, London.
Cross A. S. 1990. The biologic significance of bacterial encapsulation. Current Topics in Microbiology and Immunology 150, 87–95.
Finne J. 1985. Polysialic acid— a glycoprotein carbohydrate involved in neural adhesion and bacterial meningitis. Trends in Biochemical Science, March 129–132.
Fischetti V. A. 1991. Streptococcal M protein. Scientific American June, 32–39.
Forsberg A. Rosqvist R. Wolf-Watz H. 1994. Regulation and polarized transfer of the *Yersinia* outer proteins (Yops) involved in antiphagocytosis. Trends in Microbiology 2, 14–19.
Gomi H., Hozumi T., Hattori S. *et al* 1990. The gene sequence and some properties of protein H: a novel IgG-binding protein. Journal of Immunology, 144, 4046–4052.
Griffiss J. M. 1987. The pathogenetic basis of the distribution and epidemiology of diseases caused by encapsulated bacteria. In: Towards better carbohydrate vaccines (Eds Bell R., Torrigiani G.) World Health Organisation. J Wiley, Chichester. Chapter 11.
Jann B., Jann K. 1990. Structure and biosynthesis of the capsular antigens of *Escherichia coli*. Current Topics in Microbiology and Immunology 150, 19–42.
Jiminez-Lucho V. E., Leive L. L., Joiner K. A. 1990. Role of the O-antigen of lipopolysaccharide in *Salmonella* in protection against complement action. In: Molecular basis of bacterial pathogenesis. (Eds Iglewski B. H., Clark V. L.). Academic Press, London. Chapter 16.
Joiner K. A. 1988. Complement evasion by bacteria and parasites. Annual Review of Microbiology 42, 201–230.
Orskov F. Orskov I. 1990. The serology of capsular antigens. Current Topics in Microbiology and Immunology 150, 43–63.
Scott J. R. 1990. The M protein of group A *Streptococcus*: evolution and regulation In: Molecular basis of bacterial pathogenesis (Eds Iglewiski B. H., Clark V. L.) Academic Press, London. Chapter 9.
Silver R.P. Vimr E.R. 1990. Polysialic acid capsule of *Escherichia coli* K1. In: Molecular basis of bacterial pathogenesis (Eds Iglewski B.H., Clark V.L.). Academic Press, London. Chapter 3.

Motility and chemotaxis

Smyth C. J. 1988. Flagella: their role in virulence. In: Immunochemical and molecular genetic analysis of bacterial pathogens (Eds Owen P., Foster T.J.). Elsevier NL. Chapter 11.

8 Intracellular Invasion, Survival and Growth

INTRODUCTION

Although most bacterial pathogens inhabit the fluids and matrix between cells and tissues in the body, a few bacteria from diverse genera have adapted to intracellular growth. The ability to penetrate the host cells allows the bacteria to cross the epithelial cell layers and gain entry into the host. Examples of bacteria which use this mechanism to colonise the host are the invasive enteric pathogens such as *Salmonella* spp., respiratory pathogens such as *Legionella pneumophila* and sexually transmitted pathogens such as *Neisseria gonorrhoeae*. Such intracellular parasitism has the obvious advantage of avoiding the activities of antibody and complement molecules. However, the intracellular environment, particularly that of a professional phagocyte (e.g. neutrophil or macrophage), may be equally hostile (see Chapter 4) and requires specialised characteristics to allow survival. Bacterial inhabitation of mobile cells such as macrophages also results in the spread of the disease to many sites in the body and the multiple foci of infection which are characteristic of, for example, *Salmonella typhi* and *Mycobacterium tuberculosis*. A number of common themes in the way in which pathogenic bacteria have overcome the difficulties of an intracellular existence have emerged. This suggests that convergent evolution, that is the parallel development of similar mechanisms in different bacteria to cope with similar problems, has been in action. The molecular detail, however, of the host–parasite interaction is still at an early stage of investigation. In only a few cases have the bacterial genes involved in intracellular growth been identified and only very few of the molecules involved are known. The emphasis of this chapter is therefore on work which is beginning to be done.

It is possible to group these pathogenic intracellularly parasitic bacteria on the basis of their strategies for intracellular growth; although as in most things to do with bacteria the basis for the groupings is not always clear-cut (Table 8.1).

Firstly, the bacteria can be grouped on the basis of which types of cell are infected. Bacteria such as *Mycobacterium tuberculosis, M. leprae, Listeria monocytogenes* and *Legionella pneumophila* tend to preferentially infect **professional phagocytes**, usually monocytes/macrophages and rarely poly-

Table 8.1. Survival strategies of intracellular bacteria

Bacterium	Intracellular location			Host cell infected	
	Phagosome	Phago-lysosome	Cytoplasm	Phagocyte	Other
Salmonella typhi		+		++	+
S. enteritidis					++
S. cholerae-suis					++
Shigella spp.	+		+		++
Rickettsia spp.*	+		+	+	++
*Coxiella burnetii**		+		++	
Chlamydia spp.*	+			+	++
Listeria monocytogenes			+	++	+
Legionella pneumophila	+	+		++	+
*Mycobacterium leprae**	+	+	+	++	+
M. tuberculosis	+	+		++	+
Yersinia pestis		+		++	+
Y. enterocolitica[+]	+				+
Y. pseudotuberculosis[+]	+				+
Neisseria gonorrhoeae[+]	+			+	+
Treponema pallidum[+]	+		+	+	+
Brucella abortus			+[‡]	+	+

*Obligately intracellular.
[+]Transiently intracellular.
[‡]Inhabits the rough endoplasmic reticulum.

morphonuclear leukocytes. On the other hand *Rickettsia* spp., *Chlamydia* spp., *Salmonella* spp., *Shigella* spp., *Yersinia* spp. and *E. coli* may infect **non-professional phagocytes**, that is host cells in which phagocytosis can be induced, but for which it is not a normal function. This is reflected by a need for specialised virulence determinants in order to gain entry into the relevant cells. This will be considered in the next section. The type of cell infected will also alter the route by which bacterial antigen can be presented at the host cell surface, as Class II major histocompatibility molecules are expressed primarily by B-cells, dendritic cells and monocytes/macrophages and not by other cells of the host. A full discussion of antigen presentation and the major histocompatibility complex can be found in Chapter 3.

Secondly, bacteria such as *Mycobacterium leprae* and *Chlamydia psittaci* are **obligately intracellular** pathogens. They do not grow in synthetic media, whereas **facultatively intracellular** parasites such as *E. coli*, *Salmonella*, *Shigella* and *Yersinia* spp. have relatively simple nutritional requirements in comparison. As the exact nutritional requirements of the obligately intracellular bacteria are eventually determined it is likely that the division will be one between those with simple and those with exacting nutritional requirements. In relation to infection, both types generally grow intracellularly when in vivo. Therefore the categories are more important when considering survival of the pathogen away from the host.

Thirdly, intracellular bacteria can be divided into those which remain inside a **vacuole** in the host cell and those which move into the **cytoplasm**. It is possible to speculate that this may have implications on how antigens are presented at the host cell surface, whether antigens are presented in association with Class I or Class II major histocompatibility molecules and the subsequent cellular immune response. One of the many unanswered questions is, 'at what stage does the host cell consider the bacterium and molecules of bacterial origin to be an exogenous or endogenous antigen?'

The mechanisms of bacterial entry and the strategies of survival will be considered in this chapter, using examples from the various groups summarised above.

ENTRY MECHANISMS

Entry into cells such as macrophages is relatively easy for the bacterium as these are the **professional phagocytes** of the host and have evolved the means to engulf bacteria by the process of phagocytosis. This involves the movement of the host cell around the bacterium, with the formation of processes of the host cell, known as pseudopodia, which entirely surround the bacterium (Chapter 4, and Figure 8.1). The process of phagocytosis is not always normal, as some strains of *Legionella pneumophila* enter human monocytes and alveolar macrophages by a process known as coiling phagocytosis. As the bacterium is taken up, the pseudopods of the host cell can be seen to coil around the bacterial cell. The bacterium ends up in an abnormal phagosome which is surrounded by ribosomes and which does not fuse with the lysosome. Uptake is probably mediated by complement receptors on the surface of the phagocyte, namely CR1 and CR3 which are receptors for C3b and iC3b respectively (see Chapter 4). C3b and iC3b are known to bind to *L. pneumophila*. Also, antibodies raised against purified complement receptors inhibit the uptake of *L. pneumophila*. Binding of complement to the complement receptors CR1 and CR3 on the surface of the phagocytic cell frequently does not cause the generation of the reactive oxygen metabolites which can kill engulfed bacteria (Chapter 4). Therefore this may be a preferred route of entry for intracellular pathogens.

In contrast some cells which do not under normal conditions take up particles by a phagocytic mechanism can be induced to do so by the bacterial cell. These are sometimes termed **non-professional phagocytes**. Uptake of material into these cells normally occurs by a process of pinocytosis; pinocytosis is the term used for both the continuous non-specific uptake of liquid from the surrounding extracellular environment into intracellular (endocytic) vesicles, or the more specific receptor mediated endocytosis, where the attachment of a ligand to a receptor molecule at the host

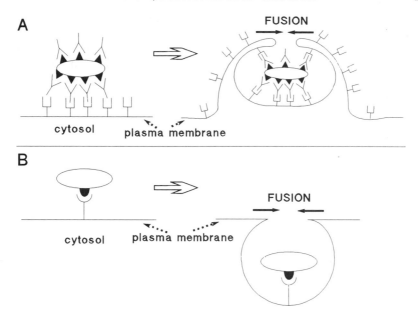

Figure 8.1. Phagocytic and pinocytic uptake of bacteria. A. Phagocytic uptake involves the polymerisation of actin filaments and the movement of the host cell outwards to surround the bacteria. The uptake may involve the binding of a ligand to the bacterial cell surface and to host cell receptors, e.g. antibody binding to antigen on the bacterial cell surface and Fc receptors on the host cell surface. B. Pinocytic uptake involves the inward pinching of vesicles into the cytoplasm. Where this is triggered by a ligand binding to a receptor it is termed receptor mediated endocytosis

cell surface triggers the uptake of the ligand into an endocytic vesicle (Figure 8.1). Both these processes occur by a mechanism of pinching vesicles off from the cytoplasmic membrane inwards into the cell, rather than the movement of the cytoplasm in pseudopods around the particle to be taken in, which occurs in phagocytic uptake. Therefore for the bacterium to gain entry into the non-professional phagocyte the host cell has to somehow be induced or 'duped' into bacterial uptake. It is now becoming apparent that bacteria not only enter non-professional phagocytes by receptor mediated endocytosis, but may also induce a phagocytic mechanism of uptake which does not occur in the normal cell; sometimes call parasite **directed** phagocytosis.

The choice of the host cell infected by a bacterium is, therefore, partly based on the ability to recognise host cell surface molecules or receptors about which little detail is yet known. The molecules of the bacterial surface involved in both attachment and entry into host cells will have evolved as a gradual selction of surface molecules with an affinity for host cell glycoproteins. Identification of the particular host cell surface receptor molecules involved in bacterial entry is beginning to shed some light on why some bacteria simply remain attached to the host cell surface and others gain entry. Therefore in general bacteria are parasitising the host receptors and functions and using them to their own ends. The only host cells to have evolved their receptors under the same selective pressures are the professional phagocytes. Some information about the genetic control and the bacterial surface proteins involved in invasion is now available for facultatively intracellular bacteria. Such information is, however, still sparse for obligately intracellular bacteria because of the inherent difficulties in culturing them outside the host.

Initially the bacterium must be able to attach to the relevant cell type. In some instances the bacteria may actively mediate their own uptake. In such cases output of energy and the expression of specialised virulence determinants by the bacterium is essential for their uptake. Examples of the different mechanisms adopted by bacteria to overcome the problem of entry into non-profesional phagocytes will now be considered.

ENTRY OF FACULTATIVELY INTRACELLULAR BACTERIA

Facultatively intracellular bacteria are capable of surviving both inside and outside the host cell. The enteric bacteria *Salmonella* spp. and *Shigella* spp. are included in this group and some detail is known of strategies used by these bacteria to invade eukaryotic cells. These mechanisms will be considered below.

Bacteria such as *Neisseria gonorrhoeae, Treponema pallidum* and *Yersinia enterocolitica* are not strictly considered to be intracellular pathogens as the majority of the bacteria growing during an infection are not intracellular. They can, however, invade host cells and use this as a means both to enter into the host and to move through host tissue. They are possibly representative of a stage in evolution somewhere between an extracellular and intracellular existence and can be termed transiently intracellular.

Neisseria gonorrhoeae attaches very firmly to the columnar epithelial cells of the genital tract. This is an example of a bacterium for which the primary host cell recognition event is to enable the bacterium to attach to the host cell surface. Once attached the bacteria proliferate at the cell surface. There is a lot of information available about the bacterial structures involved in mediating this attachment (see Chapters 7 and 9). A small proportion of the attached bacteria are taken into these epithelial cells by a process of non-professional phagocytosis. It is thought the PI outer membrane porin protein is involved in this process. The PI porin does not undergo antigenic variation as does the PII. It forms an anion selective pore in the outer membrane. It can, however, transfer directly from the *Neisseria* outer membrane into other membranes, such as that of a host cell (Figure 8.2). It is possible

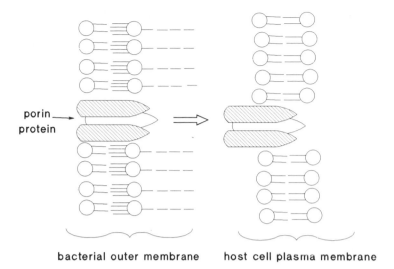

porin protein

bacterial outer membrane   host cell plasma membrane

Figure 8.2. Interaction of *Neisseria gonorrhoeae* porin protein, PI, with host cell membranes. The PI protein can transfer from the bacterial outer membrane to the host cell membrane. This is thought to trigger uptake of the *N. gonorrhoeae* into the host cell

that the incorporation of a major ionophoric protein channel in the membrane of an epithelial cell might alter the ionic/nutrient balance or membrane potential in such a way as to trigger endocytosis of the bacterium. Some of the porin proteins of *N. meningitidis* may have a similar function. Once inside the cell, the bacteria migrate inside membrane bound vacuoles to the inner side of the epithelial layer. There they are released from the host cell by either cell lysis or extrusion of the vacuoles. There is also evidence that *N. gonorrhoeae* can multiply within neutrophils.

Treponema pallidum, the spirochaete which causes syphilis, is another bacterium in which attachment to host cells may be important in its virulence. Although the majority of these bacteria exist extracellularly during an infection, they have also been observed within cytoplasmic vacuoles of a variety of cells, such as fibroblasts, endothelial and epithelial cells, as well as macrophages, neutrophils and plasma cells. Three treponema surface proteins of 89, 37 and 32 kDa have been described which bind to fibronectin. Fibronectin is one of the host protein molecules which contains the three amino acids sequence arginine, glycine, aspartic acid (RGD) which is known to be important in binding to the integrin cell surface adhesion molecules (see below). The treponema proteins also bind to this site as other peptides which contain this RGD sequence block binding of treponemes to fibronectin. It will also bind to other RGD containing extracellular matrix proteins, such as collagen I (see Chapter 5 for details of the components of the extracellular matrix). Whether or not *T. pallidum* expresses molecules which can bind directly to host cell surface receptor molecules, or not, remains to be seen. It does seem, however, that the primary method by which *T. pallidum* penetrates epithelial and endothelial cell layers is by invading between the cell junctions rather than passing through the cytoplasm, a process which has been termed intervasion. Thus *Neisseria* spp. and *Treponema pallidum* are not strictly intracellular pathogens. They only remain transiently within host cells during an infection. *Yersinia enterocolitica* also falls into this category; however, it is considered below along with *Salmonella* and *Shigella* spp. because all three types of bacteria invade through the gut mucosa. In general, truly intracellular bacteria may be defined as those which preferentially live inside cells during an infection.

The invasive enteric bacteria such as *Salmonella* and *Shigella* spp. penetrate the cells of the host intestinal mucosa and use this as a rapid means to gain direct entry into the host. From there they may infect macrophages resulting in bacteraemia and colonisation of the submucosal lymphoid tissue of the small intestine. They can cross the mucosal epithelium either be entering the microvillus-bearing **enterocytes**, or by making use of the transcytotic mechanism of the **phagocytic M cells** (see Chapter 3). Although the major role of the M cells is to enable an efficient immune response to antigens present at the mucosal surface, in a non-immune host it may take about a week before specific IgA is produced in quantity. By this time the invading bacterium may be long gone. In the case of *Salmonella typhi* the infection may well have already been spread to the liver or spleen by infected macrophages.

The interaction of *Salmonella* with the tips of the epithelial microvilli, found on enterocytes of the small intestine, results in entry via membrane-bound vacuoles from where the bacteria pass to the inside of the host. The attachment occurs in two phases, as a weak reversible and stronger irreversible stage. During the uptake, the microvilli of the intestinal brush border are destroyed. Protrusions (called ruffles or splashes because of their appearance by microscopy) filled with actin filaments surround the bacteria, and as these protrusions fold back and resorb onto the host cell surface, the bacteria are trapped within vacuoles. Activation by *S. tymphimurium* of the receptor for the cytokine epidermal growth factor is thought to be involved in the induction of the membrane ruffles.

The bacterial genes involved in the invasion by the enteric pathogens *Salmonella* spp., *Shigella* spp. and *Yersinia* spp. and the factors which control the expression of these genes are discussed below.

Invasion by *Salmonella* spp.

Detailed attachment studies have been carried out with *S. cholerae-suis* and *S. typhimurium* and a canine kidney epithelial cell line. This is often used to model epithelium as it retains the polarity and characteristics of epithelium even in culture. It appears that the initial weak interaction is dependent on recognition of a glycoprotein on the epithelial cell surface. This results in the production of six or more bacterial proteins. These are required for strong attachment to the host cell and the penetration of the epithelial cell. Their expression is only induced in the presence of the epithelial cells. It therefore seems that some aspect of the process of **attachment** is the environmental signal which controls expression of the genes required for uptake. Each of the following three treatments of the epithelial cells blocked the host cell induced protein induction in the *Salmonella*: protease trypsin; periodate, which selectiely oxidises unsubstituted hydroxy groups (adjacent in the sugar ring) to carbonyl groups, thus opening the sugar ring (see Appendix Figure A17) and making oligosaccharides or polysaccharides susceptible to cleavage by mild acid; and a neuraminidase enzyme which removes sialic acid residues from glycoproteins. This suggests that there may be molecular triggering of the bacteria by interaction with specific host cell glycoprotein molecules. Bacteria will also adhere to host cells previously fixed with glutaraldehyde. This suggests that the bacteria are making use of a host receptor already present on the cell and that the bacteria are not causing the expression of the host cell receptor.

Entry into host cells is an active event as *de novo* RNA and protein synthesis by the bacteria are necessary for invasion. The proteins induced by attachment are not the same as the family of proteins which are produced in elevated amounts in response to a variety of environmental stresses, such as intracellular growth, temperature changes etc., and which are known as the heat shock proteins (see Chapters 3 and 9). Nor are these proteins encoded on the large Vir plasmid which is associated with other virulence determinants. Genetic studies indicate that as many as nine chromosomal loci are involved in efficient host cell invasion by *Salmonella*.

It seems that adaptation to this particular niche within the host is under the control of an operon which is responding to environmental signals, in this instance attachment to a host receptor molecule. This is a common phenomenon in bacterial systems and will be discussed in detail in Chapter 9.

Invasion by *Shigella* spp.

Shigella spp. actively involve the host in their uptake and this requires the products of a number of bacterial chromosomal and plasmid gene loci. These have been the subject of some very elegant genetic analyses. Regulation of the invasion genes in *Shigella* involes **temperature sensitive regulator genes**, which reversibly control the expression of a number of virulence determinants. The bacterial genes involved in invasion are transcribed at 37 °C and not at 30 °C. Thus the virulence determinants required for invasion are only expressed when the bacterium is infecting the host, for example in the intestines, and are not expressed outside the host at lower environmental temperatures. Invasive *Shigella* spp. and also some entero-invasive *E. coli* strains carry large plasmids (180–220 kb) which encode a number of virulence determinants including the genes involved in invasion (invasion plasmid antigens — *ipaA, B, C* and *D*), haemolysin production and iron uptake. The expression of all of these genes is switched on and off by changes in temperature. The temperature sensitive regulatory gene is not encoded on the virulence plasmid but has been mapped to a chromo-somal site by obtaining mutants which constitutively express the virulence genes on the plasmid. A number of different controlling genes (e.g. *virB, F, G* and *R*) form a complex regulatory cascade. It seems that although expression of virulence factors may be determined by several genes, which are not necessarily associated, they are under common control which is conserved to a certain extent between different species of *Shigella*. There are also some similarities with the regulation of virulence gene expression in *Yersinia*. This complex genetic regulation is the subject of much current work (see Chapter 9).

Genetic analyses of the plasmid genes under the control of these regu-lators have been carried out using invasion of HeLa cells as a model. There is evidence that *Shigella flexneri* mutants in the *ipaB* gene adhere to the sur-face of HeLa cells but do not trigger actin polymerisation. As these mutants are non-invasive this suggests that adhesion and invasion are mediated by two separate bacterial surface molecules. The bacterial adhesin has not been identified but the IpaB protein, present on the surface of *S. flexneri*, acts as a contact haemolysin and is thought to mediate lysis of the phagocytic vacu-ole. It is therefore likely that the IpaB protein mediates invasion. The IpaA, B, C and D proteins, plus another 140 kDa plasmid encoded polypeptide antigen, are the predominant antigens recognised by the specific immune response detected by analysis of sera from patients who have recovered from an infection (convalescent sera). The bacteria are taken up by phago-cytosis, but the nature of transmembrane signal which triggers the phago-cytic process is not known. It is, however, possible that integrin molecules are involved. Clearly the uptake process requires the expression of several different genes making the mechanism of entry very complex.

Invasion by *Yersinia* spp.

Studies of the invasion of host cells by the two species *Y. enterocolitica* and *Y. pseudotuberculosis* have highlighted some similarities with *Shigella* spp. which will be discussed below, although the virulence of *Yersinia* spp. appears to be on the whole more complex. *Y. enterocolitica* is a foodborne human pathogen which crosses the intestinal epithelium and multiplies primarily in the underlying lymphoid tissues. *Y. pseudotuberculosis* is a rodent pathogen with a similar pathogenesis. Although these bacteria invade through the intestinal epithelium, once inside the host their major virulence determinants are related to avoidance of phagocytosis and complement mediated killing, rather than a continued intracellular existence. They are therefore not truly intracellular but are similar to *Neisseria gonorrhoea* (see above), having a transiently intracellular existence. The related *Y. pestis*, which causes plague, infects both rodents and humans and is transmitted by either flea bites or inhalation.

Yersinia spp. do not apparently require protein synthesis for invasion as they are taken up in the presence of inhibitors of bacterial RNA and protein synthesis such as rifampicin and chloramphenicol. This suggests that genes involved in invasion are not induced as a result of attaching to the host cell, as is the case for *Salmonella* spp. There is now evidence which suggests that *Yersinia* spp. hijack the normal host cell mechanisms for movement and effectively induce phagocytic uptake.

Two genes are implicated in the entry of *Yersinia* spp. into tissue culture cells, such as HeLa cells, both of which are chromosomally located. Each of these has been cloned and expressed in a non-invasive strain of *E. coli* on which they confer the ability to attach to and invade host cells.

The chromosomally located *inv*, or invasion gene, is present in both *Y. enterocolitica* and *Y. pseudotuberculosis*. This encodes for a 103 kDa outer membrane protein, called **invasin**. This protein binds to the host cell surface by a 192 amino acid region at the C-terminal end. Monoclonal antibodies specific for this outer membrane protein will block attachment. Mutations in the *inv* gene render the *Y. pseudotuberculosis* incapable of invading HeLa cells. These mutants are also less virulent when mice are challenged with them orally. The *inv* gene product is not, however, important when mice are challenged intraperitoneally when, paradoxically, mutants lacking in a functioning invasin protein are as virulent as the wild-type. The invasin protein may also be acting in association with other outer membrane proteins, and it seems likely that the relative importance of these proteins as virulence determinants may depend on, amongst other things, the route of entry into the host. There is also histological evidence that *Y. enterocolitica* can invade through the mouse gut epithelium via the phagocytic M cells, and not through the enterocytes. This point will be returned to later in the chapter, as it appears that intracellular penetration and its relationship with virulence in *Yersinia* spp. is a complex phenomenon, at present still poorly understood.

Bearing this in mind, study of the interaction of the invasion protein with host cells, albeit in tissue culture, has yielded very interesting results. The host membrane receptors for the invasin protein of *Y. pseudotuberculosis* have been identified as belonging to the **integrin** superfamily of cell adhesion molecules. The integrins are a complex group of transmembrane molecules which interact with other cells, the extracellular matrix outside the cell and the cytoskeleton inside the cell (Figure 8.3). They are therefore thought to be important in cell–extracellular matrix and cell–cell adhesion. The integrins are large surface molecules which form heterodimers with one β peptide chain being associated with a number of possible α peptide chains. For example members of the group with the same β 1 chain include α2-β1 integrin, which is a receptor for collagen, and α5-β1, which is a receptor for fibronectin. (These are also termed VLA 2 and 5 for *very late antigen*). The specifity of binding of some of these molecules may vary, as for example fibronectin may have binding sites for more than one integrin. Included in the family of integrins is complement receptor CR3 (also known as MAC 1) which is important in normal phagocytic uptake of opsonised bacteria (Chapter 4) and has sequence homology with α5-β1 integrin mentioned above. The invasin protein of *Y. pseudotuberculosis* has a particular affinity for the β1 containing integrins including α3-β1 (VLA-3), α4-β1 (VLA-4), α5-β1 (VLA-5), α6-β1 (VLA-6), but not to integrins with the β2 or 3 chains. This affinity is dependent on the presence of divalent cations such as magnesium and calcium. Antibodies to the integrin receptors prevent attachment of bacteria to HEp-2 cells (derived from larynx epithelium) and K562 cells (myeloid leukaemia lymphoblasts which are closely related to phagocytes).

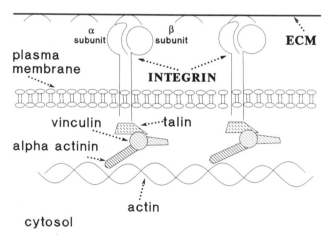

Figure 8.3. Model of the interactions between integrins and the host cell cytoskeleton. The transmembrane α and β subunits of the integrin molecules bind to components of the extracellular matrix (ECM) such as fibronectin. Inside the cell they are associated with components of the cytoskeleton such as talin, vinculin and α actinin. These in turn associate with actin filaments which controls the movement of the cell. By binding to integrins via the invasin protein, *Yersinia pseudotuberculosis* is thought to trigger cell movement in such a way that it is engulfed by the host cell. From Geiger B. 1989. Cytoskeleton-associated cell contacts. *Current Opinion in Cell Biology*, Volume 1, pages 103–109. Reproduced by permission of Current Science, Ltd

Several of the integrins bind to proteins with the common attachment amino acid sequence arginine, glycine, aspartic acid (RGD). Although invasin itself lacks the RGD sequence, it may still bind close to the normal binding domain on the integrin, and after binding transmit an intracellular signal which triggers phagocytic (as opposed to receptor mediated endocytic) uptake by a cell which would not normally be able to phagocytose a bacterium. At present the details of this are not clear. However, consideration of the normal cellular function of some of the integrins raises a possible explanation. In non-professional phagocytes (i.e. host cells which normally lack the ability to phagocytose), binding of molecules in the extracellular matrix to integrins is thought to trigger the formation of focal points of adhesion. At these focal points, the integrins interact with the actin and other cytoskeletal proteins associated with the intracellular network of actin filaments, such as talin, inside the cell (Figure 8.3). This triggering or activation can result in the polymerisation of actin filaments and is thought to be an important mechanism in the movement and spreading of cells on the extracellular matrix. The attachment of the bacterium under these circumstances is therefore radically different from that of fimbrial mediated adherence to host cells (see Chapter 7). When the invasin protein binds to the integrin it may be triggering a process similar to spreading of host cells, but which ultimately results in phagocytosis of the bacterium instead. Evidence for this is at present sparse, although actin microfilament formation is associated with the binding of invasin protein to the integrin receptor. Treatment of host cells with the drug cytochalasin B, which inhibits microfilament formation, also prevents uptake of bacteria. This raises the intriguing possibility of the bacterium having evolved a way of subverting the normal cell mechanisms for movement and spreading, thus converting a non-professional phagocyte into a phagocyte.

Interestingly invasin also binds to α4-β1, normally present on T-lymphocytes and not usually associated with epithelial or connective tissue cells. This integrin is part of a molecular complex of T-cells involved in 'homing' or trafficking of the T-cells (see Chapters 3 and 5 for further discussion of lymphocyte homing) to the lymphoid aggregates associated with the intestine known as Peyer's patches. It is perhaps no surprise that *Yersinia* spp. frequently colonise Peyer's patches during the course of an infection as has been demonstrated in mice. It is thought that the binding of *Yersinia* to T-cells may also in some way be involved in *Yersinia*-induced arthritis.

The second chromosomally encoded outer membrane protein is coded by the *ail* gene (*a*ttachment *i*nvasion *l*ocus) which has been identified in *Y. enterocolitica*. This chromosomal gene is 650 base pairs in length and codes for a 15 kDa surface protein which is different from the *inv* gene product. As with the invasin protein, the Ail protein confers invasive properties when cloned into non-invasive *E. coli*.

The Yad (for *Yersinia adhesin*; previously called YopA and P1) is a major outer membrane protein which is induced as 37 °C and forms a fibrillar network around *Y. enterocolitica* and *Y. pseudotuberculosis*. This protein is involved in colonisation of the gut epithelium and attachment to host cells. It may also be involved in resistance to complement mediated killing. Paradoxically, *inv* and *yad* double mutants of *Y. pseudotuberculosis* were more virulent than the wild-type strains when mice were challenged both orally and intraperitoneally. It therefore seems that the virulence determinants of *Y. pseudotuberculosis* are quite complex and suggests that at the moment we only know a very small part of the story. Neither of these gene products can be ruled out as virulence determinants until more is known. This also highlights the problems of interpreting results from both in vitro and in vivo assays of virulence and relating them to pathogens which may have very specific interactions with host cell molecules, which may only be present on a limited number of cells.

The story becomes even more complex when *Y. pestis* is examined. *Y. pestis* usually infects man via the blood after flea bites, or by the respiratory route in the case of pneumonic plague, rather than through the intestine as would *Y. enterocolitica* or *Y. pseudotuberculosis*. Virulent *Y. pestis* strains cannot invade HeLa cells and do not express either the *inv* or *yad* gene products; although they express a number of other virulence determinants absent in the other two species. The *inv* gene is apparently totally absent from the *Y. pestis* chromosome, as shown by DNA hybridisation studies; however, regions of homology with the *yad* gene were found on a *Y. pestis* plasmid. Sequencing of the DNA from this region revealed a point mutation in the *Y. pestis* derived gene which caused a reading frame shift in the *yad* gene resulting in the formation of a non-functional truncated gene product. It is thought that downstream of the *yad* gene there is a transcriptional terminator. Therefore only the *yad* gene is affected by the frameshift in *Y. pestis*. The mutation is in a region high in deoxyadenine residues (i.e. it is AT rich). Such regions are known in other bacteria, such as *E. coli*, to be subject to a higher mutation rate than other DNA sequences and are known as 'hot-spots' of mutation. AT-rich sequences are also 'hot-spots' for the insertion of some insertion sequences such as IS1, which is found in *Yersinia* spp., *E. coli* and other enterobacteriaceae. The insertion and deletion of sequences such as this may occur frequently (see Chapter 9). The next question is, therefore, what happens to the virulence of *Y. pestis* if it has a fully functioning Yad protein? Introduction of a plasmid carrying a functioning *yad* gene from *Y. pseudotuberculosis* resulted in **reduced** virulence of *Y. pestis* in mice challenged intraperitoneally. It has been suggested that mutations in regions such as this, leading to radical alterations in the potential virulence of the bacterium, could partly explain the waves of plague which have spread across Europe in past centuries. That is, a frameshift mutation in the AT-rich region of the *yad* gene could lead to the spread of a particularly virulent strain of *Y. pestis*.

Yersinia spp. also secrete a number of proteins into the supernatant in quantity where they are either soluble or aggregate to form filaments. They were originally designated YOP, for Yersinia *o*uter membrane *p*rotein but are now termed Yops as it is clear that they are secreted and not membrane associated. These secreted proteins can constitute up to 10% of the total bacterial protein mass. The Yops, like the other virulence determinants of *Yersinia*, are induced by an increase in temperature to 37°C, but unlike the other virulence determinants, they are also induced by low calcium concentration. At 37°C, coupled with sub-millimolar concentrations of calcium, the growth of *Yersinia* is restricted and this induces the massive production of the Yops. Therefore restricted growth induces Yop expression. How this relates to the virulence of *Yersinia* is not clear. These proteins are encoded on the same plasmid as the *yad* gene. Interestingly, it was initially difficult to isolate Yops from the culture supernatant of *Y. pestis* until it was discovered that the *Y. pestis* Yops were subject to proteolytic degradation. By using a mutant *Y. pestis* with reduced proteolytic activity a better yield of Yops was obtained. Eleven proteins have been identified in *Y. enterocolitica*, but as yet the precise function of these molecules in relation to virulence is not known. Some of the Yops are associated with cytotoxicity and others with anti-phagocytic activity. Although they are probably not related to invasion of host cells, they will be considered in this chapter because of the manner in which their expression is controlled. Genetic mapping has allowed the identification of the regions involved in the control of Yop expression. The temperature sensitivity of expression is associated with a chromosomal gene, *ymoA* (*y*ersinia *mo*dulator), which encodes for a histone-like protein. This suggests that the temperature dependent induction of gene expression is dependent upon changes in DNA topology and chromatin structure, such as DNA supercoiling (see Chapter 9). One of the genes which is subject to this control is the transcriptional activator *virF*, present on the *Yersinia* plasmid. The *virF* of *Yersinia* encodes a 31kDa protein which exists as a dimer and binds to a 28–30 nucleotide sequence upstream of the *yop* genes. It thus activates transcription of the *yop* genes. Transcription of *virF* is not regulated by calcium concentration. Similar types of thermoregulators have been identified in *Shigella* where the HNS or H1 histone-like protein negatively controls the transcriptional activator *virB*. In *Shigella* VirF controls *virG* (also called *icsA*) which is involved in intercellular bacterial spread as well as *virB* (also known as *ipaR*) which in turn positively regulates the *ipa* genes (see Figure 8.4 and above). The elevated temperature is not only required for the activity of the histone-like proteins on the *virF* gene, but also for the action of the VirF protein at the sites of transcriptional activation. The VirF transcriptional activators belong to a family of regulators known as the AraC family which are also found in other bacteria (e.g. *E. coli, Pseudomonas putida*). The similarities between some of the virulence genes of *Yersinia* and *Shigella* and the fact that they share a common

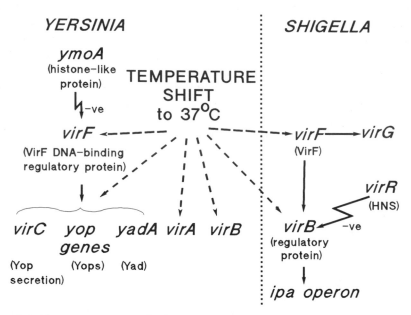

Figure 8.4. Temperature control of virulence gene expression in *Yersinia* and *Shigella*: a regulatory cascade. A temperature shift to 37 °C triggers the transcription of a number of different gene loci (italics) and the subsequent expression of regulatory proteins and specialist virulence determinants (in brackets). The temperature sensitive chromosomal locus in both *Yersinia* and *Shigella* encodes proteins which are thought to be involved in the control of DNA topology and chromatin structure (histone-like protein and HNS). These negatively control the expression of transcriptional activators (e.g. *virF* or *virB*) which activate the transcription of genes encoding virulence determinants such as adhesion proteins, proteins required for Yop secretion and Yops themselves. In *Shigella*, VirF positively controls a second transcriptional regulator, *virB*, which in turn activates transcription of proteins necessary for host cell invasion (*ipa*). A temperature of 37°C is also necessary for the activity of VirF. This suggests that the chromatin structure is modified by the temperature change and that this is necessary, along with VirF, to initiate transcription. Many aspects of the regulatory cascade remain to be fully understood

region encoding the replication of the virulence plasmid suggest that these plasmids may have been derived from a common ancestral plasmid. In *Yersinia*, VirF also controls the *virC* operon which is thought to encode the genes involved in the secretion of the Yops. Two other loci, *virA* and *virB*, are also thermoregulated, but are not influenced by VirF. There must therefore be other factors involved in the thermoregulation.

Genes involved in the calcium regulation of Yop production have been mapped on the plasmid. Included in this region are the *low* calcium response (*lcr*) and *ca*lcium *r*egulation (*car*) genes. In spite of this the complex mechanism by which the signal of low calcium concentration triggers Yop production remains to be understood.

It is thus apparent that *Yersinia* spp. are complex and intriguing pathogens.

ENTRY OF OBLIGATELY INTRACELLULAR BACTERIA

In comparison, relatively little is known about the mode of entry of obligately intracellular bacterial pathogens into host cells. In particular there is little known about the genetic control of invasion, not least because they cannot be cultured independently of the host cells. Such information that has been gleaned from the molecules involved relates largely to an analysis of how invasion may be inhibited and has often led to conflicting results.

Chlamydia spp. are one group of obligately intracellular pathogens. The most common species are *C. psittaci*, which commonly infects birds, *C. trachomatis*, which infects humans and mice causing infections at sites including the eye, urogenital tract and respiratory tract, and *C. pneumoniae*, which causes pneumonia in humans. Chlamydial infection is spread by a non-dividing cell, termed the elementary body, which after entry into the host cell multiplies and forms what are known as reticulate bodies. Elementary bodies are taken up into membrane bound vesicles by both professional and non-professional phagocytes. Attachment to host surface glycoproteins probably plays an important role in the uptake of *C. psittaci* by host cells. Treatment of the cells with proteases such as trypsin and polysaccharide hydrolysis with periodate inhibits the uptake of bacteria. This suggests that a largely intact host cell surface glycoprotein molecule acts as a receptor for chlamydial uptake.

C. trachomatis has a narrower host and cell range than *C. psittaci*, infecting mostly columnar epithelial cells of the eye, urogenital tract and respiratory tract. There is evidence that *C. psittaci* enters cells by receptor mediated endocytosis into clathrin coated pits. *C. trachomatis* may also enter cells by this mechanism, by microfilament mediated phagocytosis or indeed by either mechanism. Entry into the host cell does not depend on the *de novo* synthesis of macromolecules by *Chlamydia*, as inhibitors of bacterial RNA and protein synthesis have no effect on uptake. Therefore this parasite may be triggering the normal phagocytic process of the host in a similar manner to *Yersinia* spp., however, this remains to be fully determined. The chlamydial cell envelope is similar to that of Gram negative bacteria, but lacks peptidoglycan. Disulphide bonding of cross-linked outer membrane proteins is thought to confer rigidity to the elementary body. Possible mediators of adhesion to host cells include a major outer membrane protein of 40kDa and a 31kDa protein. the gene for the 31kDa protein has been cloned and expressed in *E. coli*. A heparin-like molecule, produced by the bacterium, has also been implicated in attachment to host cells.

In contrast to *Chlamydia* spp., *Rickettsia* spp. take a much more active part in uptake. *Rickettsia* spp. are small Gram negative bacteria which only grow inside host cells and are usually transmitted via arthropod vectors. In general they inhabit endothelial cells which line the small blood vessels. The growth of *R. tsutsugamushi*, which causes scrub typhus, has been studied in mouse lymphoblasts and *R. prowazekii*, which causes louse borne typhus, in mouse fibroblasts. It appears that they enter both professional and non-professional phagocytes by a phagocytic mechanism which is initiated by the bacterium. They then enter into a phagosome from which they rapidly move to the cytoplasm. Evidence for the bacterial mediation of this uptake includes a lack of uptake if the rickettsial metabolism is inhibited in some way. For example, glutamine is used by *Rickettsia* as an energy source and uptake does not occur if it is omitted from the culture medium. Some light has been shed on the mechanism of bacterial induced uptake by studying the haemolytic activity of *Rickettsia* spp. *Rickettsia* with the ability to lyse erythrocytes only do so after direct cell–cell contact. The bacteria attach to an erythrocyte receptor which has a cholesterol component. The lytic mechanism also involves phospholipase A activity as free fatty acids are released. Whether this activity originates from the host cell or the bacterium is not clear. Inhibitors of haemolysis also inhibit host cell entry. This suggests that haemolysis and uptake may share part of a common mechanism. The difference between the outcome of the two mechanisms may be one of control, in which haemolysis is sufficiently limited to enable the bacterium to enter the cell without completely lysing it. The haemolytic activity is probably also related to, or analogous with, the mechamism by which the bacteria escape from the vacuole and enter the cytoplasm.

Bacteria can therefore either be actively involved in host cell invasion resulting in bacterial mediated uptake, or after an initial molecular recognition event, will passively allow the host cell to take them in.

It is therefore clear from these few examples that bacteria have developed diverse mechanisms for entry into host cells. In the next section we will see that the mechanisms for survival once inside the host cell are equally diverse.

INTRACELLULAR GROWTH AND SURVIVAL

In the normal course of events in both profesional and non-professional phagocytes, the endocytic or phagocytic vacuole containing the bacteria fuses with a second type of vacuole. This second vacuole is called a lysosome and contains a range of antibacterial molecules. Fusion of the endocytic vacuole with the lysosome leads to a single vacuole called the phagolysosome. The lysosomes or lysosomal vacuoles of the non-professional phagocytes generally only contain lysosomal enzymes, whereas those of the professional phagocytes have a more extensive 'arsenal' of antibacterial molecules. These include defensins and the potential for generation of free radicals (see Chapter 4). Although this makes the macrophage a potentially more hazardous cell to parasitise, a number of bacteria are able to successfully avoid the destruction which kills other bacteria. Indeed some bacteria preferentially invade and infect macrophages.

Bacteria have evolved three different mechanisms or strategies for enhancing intracellular survival. In general these mechanisms still await a detailed molecular characterisation.

These mechanisms are: (1) resistance to the killing action of the lysosomal molecules, (2) rapid escape from the phagocytic vacuole into the cytoplasm and (3) prevention of phagolysosomal fusion. One bacterium which does not fall into these categories is *Brucella abortus* which inhabits the cisternae of the rough endoplasmic reticulum.

Resistance to intracellular killing by lysosomal molecules

Salmonella spp. are one of the few types of bacteria where a number of the genes involved in the resistance to the varied stresses of intracellular life are beginning to be unravelled. The monocyte/macrophage is the primary cell infected by *Salmonella* after they have invaded and passed through the epithelial cells. The *Salmonella* survive within the intracellular vacuole even after fusion with the potentially lethal lysosome.

Two classes of *Salmonella* spp. mutant have been obtained by transposon mutagenesis, one with increased senstivity to oxidising agents, while the other has increased sensitivity to the defensins. This suggests that there are two independent sets of genes which allow the *Salmonella* spp. to survive both the oxygen dependent and oxygen independent killing mechanisms. This is perhaps not surprising as the two killing mechanisms work in different ways (see Chapter 4). In fact it might be expected that entry into a macrophage would induce a range of bacterial genes required by the bacterium to cope with life in the intracellular environment. Indeed, after internalisation *S. typhimurium* increases the synthesis of over 30 different bacterial proteins which are located within multiple regulatory networks. These are termed MIPs or macrophage induced proteins.

The oxygen independent resistance mechanism of *S. typhimurium* has been further investigated and the genetic regulatory locus *phoP* has been shown to control the expression of at least nine macrophage induced proteins. Included in these are genes necessary for increased resistance to the oxygen independent killing activities of the macrophage cationic proteins and peptides. Mutations in these genes resulted in sensitivity to the activities of for example the NP-1 defensins which form anion specific channels in lipid bilayers of susceptible bacteria. The *phoP* gene sequence indicates that it is very similar in nature to other DNA binding regulatory proteins. These proteins form part of a two component system which senses environmental changes and transmits a signal via protein phosphorylation to a transcriptional regulatory protein (see Chapter 9). A second regulatory gene, *phoQ*, was found to be similar to the phosphorylating protein kinases of these two component systems. The mechanism of action is probably one whereby PhoQ, after sensing an environmental stimulus, phosphorylates the *phoP* gene product which, once phosphorylated, binds to DNA and positively regulates or switches on the expression of other macrophage induced proteins (Figure 8.5). Another environmental sensor/regulator identified in *Salmonella* is EnvZ which senses changes in osmolarity and is coupled to the transcriptional activator OmpR. Environmental control of gene expression is covered in detail in Chapter 9. It is thought that OmpR regulates genes which play a part in the early stages of *Salmonella* colonisation of the host.

The genes under the control of the PhoP/Q regulatory system include *phoN*, which encodes for a non-specific acid phosphatase enzyme and is induced when *Salmonella* are starved of nutrients such as carbon, phosphorus, nitrogen and sulphur. Little is known about the proteins involved in the resistance to the activity of the defensins although the product of gene *pagC* (PhoP activated gene) is an envelope protein which is also known to be required for virulence. Other genes positively controlled by the *phoP/Q* genes include *psiD, pagA* and *pagB* which are of unknown function.

A number of genes known as the *prg* (PhoP repressed gene) genes are negatively controlled by PhoP; however, paradoxically the Prg proteins are also necessary for intramacrophage survival. In order to explain this, it has been suggested that the *pag* and *prg* gene products help the *Salmonella* to

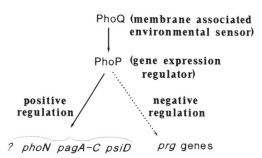

Figure 8.5. Intracellular survival of *Salmonella*; control of gene expression. Environmental signals in the macrophage trigger the membrane associated protein PhoQ, which auto-phosphorylates and catalyses the phosphorylation of PhoP. In the phosphorylated form, PhoP activates gene expression at a number of loci. Some of these may not be involved in virulence; e.g. *PhoN* codes for a cytoplasmic acid phosphatase; *psiD, pagA* and *B*, are of unknown function. *PagC* is related to virulence. Other virulence genes which remain to be identified are also positively regulated (?). PhoP prevents the expression of the *prg* genes. These genes are thought to be necessary for intracellular survival at a later stage

survive either in different types of intracellular environments, or are required at different times during the infectious process. It has been speculated that the *pag* gene products which are required for resistance to defensins are important during the early stages of uptake, immediately after phagolysosomal fusion, when the defensin will be most active. After phagolysosomal fusion, as the pH decreases, the defensins become less active. It may be at this later stage that the *prg* gene products are required. The physiological stimuli present in the macrophage phagolysosome which trigger the action of the *pho* genes are not known, but phosphate concentration and pH may be involved. The molecular detail of the interactions of the gene products with the defensins is at present the subject of much study. A second, as yet uncharacterised, regulatory gene influences the expression of six other unrelated macrophage induced proteins of unknown function.

Other macrophage induced proteins, whose production is not apparently controlled by either of these two regulators, include the heat shock proteins GroEL and DnaK. These proteins were not induced in the *Salmonella* when they infected epithelial cells. In contrast, GroEL in *Escherichia coli* is essential for normal growth and is involved in RNA, DNA and protein synthesis; DnaK has multiple effects which include initiation of DNA replication and cell division. The heat shock proteins are the immunodominant antigens of a number of bacteria that grow intracellularly, including *S. tymphimurium*, *Mycobacterium leprae*, *M. tuberculosis*, *Coxiella burnetii* and *Legionella pneumophila*. Not all the bacteria within the phagocytic vacuole survive and it is probable that their components, as well as any bacterial molecules secreted from live bacteria, are presented at the macrophage surface. The GroEL and DnaK proteins are the most abundant produced by the *Salmonella* spp. during growth in macrophages and their immunodominance may partly be due to their presence within an antigen presenting cell. The precise role of these heat shock proteins in intracellular survival is not known. A general description of heat shock proteins is given in Chapter 3.

Mycobacterium leprae inhabit Schwann cells and macrophages. They are resistant to the oxidative killing mechanism of macrophages. Resistance has been related to the presence of a phenolic glycolipid which can constitute up to 2% of the bacterial mass. The glycolipid is composed of a trisaccharide of 3,6-di-O-methylglucose, α1-4 2,3 di-O-methylrhamnose, β1-2 3-O-methylrhamnose, glycosidically linked to phenol, which is itself linked to a 29-carbon hydrocarbon with attached fatty acids (see Appendix Figure A7). It is thought that this molecule forms a protective lipid capsule around the bacterium which scavenges the reactive oxygen species produced by the peroxidase, hydrogen-peroxide-halide system of phagocytic cells.

In contrast, the details of how *Coxiella burnetii*, the agent of Q fever, survives inside both professional and non-professional phagocytes after phagolysosomal fusion are not well understood. This bacterium is an obligately intracellular parasite which manages to multiply in phagosomes containing lysosomal enzymes such as acid phosphatase and 5'nucleotidase at pH 5. The lack of detailed molecular information reflects partly the difficulties in studying the growth and survival of obligately intracellular bacteria.

Escape from vacuoles into the cytoplasm

The agent of scrub typhus, *Rickettsia tsutsugamushi*, inhabits either peritoneal mesothelial cells or neutrophils and escapes into the cytoplasm within 30 minutes of entry into these cells. Phopholipase A activity of the bacterium may facilitate entry. This may also bring about dissolution of the phagosomal membrane and escape of the bacterium into the cytoplasm.

Shigella flexneri and *S. dysenteriae* have plasmid encoded haemolysin activity on contact with erythrocytes. The gene product or products involved in haemolysis are also known to bring about entry into host cells, although the molecules involved have not been characterised. Transfer of the plasmid from *Shigella* spp. to *E. coli* K12 transformed this normally non-pathogenic strain of *E. coli* into an intracellular bacterium with the same ability to multiply within the host cell as the *Shigella* spp. The production of other virulence determinants, such as Shiga toxin (Chapter 6) or the iron chelating agent aerobactin (Chapter 5), is not necessary for the process of escape from the phagosomes. The end-result of *Shigella* invasion and subsequent multiplication in the cytoplasm is the rapid killing of the infected macrophage. The precise molecular basis of the means by which the bacteria interfere with host cell metabolism, which leads to macrophage death, is not known. The intracellular bacterial growth, however, apparently inhibits host cell respiration and fermentation pathways as measured by a decrease in intracellular levels of ATP and lactate production and an increase in pyruvate levels. Recent evidence suggests that *S. flexneri* induces programmed cell death (apoptosis) in macrophages. It is thought that the movement of *S. flexneri* through the cytoplasm occurs by a similar mechanism to that of *Listeria monocytogenes* (see below). The *icsA* gene present on a plasmid is inolved in the interaction of the *Shigella* with filamentous actin.

Some detail is known about the escape of *Listeria monocytogenes* from the vacuole. This has been associated with haemolytic activity of the bacteria. The molecule involved is the haemolysin, listeriolysin O (LLO), a member of the thiol-activated family of cytolysins (see Chapter 5). Cytolysins similar to listeriolysin are produced by a number of other Gram positive bacteria including *Clostridium* spp. and *Streptococcus* spp. It is therefore interesting to speculate that pathogens such as *S. pyogenes, S. pneumoniae, C. perfringens* and *C. tetani* may have the potential for intracellular growth.

LLO is encoded by the gene *hly* (also designated *hlyA* and *lisA*). When this gene was cloned into the common soil bacterium *Bacillus subtilis*, it grew rapidly intracellularly in the cytoplasm of a macrophage-like cell line after disrupting the phagosomal membrane. This is a habitat normally very alien to *B. subtilis*. That a single gene product could confer such a potential on a non-pathogen suggests that rapid escape from the vacuole is one of the most important aspects of intracellular survival of *L. monocytogenes*. The *B. subtilis*, however, did not display all the characteristics of intracellular growth of *L. monocytogenes* and was not capable of moving from one cell to another. *L. monocytogenes* growing in the cytoplasm is normally associated with a surrounding 'cloud' of polymerised actin filaments. This cloud then reorganises to form a tail up to 5μm long as the *L. monocytogenes* migrates towards the cell surface. At the cell surface the *L. monocytogenes* is inside a long pseudopod, which is then phagocytosed by a neighbouring host cell. The *L. monocytogenes* within the second cell is now surrounded by a double membrane, that of the first cell, surrounded by that of the second. The bacterium then escapes from both of these membranes and the cycle is repeated (see Figure 8.6). It is now clear that the polymerisation of the actin is not the host cell responding to the cytoplasmic invasion of the

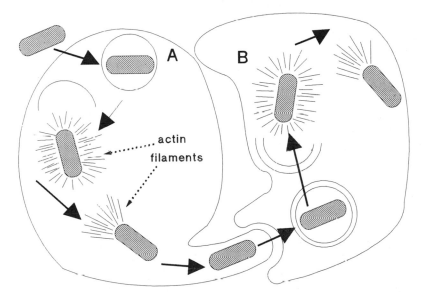

Figure 8.6. Host cell invasion by *Listeria monocytogenes*. After entering into either professional or non-professional phagocytes, *L. monocytogenes* breaks out of the vacuole into the cytoplasm (cell A). Initially the bacterium is surrounded by a cloud of polymerised actin filaments. Subsequently the actin filaments rearrange into a 'comet-tail' and the bacterium moves through the cytoplasm at rates of up to 0.4 μm per second. The propulsive force is thought to be generated by the continuous polymerisation and release of actin at the bacterial cell surface. The movement of the bacterium causes the formation of long protrusions or pseudopods from the host cell. These pseudopods are phagocytosed by neighbouring cells (cell B). Thus the *L. monocytogenes* enters another cell, this time inside a double vacuole. The bacterium again escapes into the cytoplasm

bacterium, by attempting to enclose it in a 'wall' of actin, but direct parasitism of the host cell movement mechanism by the bacterium. The material which nucleates the actin filaments is thought to be secreted from the *L. monocytogenes* (see below). Mutants of *L. monocytogenes* have been found which do not induce the formation of either the cloud or tail of actin filaments. Also, the antibiotic chloramphenicol, which will inhibit bacterial protein synthesis, but not that of the host cell, also stops actin polymerisation. No actin polymerisation was observed with the *B. subtilis* which contained the *hly*, nor did the *B. subtilis* move to the periphery of the infected cell and spread to other cells. Therefore, as might be expected, *L. monocytogenes* has other characteristics which play a part in its parasitic existence. The *plcB* gene (also designated *prtC*) encodes a phospholipase C (lecithinase) which hydrolyses phosphatidyl choline. Mutants in this gene are defective in the lysis of the double membrane vacuole which is formed when the *Listeria* move from one cell to another. A number of other genes have been mapped in *L. monocytogenes* and mutants in these genes show reduced virulence, although the gene products are for the most part only partially characterised. Nevertheless, the information obtained by these genetic studies has allowed the identification of some of the genes involved in the various stages of host cell infection, for example: *inlA*, involved in attachment to host cells; *hyl*, involved in escape from the vacuole (see above); *actA*, involved in nucleation of actin filaments; and *plcB*, involved in cell to cell movement.

It is interesting that *Shigella, Listeria* and *R. tsutsugamushi*, although distant in evolutionary terms, infect host cells in a markedly similar manner. It appears that a general strategy within this group of cytoplasm colonising bacteria is the rapid exit from the phagosome mediated by controlled contact lysis of the membrane.

Prevention of phagolysosomal fusion

Those bacteria which prevent fusion of the endocytic vacuole with the lysosome include *Mycobacterium tuberculosis* which preferentially infects macrophages. If, however, the phagocytosed *M. tuberculosis* are coated with antibody phagolysosomal fusion does take place, but the bacteria continue to multiply. Therefore this bacterium is also resistant to the antibacterial agents of the macrophage and this is probably related to the structure of the mycobacterial cell envelope which contains peptidoglycolipids and hydrocarbons not found in the more common Gram positive envelope. The mycobacteria produce sulphatides and polyanionic trehalose glycolipids which seem to interact specifically with the lysosomal membrane causing a reduction in their mobility within the cytoplasm. This reduces the chances of lysosome and phagosome meeting.

Chalmydia psittaci have the characteristics necessary to inhibit the fusion process upon entry into the host cell prior to uptake. Fusion still does not occur even after treatment with the antibiotic chloramphenicol at concentrations which inhibit bacterial multiplication within the host cell. In experiments where cells were infected with both *C. psittaci* and another organism such as *E. coli* or a yeast, only vacuoles containing the *Chlamydia* did not fuse. The inference is that a molecule or molecules present in the resting stage or elementary body of the *C. psittaci* wall modify the phagosome membrane and prevent fusion.

Legionella pneumophila has been examined growing in human peripheral blood moncytes, where it multiplies within a phagosome. Within 4–8 h the phagosome is surrounded by ribosomes. Viable bacteria are required for this to occur as formalin killed bacteria do not have this effect. This may be another case of the bacteria or bacterial products influencing host cell mechanisms.

Brucella abortus colonises the chorioallantoic trophoblastic epithelial tissue in cattle, causing abortion. This bacterium is unusual in that it inhabits the rough endoplasmic reticulum and not the phagosome or phagolysosome. The mechanisms of invasion and survival of *B. abortus*, however, remain to be determined in detail.

Bacterial metabolism within the host cell

Intrinsic to survival and growth of these intracellular bacteria is efficient metabolism within the host cell. The different types of bacteria vary in how much their metabolism is dependent on the host's.

Rickettsia spp. either generate their own ATP by oxidative phosphorylation of glutamate via the tricarboxylic acid (TCA) cycle or take up host ATP by an ATP–ADP transport system. This membrane transport system moves ATP into the bacterium and ADP out and is similar to the mechanism used by mitochondria. The pathway for ATP generation used is thought to be regulated by the citrate synthetase enzyme which is one of the key enzymes of the TCA cycle. This enzyme is inhibited by high levels of ATP. Therefore outside the host cell under conditions of low ATP the *Rickettsia* generate their own ATP from glutamate, whereas inside the cell they use the host's.

Chlamydia spp. on the other hand have lost the ability to generate their own energy needs. They have no cytochrome respiratory enzymes and cannot successfully produce energy from the catabolism of glutamate, glucose or pyruvate. They are therefore wholly dependent on uptake of the host's ATP by the ATP–ADP membrane translocase system. *Chlamydia* spp. are unusual in that they do not have peptidoglycan in the cell envelope. The rigidity of the elementary bodies is due to large disulphide bond linked complexes of a major outer membrane protein. Once inside the host cell the disulphide bonds are broken and the proteins reduced to monomers.

Treatment of *Chlamydia* spp. extracellularly with mercaptoethanol (which breaks disulphide bonds) results in the uptake of nucleoside triphospates and RNA synthesis. Therefore this change in the molecular bonding of the cell envelope is thought to increase the permeability of the bacterium to ATP and other molecules.

Coxiella burnetii is adapted to growth at pH 5, the pH of the fused phago-lysosome. ATP is generated from glutamate and glucose using the TCA cycle; however, this bacterium makes use of host molecules to a certain extent for RNA, DNA and protein synthesis. Although it has the capability of carrying out each process it cannot successfully perform all three at once independently of the host cell metabolism.

In contrast, the facultative parasites are dependent on their own meta-bolic plasticity for intracellular survival. For example the ability of *Shigella* spp. to synthesise molecules not normally present in the host cell such as the aromatic amino acids is thought to be important for their survival intra-cellularly as some auxotrophic mutants do not survive. *Salmonella typhimur-ium* is also capable of synthesising all its necessary amino acids and nucleo-tides itself which again is thought to contribute to its intracellular survival. This has been put to use in the construction of attenuated strains which could be suitable for use as live vaccines. *Salmonella* mutants in the *aro* genes which encode the enzymes necessary for the biosynthetic pathway for the production of aromatic compounds produce a limited infection, but stimulate a protective immune response when given orally.

FURTHER READING

General

Alberts B., Bray D., Lewis J. *et al* 1994. Molecular biology of the cell, (3rd Edn). Garland Publishing, New York, USA.

Britton W. J. 1993. Immunology of leprosy. Transactions of the Royal Society of Tropical Medicine and Hygiene; 87, 508–514.

Darnell J., Lodish H., Baltimore D. 1986. Molecular cell biology. Scientific American Books, New York, USA.

Dorman C. J., niBhriain N. 1993. DNA topology and bacterial virulence gene regu-lation. Trends in Microbiology 1, 92–99.

Kaufmann S. H. R., Reddehase M. J. 1989. Infection of phagocytic cells. Current Opinion in Immunology 2, 43–49.

McGee Z. A., Gorby G. L., Wyrick P. B. *et al.* 1988. Parasite-directed endocytosis. Reviews of Infectious Diseases 10, S311–S316.

Piggot R., Power C. 1993. The adhesion molecule facts book. Academic Press, Lon-don.

Theriot J. A. 1992. Bacterial pathogens caught in the actin; cytoskeleton dynamics. Current Biology 2, 649–651.

Wick M. J., Madara J. L., Fields B. N. *et al.* 1991. Molecular cross talk between epi-thelial cells and pathogenic microorganisms. Cell 67, 651–659.

Invasion

Geiger B. 1989. Cytoskeleton-associated cell contacts. Current Opinion in Cell Biology 1, 103–109.

Haake D. A., Lovett M. A. 1990. Interjunctional invasion of endothelial monolayers by *Treponema pallidum*. In: Molecular basis of bacterial pathogenesis (Eds Iglewski B. H., Clark V. L.). Academic Press, London. Chapter 14.

Isberg R. R., van Nhieu G. T. 1994. Binding and internalization of microorganisms by integrin receptors. Trends in Microbiology 2, 10–14.

Neutra M. R., Kraehenbuhl J-P. 1992. Transepithelial transport and mucosal defence I: the role of M cells. Trends in Cell Biology 2, 134–174.

Salmonella

Finlay B. B., Fry J., Rock E. P. *et al.* 1989. Passage of *Salmonella* through polarized epithelial cells; role of the host and bacterium. Journal of Cell Science Supplement 11, 99–107.

Finlay B. B., Heffron F., Falkow S. 1989. Epithelial surfaces induce *Salmonella* proteins required for bacterial adherence and invasion. Science 243, 940–943.

Francis C. L., Ryan T. A., Jones B. D. *et al.* 1993. Ruffles induced by *Salmonella* and other stimuli direct macropinocytosis of bacteria. Nature 364, 639–642.

Yersinia

Cornelis G., Biot T., de Rouvroit L. *et al.* 1991. Genetics of Yop production in *Yersinia enterocolitica*. In: Microbial surface components and toxins in relation to pathogenesis (Eds Ron E. Z., Rottem S.). Plenum Press, USA. pp 191–199.

Cornelis G. R. 1992. Yersiniae, finely tuned pathogens. In: Molecular biology of bacterial infection. Current Status and Future Perspectives. Society for General Microbiology Symposium 49 (Eds Hormaeche C. E., Penn C. W., Smyth C. J.). Cambridge Unversity Press, Cambridge, UK. pp 231–265.

Forsberg A. Rosqvist R. Wolf-Watz H. 1994. Regulation and polarized transfer of the *Yersinia* outer proteins (Yops) involved in antiphagocytosis. Trends in Microbiology 2, 14–19.

Isberg R. R., Leong J. M., 1990. Multiple beta 1 chain integrins are receptors for invasin, a protein that promotes bacterial penetration into mammalian cells. Cell 60, 861–871.

Rosqvist R., Skurnik M., Wolf-Watz H. 1988. Increased virulence of *Yersinia pseudotuberculosis* by two independent mutations. Nature 334, 522–525.

Young V. B., Falkow S., Schoolnik G. K. 1992. The invasin protein of *Yersinia enterocolitica*: internalisation of invasin-bearing bacteria by eukaryotic cells is associated with reorganization of the cytoskeleton. Journal of Cell Biology 116, 197–207.

Shigella

Maurelli A. T., Sansonetti P. J. 1988. Genetic determinants of *Shigella* pathogenicity. Annual Review of Microbiology 42, 127–150.

Sansonetti P. J., 1992. Molecular and cellular biology of epithelial invasion by *Shigella flexneri* and other enteroinvasive pathogens. In: Molecular biology of bacterial infection. Current status and future perspectives. Society for General Microbiology Symposium 49 (Eds Hormaeche C.E., Penn C. W., Smyth C. J.). Cambridge University Press, UK. pp 47–60.

Intracellular survival and growth

Salmonella

Buchmeier N. A., Heffron F. 1990. Induction of *Salmonella* stress proteins upon infection of macrophages. Science 248, 730–732.

Chatfield S, Li J. L., Sydenham M. *et al*. 1992. *Salmonella* genetics and vaccine development. In: Molecular Biology of Bacterial Infection. Current Status and Future Perspectives. Society for General Microbiology Symposium 49 (Eds Hormaeche C. E., Penn C. W., Smyth C. J.). Cambridge University Press, UK. pp 299–312.

Groisman E. A., Fields P. I., Heffron F. 1990. Molecular biology of *Salmonella* pathogenesis. In: Molecular basis of bacterial pathogenesis (Eds Iglewski B. H., Clark V. L.). Academic Press, London. Chapter 12.

Groisman E. A., Saier M. H. 1990. *Salmonella* virulence: new clues to intramacrophage survival. Trends in Biochemical Sciences 15, 30–33.

Miller S.I., Mekalanos J.J. 1990. Constitutive expression of the PhoP regulon attenuates *Salmonella* virulence and survival within macrophages. Journal of Bacteriology 172, 2485–2490.

Chlamydia

Bavoil P. 1990. Invasion and intracellular growth of *Chlamydia* species. In: Molecular basis of bacterial pathogenesis (Eds Iglewski B.H., Clark V.L.) Academic Press, London. Chapter 13, pp. 273–296.

Moulder J.W. 1991. Interaction of chlamydiae and host cells in vitro. Microbiological Reviews 55, 143–190.

Stephens R. S. 1994. Molecular mimicry and *Chlamydia trachomatis* infection of eukaryotic cells. Trends in Microbiology 2, 99–101.

Legionella

Dowling J. N., Saha A. K., Glew R. H. 1992. Virulence factors of the family *Legionellaceae*. Microbiological Reviews 56, 32–60.

Listeria

Portnoy D. A., Chakraborty T., Goebel W. *et al*. 1992. Molecular determinants of *Listeria monocytogenes* pathogenesis. Infection and Immunity 60, 1263–1267.

Theriot J. R., Mitchison T. J., Tilney L. G. *et al.*. 1992. The rate of actin-based motility of intracellular *Listeria monocytogenes* equals the rate of actin polymerization. Nature 357, 257–260.

Mycobacterium

Britton W. J., Roche P. W., Winter N. 1994. Mechanisms of persistence of mycobacteria. Trends in Microbiology 2, 284–288.

Neill M. A., Klebanoff S. J. 1988. The effect of phenolic glycoplipid-1 from *Mycobacterium leprae* on the antimicrobial activity of human macrophages. Journal of Experimental Medicine 167, 30–42.

Sibley L. D., Hunter S. W., Brennan P. J. *et al* 1988. Mycobacterial lipoarabinomannan inhibits gamma interferon-mediated activation of macrophages. Infection and Immunity 56, 1232–1236.

Other

Detilleux P. G., Deyoe B. Y., Cheville N. F. 1990. Penetration and intracellular growth of *Brucella abortus* in nonphagocytic cells in vitro. Infection and Immunity 58, 2320–2328.

Dougan G. 1989. Molecular charcterization of bacterial virulence factors and the consequences for vaccine design. Journal of General Microbiology 135, 1397–1406.

9 Genetic Variation and Regulation of Virulence Determinants

INTRODUCTION

A common aspect of the many strategies adopted by bacteria which colonise the host is the ability to vary the expression of the molecules and structures involved in virulence by either the induction/repression of gene expression or DNA rearrangements. Within-strain variation in the expression of capsular polysaccharide is illustrated in Figure 9.1. The major selective pressures which favour a rapid and reversible variation of characteristics are the colonisation of more than one type of environment and the colonisation of a rapidly changing environment. To have only those characteristics necessary for survival within a given environment, but at the same time retain the genetic information necessary for survival in

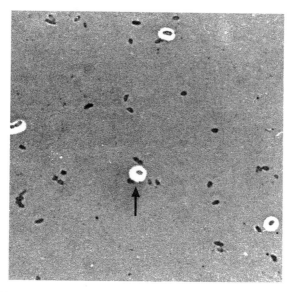

Figure 9.1. Within-strain variation in capsule expression in *Bacteroides fragilis*. Light micrograph of negatively stained bacteria. Only some of the bacteria within the population have large extracellular polysaccharide capsules (arrow)

other environments, is economical from the point of view of the general metabolism of the bacterium. Also, characteristics which may confer an advantage in one environment may be a disadvantage in another. Pathogenic bacteria are faced with the further complication of a living environment which has an immune system dedicated to the prevention of microbial colonisation.

The types of environment which pathogenic bacteria colonise include those outside the host as well as within the host. Inside the host, if the bacteria colonise more than one type of tissue the variation of bacterial surface structures which mediate **attachment** to tissue specific host receptors (Chapter 7) would be an advantage. The **avoidance** of attachment to host phagocytic cells may also be important at particular stages of infection (Chapter 7). For example a bacterium which infects the urinary tract must be able to attach to the urinary epithelium to avoid being washed away by the urine flow. If the infecting bacterium ascends to the kidneys the structures mediating attachment to host cells (e.g. fimbriae) could make the bacterium attach more readily to phagocytes and therefore more susceptible to phagocytic killing. The ability of at least a proportion of the bacterial population to change between expression of fimbriae and an anti-phagocytic capsule would be an obvious advantage. There is evidence that this pattern of events occurs during infection with *Proteus mirabilis* in a rat model of ascending pyelonephritis. Bacteria which can grow within the host both extracellularly and **intracellularly** (Chapter 8) also cope with two very different types of environment.

The type of variation necessary for survival in different and changing environments is, by and large, the presence or absence of a particular component or characteristic of the bacterium. Where these changes occur as a result of an environmental stimulus triggering gene induction or repression (essentially phenotypic variation) this can be called **environmental modulation**. If the change involves DNA rearrangement (genotypic variation) it is normally referred to as **phase variation** (see below).

The specific immune response, in particular the production of high affinity antibody molecules, has driven the evolution of bacterial mechanisms for variation a step further. A number of bacteria can rapidly generate a succession of bacterial components of similar structure, but of different antigenic type. This is termed **antigenic variation**, and as with phase variation, involves DNA rearrangement. Antigenic variation is particularly advantageous to the pathogenic bacterium as the population of bacterial cells within the host is derived from a small number of clones of infecting cells. (It should be noted that the definitions of the terms environmental modulation, phase variation and antigenic variation as stated above are not adhered to by all authors. In particular, in older publications the term phase variation has been used for both antigenic variation and environmental modulation.)

One of the simplest mechanisms for the generation of variation in bacteria is the slow accumulation of point mutations within the genome. Where these mutations occur in structural genes this results in **antigenic drift**. This occurs in **all** bacteria and is not unique to pathogenic bacteria. Therefore as a result of antigenic drift, prior exposure of the host to one clonal variant does not mean that the immune system will recognise another. It is interesting, however, that in general the infection of a host by a species of bacterial pathogen seems to be limited to a small number of variants or clones of the total number possible.

Both antigenic and phase variation, however, generate variants not only at a higher rate than antigenic drift, but also the changes are in general **reversible**. The DNA rearrangement can occur either within an **individual** bacterium or between bacteria in a **population** of clones. In an individual bacterium, the mechanisms may include homologous DNA recombination and the reassortment of elements of mobile DNA which recombine without obvious DNA homology. Within a bacterial population, there is the potential for horizontal or cell to cell transfer of information necessary for a bacterium to be pathogenic, as the genes for the virulence determinants are frequently encoded on mobile extrachromosomal genetic elements, for example plasmids and bacteriophage, frequently within the confines of transposable or mobile elements of DNA.

Genetic variation associated with bacterial pathogenesis therefore exists at two levels. Firstly, antigenic variability within the whole bacterial population, due to a combination of antigenic drift, gene transfer and DNA recombination and secondly, genetic changes during growth in the host brought about largely by phase and antigenic variation. A combination of all of the above processes has the potential to generate new variants and allow the bacterium to be effectively 'one step ahead' of the specific immune response.

Another aspect of the mechanisms that generate genetic variation is the spread of genes associated with resistance to antibiotic compounds. In recent times, resistance to antibiotics has become as much a determinant of the success of a bacterial pathogen as 'natural' virulence determinants; however, a detailed discussion of the evolution of antibiotic resistance is beyond the scope of this text.

The key processes in the generation of genetic diversity amongst pathogenic bacteria, and indeed all bacteria, are (1) the generation of mutations and (2) the recombination of DNA. In order to appreciate fully the means by which bacterial pathogens generate diversity, it is essential to understand these processes. This chapter will therefore cover the basic genetic mechanisms of recombination before discussing specific examples which relate to bacterial virulence. The environmental modulation of bacterial virulence will be·discussed at the end of the chapter.

MUTATIONS AND GENETIC RECOMBINATION IN BACTERIA

The mechanisms whereby mutations arise and recombinations of DNA take place are best understood from detailed studies with the bacterium *Escherichia coli*; however, it is fair to say that mechanisms similar to those in *E. coli* are believed to operate in many other bacteria. The frequency with which mutations arise in bacteria such as *E. coli* is closely linked to the replication and repair of damaged DNA. Also, the mechanisms of replication and repair of DNA are closely associated with, or have common points with, the mechanisms by which DNA recombines. It is therefore necessary to review these processes in order to understand fully the mechanisms known to operate in generating phase and antigenic variants in pathogenic bacteria.

The replication of DNA

Many mutations in bacteria arise as a result of infidelity of the DNA replication process and many of the recombination events that take place also involve DNA replication. The single circular chromosome of *E. coli* consists of about 4.7 million base pairs (bp) and has a contour length of about 1300 μm. Bearing in mind that the size of the *E. coli* cell is generally no more than 2.0 μm long by 0.5 μm across, it is necessary for the chromosomal DNA to be tightly packed as **supercoils** into the cell. It must be remembered here that during the course of an infection the bacteria may be growing rapidly and hence the cells are replicating their chromosome rapidly. The genome of most bacteria also contains extrachromosomal units of DNA termed **plasmids**. These will also replicate throughout an infection and, if not integrated into the chromosome, replicate independently. They can vary in size from 1 or 2 kilobase pairs to several thousand kilobase pairs, are also supercoiled and encode a range of functions from virulence determinants to antibiotic resistance. In order to achieve tight packing of all of the genomic DNA, the double stranded DNA is coiled in a series of domains each about 20 μm long. These coils are revolved around a central core of RNA. There are therefore about 65 of these domains around the central RNA core. The coiled domains are then coiled further, i.e. negatively supercoiled or super twisted, so that each supercoil is about 150 base pairs long. The 400 or so supercoils in each domain are coiled independently in each of the domains. Figure 9.2 shows how the coiling is achieved. It is worth mentioning here that the degree of supercoiling appears to be modulated by changes in environment. This in turn regulates the expression of a number of genes, including those involved in virulence. This will be discussed in more detail under 'Environmental Regulation of Virulence Determinant Expression' below. The enzyme responsible for introducing the negative supercoils into each domain in *E. coli* has been identified as DNA

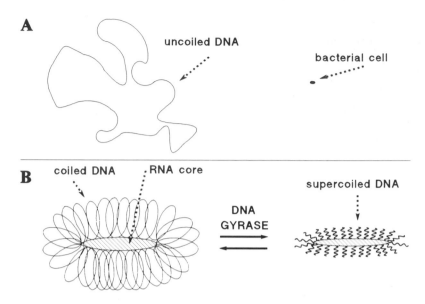

Figure 9.2. Representation of DNA structure in *Escherichia coli*. There are approximately 4–5×10^6 base pairs in the chromosome which represent a length of about 1.3 mm coiled into a cell of about 0.5×2–$3 \ \mu m$ (A). In the supercoiled DNA there are about 65 domains each $20 \ \mu m$ long wrapped around an RNA core (B). One condensed supercoil consists of about 400 bp and each domain of supercoiled DNA has 406 negative supercoils. From Greenwood D. and O'Grady F. (Eds) 1985. The Scientific Basis of Antimicrobial Chemotherapy. Reproduced by permission of The Society of General Microbiology

gyrase or DNA topoisomerase II. This enzyme consists of four subunits; two 'a' monomers (105 kDa) encoded by the *gyrA* gene in *E. coli*, and two 'b' monomers (95 kDa) encoded by the *gyrB* gene. It works during the replication of DNA by introducing nicks staggered by four base pairs, twisting the molecule and resealing the staggered nicks. The 'a' subunits are responsible for introducing the nicks and resealing whereas the 'b' subunits are necessary for twisting the DNA (Figure 9.3). Similar DNA gyrases have been found in many other bacteria and it is presumed that they all work by a similar mechanism. The complex structure and topology of the chromosome is an important factor when considering the replication and recombination mechanisms. Since the experiments of Cairns in 1963, the replication of the circular chromosome in *E. coli* has been known to be semiconservative with single points of origin and termination and two opposing replication forks (Figure 9.4). The events at the forks themselves are important in introducing errors of replication and hence mutations. The synthesis of DNA begins with the production of an RNA primer molecule near the origin of replication. The addition of deoxynucleotides then pro-

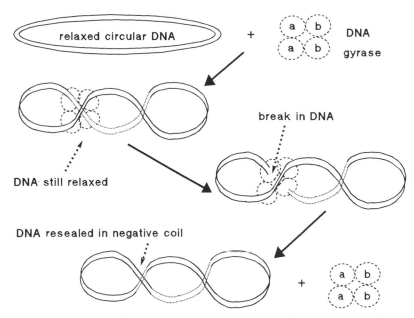

Figure 9.3. The action of type II DNA topoisomerase (DNA gyrase with a and b protein monomers) on relaxed DNA. This process requires ATP and can be reversed. DNA topoisomerase I removes negative supercoils to relax the DNA and seems to operate antagonistically with the type II enzyme to regulate the level of DNA supercoiling in the cell. Other type III and type IV topoisomerases are involved in resolving concatameric DNA and chromosome segregation

ceeds on the primer through the action of DNA polymerase I. Once the replication forks have been initiated, then the main replication enzyme, DNA polymerase III, starts to function. This enzyme synthesises a continuous complementary strand of DNA by adding deoxynucleotides to the 3'-OH end of the DNA; i.e. it synthesises DNA in the 5' to 3' direction only. The paradox is that DNA polymerase I can also only synthesise DNA in the 5' to 3' direction. This means that the only possible option is for DNA polymerase I to polymerise DNA in discontinuous strands. The existence of such strands was discovered by Reiji Okazaki in 1968. These lagging strands, called **Okazaki fragments** of DNA, are about 1000 base pairs long and are replicated on individual 5 base long RNA primers. The DNA polymerase I recognises the 3'-OH end of the RNA and begins synthesis. Eventually the primer is removed as the forks progress and the gaps sealed through the action of DNA ligase. The short primer is removed through the 5' to 3' exonuclease activity of the DNA polymerase I as it catches up with the preceding strand or Okazaki fragment. The overall process at the replication forks is illustrated in Figure 9.5.

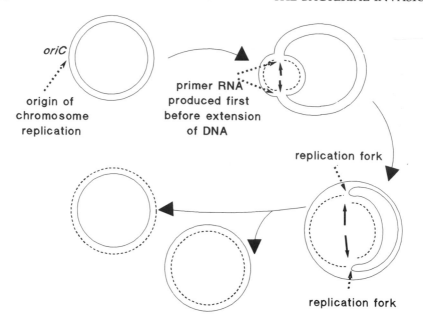

Figure 9.4. Bidirectional and semi-conservative replication of *Escherichia coli* chromosomal DNA. Solid lines represent the parent DNA template and dotted lines the newly synthesised DNA

The enzymes involved in DNA replication

Both DNA polymerases I and III catalyse the same basic polymerisation reactions and they both have an absolute requirement for an opposing strand DNA template. The reactions are shown in Figure 9.6. The addition of nucleotide triphosphate (dNTP) to the 3′-OH end leads to the production of pyrophosphate. This must be removed through the action of pyrophosphatase, otherwise the polymerisation reaction will be reversed. Spontaneous hydrolysis of the phosphodiester bonds can also occur and the action of DNA ligase is required to mend the breaks. In addition to the polymerisation reactions, Figure 9.6 also shows the exonuclease activities of both DNA polymerases. Both can digest DNA from the 3′-OH end and reverse the polymerisation process. This serves an important function in the editing of DNA during replication. Only DNA polymerase I can also digest DNA in the 5′ to 3′ direction. DNA polymerase I is a relatively simple enzyme encoded by the *polA* gene in *E. coli*. It has an important function in that it can polymerise DNA, starting from single strand nicks, and displace a strand; this is important in various repair and recombination mechanisms (see below). DNA polymerase III is a complex enzyme and there are at least nine proteins in the holoenzyme. These are encoded by the *dna*

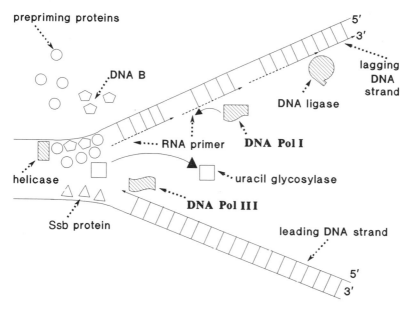

Figure 9.5. A simplified view of the biochemical events taking place at the DNA replication fork in *Escherichia coli*. Ssb is single strand DNA-binding protein

genes in *E. coli*, with *dnaE* encoding the main polymerase. Unlike DNA polymerase I, this enzyme only polymerises DNA in short gaps of about 100 nucleotides long; which is about the length of the replication fork itself. It cannot nick DNA and replicate by displacing a strand. The precise function of all of the components of the DNA polymerase III holoenzyme are not known; however, it is undoubtedly true that some, such as the *dnaQ* product, are necessary for editing the DNA. DNA ligase is another important enzyme in the system. It can join a 3'-OH group to a 5' group as long as there is no gap and that the substrate is double stranded. Other proteins involved are: the Rep protein (encoded by *rep* in *E. coli*) which assists in unwinding the DNA at the replication fork; single-strand binding protein (encoded by *ssb* in *E. coli*) which protects single stranded DNA from nuclease action. A summary of the enzymes involved is outlined in Table 9.1. It is worth re-emphasising that many of these enzymes are involved in the repair and recombination processes which will be outlined below.

Mutations and the repair of DNA

Changes in the expected genetic sequence, or **mutations**, occur due to errors in the replication of DNA by the DNA polymerases. Mutations will be

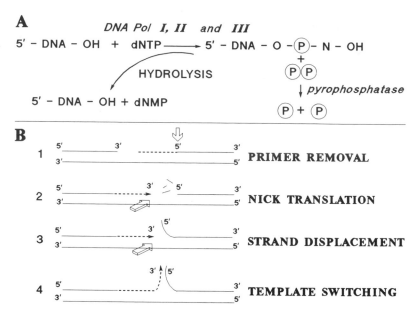

Figure 9.6. The polymerisation reactions for DNA synthesis. A. Reactions catalysed by DNA polymerases. Removal of pyrophosphate by pyrophosphatase enables the reaction to proceed. B. Reactions catalysed by DNA polymerase I. DNA polymerase III catalyses similar reactions except for strand displacement, 5′-3′ digestion and nick translation

defined strictly in these terms and will not include changes in sequence due to recombinational events or DNA rearrangements that occur from time to time. These will be discussed below. The replication of DNA is largely prone to error and mechanisms exist to enable the process to become more accurate. When DNA synthesis is allowed to operate without the aid of such mechanisms the rate of error due to the incorporation of a mismatched base is about one in every 100 bases. This is clearly an unacceptable load for most cellular systems and would lead to the disruption of many essential genes. The mechanisms adopted by bacteria to correct errors improve the accuracy by more than 10^7 times. This remarkable achievement is brought about by three levels of action by the cells: (a) the correct selection from the four nucleotides; (b) a proofreading process and (c) post-replication repair of mismatched bases after the replication fork has passed.

The first two mechanisms of proofreading and correct selection of nucleotides are closely associated with the polymerisation process itself and are often termed **error avoidance** mechanisms. The selection of the correct nucleotide is carried out by the polymerase itself; which has a one in four chance of getting it correct. This assumes that the nucleotides are available

Table 9.1. A summary of the enzymes involved in DNA replication and their functions

Gene	Enzyme	Function
	DNA polymerase III	
polC (dnaE)	α subunit	The main polymerase
dnaQ	ε subunit	Proofreading exonuclease
dnaN, Z, X	β, γ, δ subunits	Accessory proteins
polA	DNA polymerase I	Removal of primer Sealing of gaps
lig	DNA ligase	Seals nicks in single stranded DNA
ssb	Ssb protein	Binds and protects single stranded DNA
dnaB	DNA helicase	Unwinding of helix and priming
gyrA, B	DNA gyrase/ topoisomerase II α and β subunits	Promotes negative supercoiling of DNA

NB   There are other proteins involved in DNA replication whose function remains to be determined.

in the correct proportions. It has been shown that imbalances in the nucelotide availability will lead to more mis-incorporated bases. It is possible to insert nucleotides in any combination; however, the correct pairing of AT or CG will be the most favourable energetically. The dNTP binds first; however, screening of the nucleotide does not appear to be very efficient at this level. Instead, screening at the level of incorporation of the nucleotide monophosphate (dNMP) is more important. The production of non-complementary AGs and CTs leads to a reversal of the process and exclusion of the incorrectly selected dNMP. The presence of the mismatched bases somehow causes the polymerisation to 'stagger' long enough for the 3' to 5' exonuclease activity of the polymerase to remove the mismatch; and possibly other nucleotides incorporated prior to the mismatch. The polymerisation process then resumes. The overall steps are shown in Figure 9.7. The operation of these steps means that the error rate is improved to one in 10^6 base pairs.

The third mechanism of post-replication repair is an error correction process that catches the mismatches which slip through. This process is more complicated and is often termed **mismatch repair**. The essential steps in the process are shown in Figure 9.8. This mechanism relies on the fact that DNA is methylated at specific sites as replication proceeds. It also relies on a period of time elapsing after the replication fork has passed in which only the old template strand is methylated. The new strand still awaits

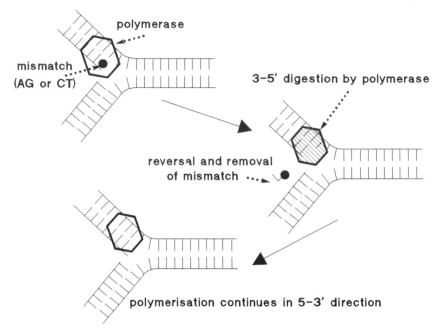

Figure 9.7. Proofreading of newly synthesised DNA by DNA polymerases

the methylase. DNA in this state is termed **hemimethylated**. An adenine methylase (Dam methylase) encoded by the *dam* gene in *E. coli* recognises the sequence GATC and adds a methyl group to the adenine. The activity of the methylase is not required for cells to grow; however, it is needed for the repair process. The *dam* gene is in a class of genes known as **mutator** genes. The other components of the repair mechanism are encoded by the *mut* (for mutator) genes. There are two possible models for the functioning of the *mut* gene products. Any mismatch sited between two hemimethylated GATC sites is first recognised by MutS and MutL. MutH recognises the hemimethylated GATC sites and cleaves a single strand on the non-methylated side. In one model cleavage occurs at both GATC sites, to excise the intervening strand of DNA with the mismatch. In the other model, MutH cuts only one GATC site and there is cleavage at the mismatch itself. The Ssb protein is there again to protect the single stranded DNA which must remain intact for repair of the gap by DNA polymerase I. Another methylase in *E. coli* (the *dcm* methylase) methylates cytosines at GGT/ACC sites. This system is not as well known. Although *dcm* mutants are not apparently mutators, like *dam* mutants, the *dcm* gene is closely associated with a gene required for very short patch DNA repair (*vsr*). The Vsr mechanism is not known.

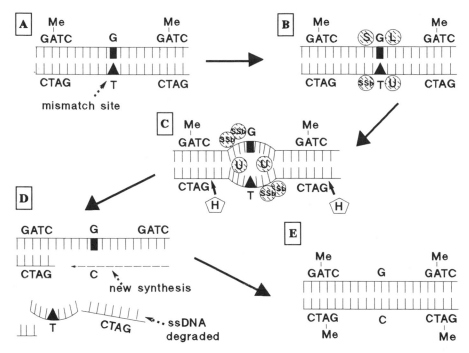

Figure 9.8. A model for mismatch repair of DNA. A. Newly synthesised DNA is hemi-methylated at the sequence GATC (A-Me) for several minutes. B. Any intervening mismatch, such as the G-T illustrated, is recognised by the gene products of the *mutS* (S), *mutL* (L), *mutU* (U) and single stranded DNA binding protein (Ssb). C. Single strand cuts are made by the *mutH* gene product (H). D. The resulting gap is repaired by DNA polymerase I and the excised DNA degraded. E. The DNA is ligated and the repair completed before full methylation by the *dam* methylase

Methylation of DNA also has a function in the regulation of gene expression and some gene rearrangements and this will be discussed in later sections.

E. coli also contains a number of repair enzymes called nucleotide glycosylases (or N-glycosylases). The best characterised is the uracil glycosylase. Although uracil is usually found in RNA, it can be mis-incorporated into DNA at a rate of about one in 12 000 bases to form an AU pairing. GU pairing can also be brought about through the deamination of cytosine. Uracil glycosylase removes the uracil base, a specific endonuclease then makes a single nucleotide gap which is repaired by DNA polymerase I and DNA ligase. The sequence CCA/TGG recognised by the *dcm* methylase is a known hot-spot for mutation involving changes from CG to AT pairing. This is because the methylated cytosine can be deaminated but is not recognised by the uracil glycosylase. It could be speculated that the Vsr mechanism associated with *dcm* is there purely to counter the mismatch directed by *dcm* methylase action.

It is well established that agents that damage or alter the chemical structure of DNA can cause mutations. These agents include chemical mutagens and ionising radiation such as UV light. Many of these agents are not directly relevant to bacterial virulence; however, it is worth noting that many strong oxidising agents, such as those found in macrophage (see Chapter 4), can damage DNA. The action of these agents will lead to the induction of some DNA repair mechanisms which are outlined below. The elements of these mechanisms are also important in regulating or modulating the recombination systems involved in generating phase and antigenic variants.

Damage to DNA caused by agents in the environment, such as chemical mutagens or ionising radiation such as UV light, is repaired at three basic levels: (a) repair that is not associated with DNA synthesis (i.e. is **pre-replicative**); (b) repair that is **post-replicative** after DNA synthesis; and (c) repair by the SOS inducible system in response to considerable DNA damage.

In the first case, the repair involves two types of mechanism that are not subject to errors (i.e. will not lead to mutations). These mechanisms work constitutively in the cells. The action of agents such as UV light leads to the formation of dimeric forms of bases, such as thymidine dimers. DNA replication cannot easily proceed past a dimer under normal conditions; thus preventing further growth of the cells so damaged. Some initiation of replication can occur beyond a dimer; however, this leaves a gap. The dimers are cleaved directly by a visible-light activated photo-lyase. Also operating constitutively at a low level is a DNA excision repair system that is mediated by the products of the *uvrA, B* and *C* genes.

In the second case, post-replicative repair is not generally prone to error and is present constitutively in the cells. Initiation of DNA synthesis takes place after dimers have formed, leaving a small gap. For the cells to continue growth, these gaps must be repaired. This is done through the action of the *recA* gene product, the RecA protein, and recombinational events. The recombination mechanisms are detailed below.

The third repair mechanism is induced by considerable damage to the DNA of the cell; as might be expected when cells are subjected to attack by phagocytes. This will involve the formation of other covalent linkages, double and single strand breaks as well as the formation of dimers. The induced activity of this repair system in *E. coli* is called the SOS response. As the repair is of extensive lesions in the DNA structure and must be rapid for the cells to survive, the replication of damaged regions of DNA appears to be done at the expense of fidelity. In other words this is an **error-prone** repair. Lower doses of for example UV light cause moderate DNA damage (e.g. formation of perhaps 30 dimers per cell) and do not lead to the full induction of the SOS response. This is largely error free and such doses of UV light do not cause an increase in mutants. Higher doses of UV light are very mutagenic due to the induction of the error-prone repair system. The control of induction of the SOS system is outlined in Figure 9.9. The activation of this response requires the presence of RecA protein, which is also required for homologous recombination (see below), and LexA. Mutants of *recA* cannot induce the SOS response and are very sensitive to UV light and other DNA damage. Mutants of *lexA* are able to recombine normally; however, they show no increased mutagenesis due to high levels of UV damage. LexA is an autoregulated repressor of a range of genes induced through the SOS response. Under normal conditions there is low expression of LexA which also represses its own synthesis as well as RecA. The presence of damaged DNA in the cell somehow activates RecA to cleave LexA by virtue of its specific protease activity. This leads to more expression of LexA repressor; however, there is also increased expression of RecA. The result is relief from repression of a range of other genes under the control of LexA. These include *uvr A, B, C, D* and *sfi*,

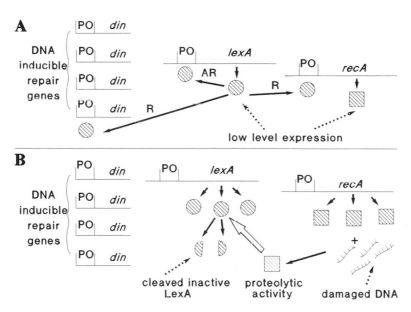

Figure 9.9. A model for SOS induction of error-prone DNA repair in *Escherichia coli*. A. Where there is no high level damage to DNA in the cell the *lexA* gene product is an autorepressor (AR) as well as a repressor (R) for *recA* expression and a wide range of inducible DNA repair genes (*din*). The promoter/operator regulatory regions are designated by PO. B. Where there is extensive damage to DNA in the cell the proteolytic activity of RecA is induced and LexA is cleaved, so relieving its autorepression and repression of *recA* and the *din* gene expression

which inhibits cell division. The result is high expression of a range of DNA repair functions.

These repair mechanisms all operate together and it is worth noting that the control of LexA expression is not purely an all or nothing response. It operates at different levels depending upon the degree of damage. Hence the rate of production of mutants can alter depending upon the damage stress in the environment of the bacterium. Although by no means proven, the stress of phagocytic attack could lead to a rapid increase in the rate of mutation and perhaps homologous recombination in the bacteria concerned. Clearly it may be that the presence of an error-prone repair system is of importance in increasing the possible number of variants in the population of bacteria.

Homologous recombination in bacteria

Recombination can be defined as the process by which sequences of DNA are broken and rejoined in such a way that a new combination of sequence is generated. This can be brought about by a variety of mechanisms in bacteria and harnessing these processes is one of the underlying means by which phase and antigenic variation mechanisms operate in bacterial pathogens. Although recombination has been mostly studied in *E. coli*, there is strong evidence that similar mechanisms operate in many other bacteria. A requirement of the process of homologous recombination is that the two sequences of DNA are of largely similar sequence; i.e. they have a high degree of homology. The extent of similar sequence must extend over at least 40 to 50 base pairs. When DNA of close homology to the bacterial DNA present is introduced into a bacterium or is present in the bacterium as plasmid DNA, then it will recombine. This is an efficient high frequency event and any DNA introduced is almost certain to be involved in one or more recombination reactions. This involves the breaking and rejoining of phosphodiester bonds on both DNA molecules so that an exchange of DNA sequence takes place. The process is enzymically mediated by the bacterium through its recombination system. If the homology is not total between the DNA strands, due to mutations or other changes of sequence, then the process will generate new sequence combinations. A number of models have been proposed to explain the mechanism that operates. The Meselson–Radding model is outlined in Figure 9.10 where one strand is nicked and assimilated into the other strand of DNA prior to digestion of the displaced single strand (or D-loop) and ligation. Another very similar model (not illustrated) is the Holliday model, where two strands are nicked. After branch migration or displacement of the branch (and possibly twisting of the whole structure to form a different isomer) the branch is nicked and rejoined to resolve the two strands again. If there is a single base pair difference in the two strands, a mismatch is produced. This is either repaired by the normal

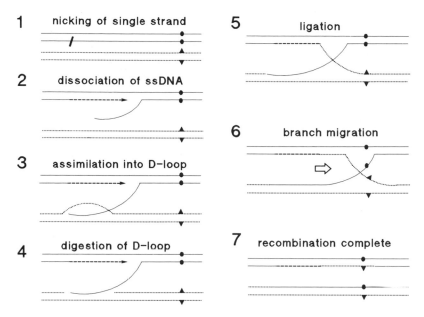

Figure 9.10. The Meselson–Radding model in seven steps for strand exchange in homologous recombination of DNA. Branch migration (6) may continue to exchange the DNA for several hundred base pairs and the structure may be twisted into another isomer before the recombination is completed (7). ssDNA, single strand DNA

mismatch repair system or there is no repair and there is segregation of the mismatches upon DNA synthesis.

The complex of enzymes involved in this process is well established in *E. coli*; however, similar systems seem to operate in other bacteria. At least 33 different genes at different locations on the *E. coli* chromosome are involved in the process and many are also involved in the repair of damaged DNA and the synthesis of DNA. Some of these genes are termed the *rec* genes and many were discovered as mutations that either failed to mediate recombination, were sensitive to UV light and DNA damage in general, or both. The two key enzyme systems in the process are RecA and the RecBCD complex or **recombinase**. The RecA protein is a remarkable protein. In addition to its protease activity against LexA (see above), it promotes the strand displacement reaction after it has bound to single stranded DNA. It requires at least 40–50 base pair homology to pair the single stranded DNA with its complementary sequence. It then slowly promotes the exchange of strands and formation of the D-loop. The RecBCD enzyme is termed the recombinase and cuts the DNA and unwinds single stranded DNA for RecA to bind to. It is composed of three proteins of 130, 120 and 60 kDa molecular mass. They bind to DNA and then unwind it until a specific sequence called a **chi** sequence (5'-GCTGGTGG-3') is encountered. This sequence is relatively short and there are about 1000 sites around the *E. coli* chromosome. Recombination appears to be stimulated at or near these sites. The RecBCD enzyme cuts the DNA at or near the chi-sequence and Ssb protein then protects the single stranded DNA from exonuclease digestion prior to RecA binding (Figure 9.11). The other genes associated with homologous recombination in *E. coli* are listed in Table 9.2. In addition, there are other possible recombination pathways that can operate if RecBCD is not functioning. The best characterised are the *recE* and *recF* pathways (Figure 9.12). These pathways operate when there are mutations in *recBCD* suppressors, termed *sbcA* and *sbcBC*, and can replace the functions normally provided by RecBCD. There have been many other such recombination genes found in *E. coli* associated with the three *rec* pathways although their precise function under normal conditions is not clear. One theory is that the three pathways are somehow involved in the different recombinational exchanges associated with transduction, conjugation, plasmid exchanges, transformation etc. In the case of conjugation and transformation, single stranded DNA is introduced into the bacterium. In plasmid conjugation, the DNA is rapidly replicated as the single stranded DNA is transferred. In the case of transduction and plasmid–plasmid or plasmid–

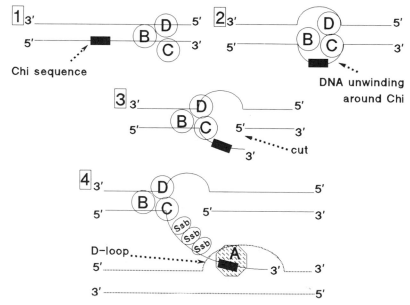

Figure 9.11. The role of RecBCD (BCD) and RecA (A) proteins in mediating homologous recombination in four steps in *Escherichia coli*. Single strand DNA binding protein (Ssb) protects the DNA being assimilated into the D-loop

Table 9.2. Some of the genes found to have an effect on and appear to be associated with homologous recombination in *Escherichia coli* K12

Gene designation	Biochemical function of gene product
recA	Binding to ssDNA and ATP-dependent assimilation into homologous DNA
recB, C, D	Forms the recombinase complex and cuts near chi sequence
recE	5'-exonuclease activity
sbcB	3'-exonuclease activity
ssb	Binds to ssDNA
lexA	Autorepressor and represses *recA* expression and expression of DNA repair genes
polA	DNA polymerase I
lig	DNA ligase
gyrA, B	DNA gyrase/topoisomerase II
topA	DNA toposiomerase I
uvrD	Helicase II unwinds dsDNA
dam	DNA adenine methylation
dcm	DNA cytosine methylation
dut	Deoxyuridine triphosphatase
rep	Separates dsDNA in presence of ssDNA
xth	dsDNA 3'-exonuclease
xseA, B	ssDNA degradation from 3' and 5' ends
mutH	Binds to hemimethylated GATC
mutS	Binds near base pair mismatches
mutL	Not known
recF/J/N/O/Q	Not known
sbcA/C	Not known
ruvA/B/C	Processes/resolves recombination intermediates
rdgB	Not known

ssDNA, single stranded DNA; dsDNA, double stranded DNA.

chromosome exchanges, recombination is between double stranded DNA molecules. The *recA* gene appears to be conserved in many bacteria (Table 9.3). The assumption is that the mechanisms present in *E. coli* operate in a similar way in these other bacteria.

Site-specific recombinations

A number of separate recombination mechanisms different to the *rec* system exist whereby the exchange of strands takes place at a very specific sequence. Examples of this include the integration of lambda phage DNA into the *E. coli* chromosome and the resolution of plasmid multimers. In

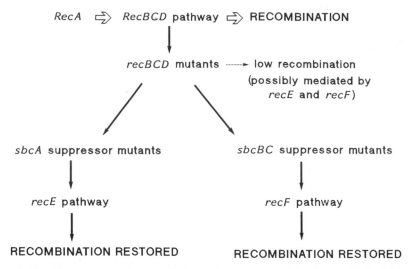

Figure 9.12. Alternative pathways for homologous recombination in *Escherichia coli*. The RecA and RecBCD pathways mediate homologous recombination. Functioning RecA is an absolute requirement; however, there is a low level of recombination in *recBCD* mutants. Mutations in suppressors (*sbcA* and *sbcBC*) can restore normal recombination via the *recE* and *recF* pathways

Table 9.3. Some bacteria for which a *recA* gene homologue has been discovered

Bordetella pertussis	*Brucella abortus*
Escherichia coli	*Haemophilus influenzae*
Klebsiella aerogenes	*Klebsiella pneumoniae*
Legionella pneumophila	*Mycoplasma* spp.
Mycobacterium tuberculosis	*Proteus mirabilis*
Neisseria gonorrhoeae	*Pseudomonas aeruginosa*
Proteus vulgaris	*Serratia marcescens*
Salmonella typhimurium	*Streptococcus mutans*
Shigella flexneri	*Vibrio cholerae*
Streptococcus pneumoniae	
Yersinia pestis	

the first case, the phage encodes a recombinase which recognises a specific attachment (*att*) site on the chromosome. The process also requires the action of the integration host factor (IHF) a two subunit protein not encoded by the lambda phage but by the *E. coli* host.

In the case of some plasmids present in the bacterium in multiple copies, there is a problem as homologous recombination may lead to the formation of multimers of the plasmid (i.e. the plasmids become joined together in one molecule). These are not segregated efficiently and this can lead to loss of the plasmid as the bacteria grow and divide. In order to counteract this effect, *E. coli* encodes a recombinase (XerC) which recognises a specific sequence called the *cer* recombination site and resolves the multimers. This has to be very efficient to maintain the plasmids as monomers. Other examples of site specific recombinations will be described later under antigenic and phase variation mechanisms.

Non-homologous recombination

There also exist many different ways in which recombinations can take place between DNA molecules where there is little or no clear extensive homology of sequence. In some cases there may be a short homologous sequence of several base pairs which would not be sufficient for the action of RecA. These recombinations fall into two basic classes: those that lead to deletions of DNA and those that lead to insertions or transpositions of DNA. A combination of these mechanisms is responsible for the numerous genomic rearrangements that occur in bacteria; some of which may be associated with virulence. It must be stressed that, unlike homologous recombination and some site specific recombinations, non-homologous recombinations take place at much lower frequencies in bacteria. For example transpositions may only occur at a frequency of between 1 in 10^4 to 10^6 per cell per generation.

DNA transposition mechanisms

The transposition of DNA is the most likely method by which plasmids have rapidly evolved, particularly in the acquisition of antibiotic resistance. Transposition is the movement of a discrete segment of DNA from one location in a genome to another location either in the same molecule of replicating DNA (or replicon) or into another replicon. In other words, this might include movement from one site on the chromosome or plasmid to another site or movement from the chromosome to a plasmid or vice versa. The combination of possibilities is very large and this has considerable implications for the evolution of genomes in general. The discrete pieces of DNA that move in this way are called **transposable elements** (sometimes called **transposons**). There is a diverse range of transposable elements in bacteria and they are too numerous to describe all of them here. Three basic classes have been identified: (a) the insertion sequences (IS elements) and their related composite transposons, (b) the Tn3-like transposons and (c) the transposing bacteriophage.

A number of features appear to be common to most transposable elements. All have distinct ends and virtually all are flanked by an inverted repeat sequence of DNA. This repeat is usually not an exact repeat but nearly exact. The inverted repeat sequences are essential for the transposition process. When the transposable element transposes or inserts into a new site, this is usually accompanied by a short direct duplication of the target site at the ends of the transposable element. Transposable elements encode a transposase which is necessary for transposition; however, the process also requires functions encoded by the host bacterium. The element may also encode functions which regulate the transposition process; usually negative regulation.

The mechanisms by which these elements move have been the subject of intense study; particularly in *E. coli*. Examples from the first two classes will be used to illustrate the two basic mechanisms that are known to mediate the transposition of DNA, namely **conservative** and **replicative** transposition.

Replicative transposition

Members of the Tn3 family of transposons replicate during the transposition process. In other words, a copy of the transposon is reproduced at the new site while the original copy remains at the old site. The basic structure of Tn3 is shown in Figure 9.13. Tn3-like elements are large transposons that carry accessory genes such as *bla* in Tn3 which codes for a β-lactamase which confers ampicillin resistance. They also encode a transposase, TnpA, a resolvase, TnpR and have an internal resolution site termed *res*. The size of these and related elements can vary greatly; however, they are not usually less than 3 kilobase pairs due to the requirement for a transposase. The overall process is summarised in Figure 9.13. It is a two-step process. The first step is the formation of a cointegrate structure whereby the two replicons become joined and there are two direct repeats of the transposon. The transposase, TnpA, binds to the direct repeats at the ends of the Tn3 and then binds to a target site. The length of inverted repeat DNA at the ends of Tn3-like elements tends to be about 38 base pairs and is conserved amongst these elements. This does not require homology between the ends of the element and the target site. It has been reported, however, that Tn3-like elements tend to show a preference for AT rich regions of DNA. Also with these elements there tends to be a very strong bias toward insertion into plasmid DNA and not chromosomal DNA. The reason for this is not known. Opposing single strand cuts are made in the target site; in the case of Tn3 the cut is staggered by 5 base pairs, and at the ends of the transposon. DNA ligase from the host bacterium repairs the cuts and, because of the proximity of the target site and the transposon ends, there is a DNA strand exchange. There is then replication of the resulting single stranded DNA gap by the host bacterium DNA polymerases. This gap extends the length of the trasposon itself and the 5 base pairs from the staggered cut at the target site. This produces a cointegrate structure which is formed by the merger of two replicons. Resolution of this structure to two separated

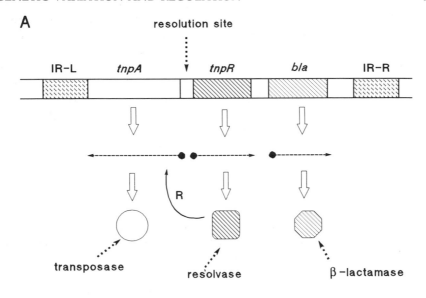

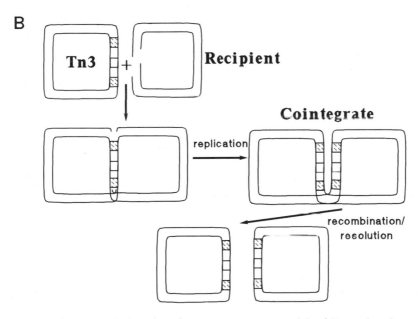

Figure 9.13. Structure (A) and replicative transposition (B) of Tn3. The element is flanked by inverted repeat sequences IR-L and IR-R which enclose the transposase (*tnpA*), resolvase/repressor (*tnpR*) and β-lactamase (*bla*) genes. The resolvase (TnpA) acts at the resolution site to complete the transposition process after the formation of a cointegrate structure involving a 5 bp target site duplication. TnpR also acts as a repressor for TnpA expression

structures is achieved through the action of the resolvase TnpR on the specific 130 base pair resolution site *res*. This is an example of a site specific recombination. This process, although efficient, is not as efficient as homologous recombination. Negative regulation of transposition is achieved by binding of TnpR to *res* which represses synthesis of TnpA. The promoter for TnpA overlaps with *res*. There is also evidence that in some elements of this type there is another regulatory gene, *tnpM*, which modulates expression of both TnpA and TnpR.

Conservative transposition

This process is very different in many respects to replicative transposition. In this case, the element moves to another site without the formation of a cointegrate intermediate and without replication of the element. This is sometimes called a **cut-patch** model for transposition. For elements that transpose exclusively via this route, there is no cointegrate intermediate and no internal resolution site in the element for the resolution of cointegrates. Despite these differences, there are still some common features to the process. The target site is still duplicated at the site of insertion, there is generally no strong target site specificity and the elements encode a transposase that is, in most cases, negatively regulated. The best characterised element which replicates exclusively via a conservative mechanism is Tn10. Although all of the studies have been done in *E. coli*, it is perhaps prudent to remember that this element was first discovered on plasmid R100; a multiple antibiotic resistance plasmid from *Salmonella*. The element Tn10 encodes a tetracycline resistance gene, *tet*, which is flanked by two inverted repeats of the insertion sequence IS10. This is a good example of a composite transposon. The transposition of Tn10 is largely mediated by expression of the transposase from the right-hand-side copy of IS10 (IS10-R). An overall model for Tn10 transposition is shown in Figure 9.14. There is a double strand cut at the ends of the element on the donor DNA molecule. There is also a staggered single strand cut at the target site. Again, there is no homology requirement for the target site as for Tn3. In the case of Tn10, the staggered cuts at the target site are 9 base pairs apart. The Tn10 is ligated into the target site and the resulting 9 base pair gaps repaired to give the direct repeats at the end of the insertion. The donor DNA molecule is very vulnerable to exonuclease digestion and it is generally assumed that it must be destroyed in the process. Negative regulation of the transposase is achieved through a number of interacting mechanisms. The promoter sequence for the transposase is inefficient and is also subject to control by two other methods: (a) adenine methylation by the *dam* methylase and (b) antisense RNA regulation (Figure 9.14). Operation of these methods limits expression of the transposase to an estimated one molecule in every four cells. When the promoter P_{in} sequence is methylated at the GATC site, bind-

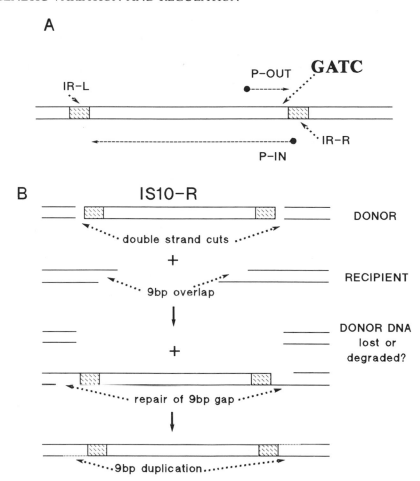

Figure 9.14. Structure (A) and conservative 'cut–paste' transposition (B) of IS10-R from transposon Tn10. The element is flanked by inverted repeat sequences IR-L and IR-R. The transposase is expressed from the promoter P-IN transcript whereas the P-OUT transcript acts as an antisense RNA repressor. The expression of transcript from P-IN is also negatively regulated by full adenine Dam methylation at the GATC sequence. Transcript is only produced when the sequence is transiently hemimethylated after a replication fork has passed

ing of the RNA polymerase and transcription is severely inhibited; however, when the DNA molecule is replicated, the adenine at the GATC site is hemimethylated for a brief period (as outlined under 'Mutations and the repair of DNA' above). Under these conditions, the RNA polymerase can bind and initiate transcription of the transposase gene. Hence, transposition of Tn10 seems to be associated with DNA replication. Control via methylation of a GATC site in the transposase promoter is common in most of the insertion sequences discovered in the Enterobacteriaceae; IS1 is perhaps one notable exception which will be discussed below. Expression of the transposase gene is also inhibited by expression of an antisense molecule of RNA from the promoter P_{out}. This effect was discovered as a multi-copy inhibition effect whereby added copies of Tn10 in the DNA of a cell inhibit further copies transposing.

Conservative and replicative transposition

The use of conservative and replicative transposition mechanisms need not be exclusive and some elements may be able to employ both routes. One example is the insertion sequence IS1. This element is present in multiple copies in the genomes of the Enterobacteriaceae and along with other insertion sequences may be responsible for many genomic rearrangements. IS1 at 768 base pairs is the smallest transposable element of its kind and like other insertion sequences does not appear to encode any genes other than those associated with transposition. No clear mechanism for negative regulation of this particular element has been determined and this may reflect its wide copy number range in various bacteria (see Table 9.5).

Other rearrangements associated with transposable DNA

In addition to mediating transposition of the element itself, many transposons and insertion sequences also bring about other genomic rearrangements. These include deletions, duplications and inversions. Deletions can be of two types: precise excision of the element itself and adjacent deletions of host DNA. Target site base pair duplications associated with many of these elements are acted upon by host recombination mechanisms to accurately excise the element. Equally, replicative transposition to a site nearby on the same molecule of DNA will lead to an extensive homologous region and subsequent deletion of the intervening sequence. IS1 is particularly active in generating adjacent deletions of DNA. These extend to 'hot-spot' sequences which appear to have some limited homology with the ends of the element.

Environmental modulation of transposition

Since all of the recombination mechanisms outlined above are mediated by enzymic systems, it is not surprising that changes in the host cell environment are seen to change the rate of transposition. Certainly the degree of DNA damage is responsible for regulating the level of LexA and in turn the rate of accumulation of point mutations. It is possible that other DNA repair mechanisms are modulated through environmental changes. The rate of transposition of Tn3-like elements is very sensitive to the growth temperature of the bacterial cell. In some cases the rate of transposition can increase from 1 in 10^6 cells to above 1 in 10^3 cells with a change in temperature from 37 °C to 30 °C. The reasons for this are unclear; however, it does not seem to be due to an increase in transcription of the transposase gene. Similarly, both transposition and deletion formation by IS1 and its composite transposons are sensitive to growth temperature. The reasons for this are not known; however, a number of host functions may be implicated.

MOBILE GENETIC ELEMENTS, PLASMIDS AND VIRULENCE

Many bacterial genes are not sited on the main chromosome but on separate circles of DNA termed **plasmids**. These replicate as **replicons** separate from the chromosomal replicon. The genes of many bacteriophage (or phage) are also encoded on DNA circles. Some of these are stably inherited in the host as **lysogens**. These **lysogenic** phage may therefore be considered as a type of plasmid. Both may replicate as either separate DNA replicons or integrate into the host chromosomal replicon. Most bacteria studied to date appear to contain plasmid DNA. The types of plasmid can range from small circles of 1 to 2 kilobase pairs to large circles of hundreds of kilobase pairs to even larger linear 'plasmid' DNA in some bacterial species. There is a wide diversity of plasmid type and it is not surprising that many pathogenic bacteria have virulence determinants and genes that aid in their survival in the host encoded on plasmids. Many plasmids encode genes which enable them to transfer from cell to cell by a process of **conjugation** and often from species to species. Many of the genes that they encode are also sited within transposable DNA elements which may move from chromosome to plasmid, from plasmid to plasmid and to various sites within the chromosome without the need for DNA homology (see above). The combination of plasmid transference from cell to cell, the ability of plasmids to interact with chromosomes through site-specific and homologous recombinations and the transposition of DNA means that populations of bacteria are diverse in their genomic rearrangements.

The insertion of phage DNA at a particular chromosomal site may alter gene expression if the insertion site is within a structural gene or controlling sequence. It is thought that phage DNA insertion alters the expression of the cytolytic β toxin of *Staphylococcus aureus* (Chapter 5). If the integrating phage also encodes another virulence determinant this can effectively cause a switch from the expression of one gene to another.

The genes encoded on plasmid DNA are usually not necessary for growth of the bacterium but provide functions which may be required when there is a specific selection pressure. Hence these genes are termed **accessory** genes. Some plasmids fail to segregate successfully when the bacterium divides when there is no selective pressure on the plasmid genes. This loss of plasmid DNA is termed **curing** and could be regarded as an off switch for virulence in those cells (see 'Mechanisms of Antigenic and Phase Variation' below). These cells can then only regain their virulence by acquiring plasmid DNA from other bacterial cells. Examples of accessory genes also include the diverse range of antibiotic resistance genes and the catabolic genes present in soil bacteria. A detailed discussion of these is, however, beyond the scope of this book.

Plasmids have been classified into groups called **incompatibility groups**. This is done on the basis of their replication mechanisms and how their replication is controlled. All plasmids have replication origin sequences which are recognised by the host DNA replication enzymes. These enzymes are largely responsible for replicating the plasmids and most plasmids do not encode their own DNA replication genes. Most plasmids possess mechanisms which enable the plasmids to be segregated efficiently when the bacterium divides. In order to reduce the burden on the bacterium, they usually also operate negative regulation mechanisms to maintain a low copy number and prevent over-replication. It is these mechanisms that determine the incompatibility group or **Inc group**. Plasmids that possess the same or similar replication and negative regulatory mechanisms inhibit each other and they eventually segregate separately. They are in effect **incompatible**. Plasmids with differing control and replication mechanisms can survive together in the same cell and are **compatible**. The IncFI plasmids can replicate in a narrow range of Gram negative bacteria from *E. coli* to *Salmonella* spp. They include the F plasmid of *E. coli*, some antibiotic resistance plasmids and the ColV plasmid mentioned below. The multiple antibiotic resistance plasmid R100 from *Salmonella* is in another incompatibility group, IncFII. Other plasmids with a very wide range of host species belong to the IncN, P, Q and W groups. For example IncP plasmids appear to be able to integrate into and mobilise chromosomal genes in virtually all the Gram negative bacteria examined to date.

Virulence plasmids and transposons

The first indication that a virulence determinant need not be encoded on the chromosome of a bacterium was when it became clear that the diphtheria toxin in *Corynebacterium diphtheriae* was encoded on a lysogenic phage. Subsequently many other examples of the encoding of virulence determinants on extrachromosomal elements have been discovered. Some of these are listed in Table 9.4.

The role of virulence plasmids in *Salmonella* spp. is now well established and has been the subject of intense study. The *vir/spv* genes needed for invasion of host cells (see Chapter 8) appear to be plasmid encoded in many strains. Although there is a diverse range of plasmids in *Shigella* spp., many contain conserved homologous regions of DNA. For example, all seem to have a highly conserved 8 kilobase pair region which encodes the *spv* genes.

Table 9.4. Some examples of virulence associated determinants which may be plasmid encoded

Organism	Virulence determinant
Corynebacterium diphtheriae	Toxin
E. coli	Haemolysin
	Heat stable toxins STI/II
	Heat labile (LT) toxin
	Shiga-like toxins
	Pili/fimbriae (K88, K99, 987P)
	Hydroxamate iron
	Chelation (aerobactin)
	OMP for aerobactin uptake
Staphylococcus aureus	Exfoliative toxins
	Toxic shock syndrome toxin 1
	Staphylococcal enterotoxins
	Staphylokinase and lipase
Clostridium tetani	Neurotoxin
Clostridium botulinum	C3 toxin
Bacillus anthracis	Toxin
Salmonella spp.	*vir/spv* genes
Streptococcus pyogenes	Streptococcal pyrogenic toxins
Vibrio cholerae	Cholera toxin
Shigella flexneri	OMP for host cell invasion
Borrelia hermsii	Variable membrane proteins
Yersinia spp.	OMP for host cell invasion secreted proteins (Yops)

OMP, outer membrane proteins.

These are not expressed by the *Shigella* when grown in broth cultures. They
are expressed when the bacteria are inside host cells and are necessary for
their survival. Genes associated with iron uptake have been discovered on
ColV plasmids in *E. coli*. These are the genes required for aerobactin
biosynthesis and synthesis of the outer membrane protein receptor for aerobactin (see Chapter 5). They are bounded by copies of the insertion
sequence IS1 and are transposable as a consequence of this. Indeed, other
virulence determinant genes associated with IS1 are found on plasmids in
Salmonella spp. Copies of IS1 have also been associated with the K88 fimbrial antigen of *E. coli* (Chapter 7). Another IS1 composite transposon is
Tn1681, which encodes the heat stable enterotoxin of *E. coli* (Chapter 6) and
has been the subject of much study.

The distribution of insertion sequences such as IS1 is therefore likely to
determine the mobility of many virulence associated genes as well as other

genes. An indication of the range of insertion sequences and their copy numbers found in some bacteria is shown in Table 9.5. IS1 is widely distributed amongst most of the Gram negative bacteria in both the chromosomes and plasmids. A close scrutiny of the genetic maps of some bacteria has revealed similar patterns of gene organisation. On one level genes of closely related function in *E. coli* appear to cluster closely together on the chromosome. On another level it appears that the genes that are most often transcribed are orientated in their transcription in the same direction as the replication forks. A comparison with the genetic maps of *Salmonella typhimurium*, *Shigella dysenteriae*, *Citrobacter freundii*, *Klebsiella pneumoniae* and *Enterobacter aerogenes* reveals striking similarities in the order of the genes. (The gene order in more distantly related bacteria such as *Bacillus subtilis* varies widely.) Blocks of genes are often arranged in the same order but the complete block may be rearranged on the chromosome. For example, the remarkable similarity in gene order between *E. coli* and *S. typhimurium* is illustrated by a region of about 10% of the *S. typhimurium* genome which is reversed in *E. coli*. This conservation in gene order and apparent rearrangement may reflect selective pressures on gene order and IS

Table 9.5. Properties of some insertion sequences and composite transposons

	Base pairs	Copy number in *E. coli* K12	Target duplication (base pairs)	Inverted repeat (base pairs)
Insertion sequences				
IS1	768	4–12*	8–11	24 (20)
IS2	1327	4–13	5	41 (32)
IS3	1400	5/6	3–4	38 (32)
IS4	1426	1/2	11–13	18 (6)
IS5	1195	10/11	4	16 (15)
IS30	1250	2–8	?	26 (23)
IS10R	1057	0	9	18
IS50R	1534	0	9	9 (8)

	Kilobase pairs	Flanking IS element	Determinant gene
Composite transposons			
Tn10	9.3	IS10 (IR)	Tet^r
Tn9	2.6	IS1 (DR)	Cam^r
Tn5	5.7	IS50 (DR)	Km^r
Tn1681	2.1	IS1 (IR)	Heat stable enterotoxin

*There may be between 0 and 30 copies of IS1 in other strains of *E. coli*. IS1 is also present as multiple copies in *Klebsiella* spp., *Serratia* spp., *Salmonella* spp., *Yersinia* spp. and up to 200 copies in *Shigella dysenteriae*. IR indicates inverted repeats and DR indicates direct repeats.
Not all inverted repeat sequences are accurately copied and the figures in parentheses indicate the number of base pairs in the inverted repeat regions that are exact copies.
Tet^r, Cam^r, Km^r; resistance to tetracycline, chloramphenicol and kanamycin.

mediated rearrangements. If two IS elements in the same DNA molecule are all that are required to make a composite transposon, then the genome might be considered to be composed of a series of linked transposons. It appears that the genes which encode some of the superantigens, for example toxic shock syndrome toxin 1 and the staphylococcal enterotoxins, are carried on transposons which have either plasmid or chromosomal locations (Chapter 2). Certainly the acquisition of transposons, many of which are composite transposons, has allowed the rapid evolution of plasmids. It is therefore perhaps not surprising that many virulence determinants are associated with transposons and are mobile in both the chromosome and plasmids.

ANTIGENIC DRIFT

Antigenic drift can be defined here as the slow accumulation of mutations in the structural genes for surface components of the bacterial pathogen. (See above for the molecular mechanisms by which such mutations arise.) All bacterial species show this interstrain variation of surface antigens; for example, variations in flagellar and lipopolysaccharide or O-antigens of *Salmonella* spp.

The interstrain surface antigen variants of bacteria are termed **serotypes** or **serovars**. Detailed studies of the serotypes associated with infections have provided useful indications of the source(s) of the outbreaks of infection. These studies are of the **epidemiology** of an infection and provide a clear basis upon which to study the genetic diversity and structure of pathogenic bacterial populations. Although the identification of a different serotype provides a convenient way of discriminating between different outbreaks of disease, it does not always imply a clonal relationship between the serotypes. A more detailed analysis of the genetic variability of different serotypes often reveals surprising results. This has been done by employing a technique known as **multilocus enzyme electrophoresis**. This technique offers a more subtle way of indicating how closely related two strains of bacteria are and involves measuring the mobility of specific enzymes upon electrophoresis. These are often common metabolic enzymes such as dehydrogenases which can be easily stained in starch and polyacrylamide gels in the presence of other proteins. Electrophoretic mobility variants (i.e. enzymes which have slightly altered amino acid sequences and hence a different overall charge) migrate to different positions on the gels. The degree of difference in mobility directly reflects changes in amino acid sequence that may have occurred. Other techniques of determining relatedness include DNA hydridisation studies, comparison of restriction endonuclease digestion patterns and direct comparison of available DNA sequences.

Three general points have emerged from such studies. Firstly, pathogen populations are largely clonal and it is unlikely that there is a large degree of recombination between various strains or clones. The variation in populations appears to have accumulated separately. An exception may be *Neisseria gonorrhoeae* where there appears to be a high degree of recombination between clones. *N. gonorrhoeae* is also unusual in that it is strictly a human pathogen which does not colonise any other environment. Secondly, the number of clones of many pathogenic bacteria isolated appears to be much lower than expected when considering the level of diversity possible at the loci examined. Thirdly, the majority of cases of infection are brought about by a small proportion of the possible clones in the overall population. In other words, there is less diversity in pathogenic strains than in non-pathogenic strains. This perhaps provides a confusing picture of variation in bacterial populations; however, it is not surprising that successful pathogens have many highly conserved functions. Instead, it appears that all of these bacteria may have evolved pre-programmed mechanisms to generate antigenic diversity. Some of these are discussed in detail below.

MECHANISMS OF ANTIGENIC AND PHASE VARIATION

Either antigenic variation, whereby the structure of an antigen is qualitatively varied or phase variation, whereby a structure is present or absent, can be brought about through genetic rearrangements. Unlike the mechanisms that are responsible for the switch on or off of virulence associated genes in response to environmental signals (environmental modulation), these changes can be said to be 'random changes'. However, since random changes are brought about by rearrangements of DNA these may be 'programmed rearrangements'. It seems that many pathogenic bacteria have evolved DNA sequences that are ordered in such a way that they are more likely to rearrange. This may involve one of four general mechanisms: (a) sequence specific recombinations, (b) additions or deletions involving oligonucleotide repeat sequences, (c) additions or deletions to homopolymeric repeat sequences and (d) RecA mediated homologous recombinations between multiple copies of related gene sequences.

It is also possible that variation may be brought about through mechanisms that do not involve DNA rearrangements. For example DNA adenine (*dam*) methylation may control phase variation of the Pap pili in *E. coli*.

Many bacteria are capable of using more than one mechanism for generating new variants and some of these are summarised in Table 9.6.

Sequence specific recombinations

In order to illustrate the possible mechanisms it is best to consider a number of examples of commonly studied pathogenic bacteria. The relative roles of each of the mechanisms will be compared for each pathogen.

Table 9.6. Some examples of molecular mechanisms for the generation of genetic variation in pathogenic bacteria

	Bacterium		Gene and determinant affected
Sequence specific recombinations	S. typhimurium	hin	H1/H2 flagella
	E. coli	fim	Fimbriae
	E. coli/pR721	pil	Pilins*
	Moraxella bovis	tfp	Pilins
Additions or deletions to oligonucleotide repeats	N. gonorrhoeae/ meningitidis	opa	Opacity proteins
	H. influenzae	lic	LPS antigens
	H. influenzae	hif	Fimbriae
	Streptococcus spp.	emm	M Protein
Additions or deletions to homopolymeric repeats	B. pertussis	bvgS	Virulence associated gene
	B. pertussis		Fimbriae
	N. gonorrhoeae	fim	Pilins
	N. meningitidis	pil	Opacity proteins
	Y. pestis	opc	Adhesin
	Mycoplasma hyorhinis	yad (yopA) vlp	Lipoprotein
RecA mediated homologous recombinations	N. gonorrhoeae		Pilins
	H. influenzae	pil cap	Capsule
DNA methylation	E. coli	pap	Pili

*Not covered in the text.

Flagellar antigenic variation in Salmonella typhimurium

This was the first such mechanism of this type to be characterised and is one of the best documented. The mechanism by which the bacterium switches between two different flagellar variants involves a site specific recombination. Historically this variation has been termed phase variation, and is still considered by some authors as an example of phase variation as there is a defined switch between expression of two flagellar types; however, the ultimate effect of this switch is a qualitative change in the flagella present at the bacterial cell surface, effectively antigenic variation. As early as 1922 it was known that clones of *Salmonella* contain two distinct flagellar serotypes, type H1 and type H2. By 1949 it was clear that, depending on the strains used, the bacteria were able to switch from H1 to H2 flagella and vice versa at frequencies 10^{-3} to 10^{-5} per cell per generation. This was an unusually high frequency of genetic variation brought about through the alternate expression of two unlinked (i.e. separated on the *Salmonella* chromosome) genes which encoded the respective H1 and H2 flagellar proteins. In the 1950s, genetic experiments involving phage transduction crosses (where *Salmonella* specific B22 bacteriophage are used to transfer DNA from one strain to another followed by homologous recombination) showed that the state of the H2 gene, or a very closely associated piece of controlling DNA, determined whether H1 or H2 genes were expressed. When H2 was expressed and the closely associated controlling element was active, then expression of H1 was repressed. Transductional transfer of the H2 gene to an H1 strain where H2 was not active resulted in recombinants which had almost all switched to H2 expression and repressed the expression of H1. The reverse experiment where H1 genes were transduced into H2 expressing cells did not result in a switch of expression from H2 to H1. Hence the H2 gene alone appeared to determine which flagellum was expressed. It was not until the late 1970s using the, then, modern molecular biology techniques that the nature of the mechanism by which H2 expression controlled H1 expression became clear. This is summarised in Figure 9.15. When the H2 gene is expressed a repressor protein (rH1) for H1 is also expressed from the same operon. The promoter which produces the polycistronic mRNA for H2 and rH1 resides in a 970 base pair sequence of DNA which can invert at a relatively high frequency. Through this inversion H2 can be switched ON or OFF. The inversion is brought about by

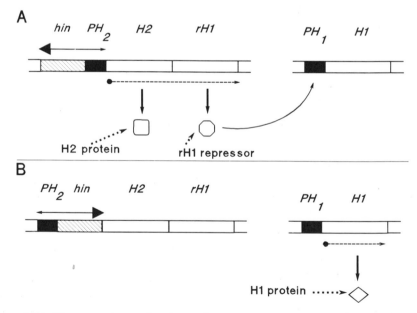

Figure 9.15. The genetic mechanism of antigenic variation in flagellar antigen expression in *Salmonella typhimurium*. When the invertible region of DNA (*hin*) is in one orientation (A) the H2 antigen is expressed along with a repressor protein (rH1) which prevents expression of the H1 protein. With *hin* in the opposite orientation (B) neither H2 nor rH1 is expressed and H1 flagellar antigen is produced

the action of the *hin* gene product, termed the **recombinase**, which recognises the 26 base pair inverted repeat ends (*hix-L* and *hix-R*) of the invertible segment of DNA. Deletions into the invertible sequence eliminated the inversion of DNA and hence the antigenic variation. Also the 26 base pair inverted repeat sequences are strictly necessary for the mechanism to work. Both the sequence of the *hin* gene and the inverted repeat sequences that the *hin* gene product recognises show a close relationship to functionally related sequences in other DNA inversion systems. For example there is a highly conserved consensus sequence in the left (L) and right (R) inverted repeat *hix*, *gix*, *cix* and *pix* sequences in the H1/H2 system and bacteriophages Mu, P1 and the defective *E. coli* prophage e14. These are compared in Table 9.7. In the case of the phages Mu and P1 the low frequency inversion of DNA sequences determines the host range of the phage. Not surprisingly, there is also a close relationship between the Hin recombinase amino acid sequence and those of the related recombinases. Between 60 and 70% of the amino acids are identical for *hin*, *gin*, *cin* and *pin*. There is also some similarity to the amino acid sequence of the TnpR resolvase of Tn3-like transposable elements (see above).

The inversion of DNA has been demonstrated on supercoiled plasmid DNA substrates in cell free systems and, in addition to the recombinase (*hin*, *gin* or *cin*), only buffer, NaCl and Mg^{2+} need to be added. It is likely that other bacterial proteins, often called (bacterial) host factors, are also involved. This is not surprising when one considers that a very specific recombination between sequences 996 base pairs apart has to be mediated by bringing the pairs of sequence into close proximity. Although recognition of a 26 base pair inverted repeat sequence by Hin is required, Table

Table 9.7. A comparison of inverted repeat sequences associated with DNA inversions in bacteria and phage

Inversion system		Inverted repeat sequence		
		−13	1+1	+13
Consensus sequence		---TT-TC--AAACCAAGGTTT	--GA-AA---	
Salmonella	*hix*-L	---TT-T----AAACCAAGGTTT	--GA-AA---	
(*hin*)	*hix*-R	---TT-TC-------AAGGTTT	--GA-AA---	
P1 phage	*cix*-L	---TT-TC--AAACCAAGGTTT	--GA------	
(*cin*)	*cix*-R	---TT-TC--AAACCAAGGTTT	--GA-aa---	
Mu phage	*gix*-L	---TT-----AAACC--GGTTT	--GA-AA---	
(*gin*)	*gix*-R	---TT-----AAACC--GGTTT	--GA-AA---	
e14 Phage	*pix*-L	---TT-TC--AAACCAAggttt	--ga-a----	
(*pin*)	*pix*-R	---TT-TC--AAACCAA---tt	--ga-a----	

Lower case a, g, t represents bases in the sequence outside the inverted repeat when in the ON configuration. Recombination occurs precisely at the −1/+1 AA bases.

9.7 clearly shows that the L and R sequences are not accurate inverted repeats. Instead there seems to be a combination of two near perfect 12 base pair repeats separated by a 2 base pair core at the centre of the recombination site. Purified Hin protein can catalyse double strand cleavage at these 2 base pairs at a low rate in cell free systems and binds to each inverted repeat sequence. Cin and Gin recombinases like Hin are hydrophobic 21 kDa proteins which form insoluble aggregates and appear to have identical functions. There is a strong dependence on orientation and only a very low level of recombination is possible between direct repeats of the sequence and sequences on different plasmids. However, other factors in addition to the direct repeat sequences are required for recombination. Deletion and insertion mutational studies have shown that a sequence within 200 base pairs of the *hix-L* inverted repeat sequence is also required for efficient inversion at the normal level. A 60 base pair sequence separated from *hix-L* is required to enhance recombination and is termed a **recombinational enhancer**. There are similar recombinational enhancer sequences in the *gin* and *cin* systems. The presence of this sequence increases the inversion rate 20-fold and in the presence of a host bacterium (in these studies *E. coli*) protein called Fis (*f*actor for *i*nversion *s*timulation) the inversion rate can be increased by up to 150-fold. The Fis protein has been purified and is shown to bind to the recombinational enhancer sequence. Mutations in the *fis* gene do not appear to affect growth of the *E. coli* cells. A clue to how Fis protein binding to the recombination enhancer sequence might increase the recombination rate probably lies in its ability to bend the DNA it binds to. The Fis protein can also bind to and bend a sequence near the lambda prophage attachment site in *E. coli* and hence stimulate excision of the lambda phage. However, there is no close homology between this sequence and the *hin* recombinational enhancer sequence and it is probable that Fis binds to a particular shape of DNA and not a specific sequence. Fis protein is similar in its interaction with DNA to the well characterised IHF (*i*ntegration *h*ost *f*actor) protein which promotes the integration of lambda phage in *E. coli*. IHF consists of two protein subunits encoded by the *E. coli hip* and *himD* genes. Like Fis, this dimeric protein can bind to and bend DNA and both proteins are thought to bring the sequences necessary for recombination into close proximity prior to the recombination reaction. Because of their apparent function both Fis and IHF feature strongly in a number of other models for recombination in *E. coli*. Another important host protein is HU, which is able to stimulate Hin-mediated recombination by 10-fold. This only works well when the recombinational enhancer sequence is at an optimal distance (100 to 350 base pairs) from the site of recombination. Hence HU does not appear to affect the inversion rate in Gin- and Cin-mediated recombinations as the recombinational enhancer sequences are less than 100 base pairs and over 400 base pairs from the recombination sites respectively. HU is a histone-like protein normally associated with *E. coli* DNA. Its function also appears to be to maintain the DNA shape necessary to bring the inverted sequences into close proximity. An overall model for this process is shown in Figure 9.16.

Antigenic and phase variation of pilus expression in Moraxella bovis and Moraxella lacunata

Moraxella bovis, which causes keratoconjunctivitis in cattle, produces two types of pilin called the Q(β) and I(α) pilins. These belong to the N-methyl-phenylalanine family of pilins commonly found in Gram negative bacteria (see Chapter 7) and are encoded by the *tfpQ* and *tfpI* genes. Switching between expression of these two types of pilin takes place through inversion of a 2.1 kilobase pair sequence of DNA. In this case expression is controlled by inversion of the sequence encoding the pilin genes and not the sequence for the promoter. In one orientation the *tfpI* gene is adjacent to the promoter whereas in the reverse orientation the *tfpQ* gene is adjacent to the promoter (antigenic variation). The end points for the inverted

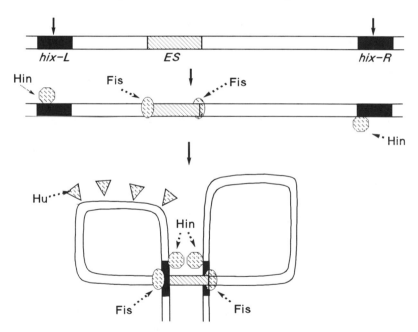

Figure 9.16. The structure and mechanism of DNA bending which mediates inversion of the invertible *hin* region in *Salmonella typhimurium*. The element is flanked by inverted repeat DNA sequences *hix-L* and *hix-R* at which the *hin* recombinase binds. The host encoded Fis protein binds at a recombinational enhancer sequence (ES) within the *hin* element and bends the DNA. This also involves binding by the histone-like protein Hu

sequence are within the pilin genes. Hence any inaccuracies in the insertion can lead to a frameshift mutation or the production of a mis-sense pilin protein. Either event could bring about the pilin minus phenotype observed in some variants (phase variation). Despite the gross differences between the *Moraxella* inversion system and that of the *Salmonella hin* system, there are remarkable similarities which suggest that there are closely related recombinational mechanisms in operation. The recombination site is located in a 26 base pair region which shows some homology to the *hixL* sequence in *S. typhimurium*. There is also a 60 base pair sequence within the invertible region of DNA which shows 50% homology to the recombinational enhancer sequence in the *cin* inversion system of phage P1 (which is in turn related to the *hin* recombinational enhancer sequence). It is likely that, although members of the *hin* family of invertible sequences are more closely related, both *hin* and the *Moraxella* inversion systems are evolutionarily related. However, genetic analysis of the similar pathogen *Moraxella lacunata*, which causes human conjunctivitis, has revealed the presence of an inversion recombinase gene termed *piv* adjacent to a similar invertible sequence of DNA. A closely related gene with 98% homology is also present immediately adjacent to the invertible sequence in *M. bovis* and both can complement each other in *trans*. Surprisingly there is no amino acid sequence similarity between the *piv* genes and the *hin* family of recombinases or the related transposon Tn3 resolvases.

Phase variation of fimbriae in E. coli

In the case of *E. coli* another inversion mechanism controls the switching ON or OFF of a single fimbrial gene, *fimA*. The overall mechanism is outlined in Figure 9.17 and is different in many respects to that operating in the *Salmonella hin* system. The *fimA* gene encodes the major protein subunit for the type 1 'mannose sensitive' fimbriae (see Chapter 7). The whole of the *fim* region has been cloned in *E. coli* plasmids and, in addition to expression of the *fimA* gene, the products of *fim* genes *C, D* (for secretion and assembly), *H* (the adhesin) and structural genes *F* and *G* are required for the production of fully functional adhering fimbriae. In the absence of *fimG* there is an increase in the rate of inversion suggesting that the product of this gene represses the recombination process. However, clones expressing *fimA* alone can produce non-functional fimbriae and this has simplified the genetic studies of the inversion mechanism. The sequence of DNA inverted is 314 base pairs and contains a promoter sequence necessary for the transcription of *fimA*. As for the *Salmonella hin* system the inverted region of DNA is also flanked by inverted repeat sequences. However, this sequence is only 9 base pairs and there is no sequence homology with the longer *Salmonella* inverted repeat sequence. This indicates the likelihood of a different recombination mechanism. Indeed, unlike the invertible

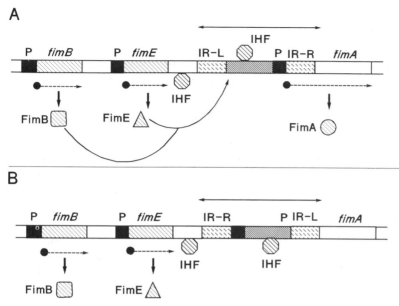

Figure 9.17. The genetic mechanism of ON/OFF phase variation in expression of fimbriae in *Escherichia coli*. An invertible sequence of DNA bounded by inverted repeats IR-L and IR-R in one orientation (A) leads to expression of the major fimbrial protein FimA. In the other orientation (B) FimA is not expressed. Inversion is mediated by FimE and FimB proteins expressed by genes outside the invertible DNA sequence. Binding of bacterial encoded integration host factor (IHF) protein enhances the recombination by bending the DNA

sequence in *Salmonella*, there is no internal *hin* like gene, *hin* cannot complement the functions of *fimE* or *fimB* which are responsible for mediating the inversion and which show no homology to *hin*. In one orientation, the *fimA* gene is transcribed and fimbriae are produced. In the opposite orientation the genes *fimE* and *fimB* are transcribed and fimbriae expression is switched off. Along with the two subunits of integration host factor (IHF), both *fimE* and *fimB* are required for the inversion to take place. The action of the genes *fimA* and *fimB* determines the orientation of the switch. In the absence of both genes there is no inversion and *fimA* expression is either permanently ON or OFF. When only *fimE* is functioning and *fimB* is inactivated, then the switch can only go in the direction of *fimA* ON to *fimA* OFF. The protein sequences of the *fimA* and *E* genes show 48% identity to each other and are also significantly similar to a number of integrase proteins responsible for mediating integration of lambda phage DNA into the *E. coli* chromosome. This strongly implies that both *fimA* and *fimE* are recombinases. However, it is possible that these genes, unlike *hin*, are responsible for directing the action of a bacterial recombination function. Certainly both *fimE* and *fimB* appear to play another non-recombinational role in regulating the level of expression of *fimA* and production of fimbriae. Mutations in the *fimE* gene lead to a higher level of expression of fimbriae per cell (hyper-fimbriation) whereas there are fewer fimbriae per cell in *fimB* mutants. Hence the *fimE* product represses the *fimA* promoter in the invertible region whereas the *fimB* product is an activator.

Additions or deletions involving oligonucleotide repeat sequences

The addition or deletion of a variable number of tandemly repeated short sequences of DNA situated upstream of structural genes (at the 5' end) is a mechanism by which the antigenicity of cell surface proteins and LPS can be varied in a range of pathogenic bacteria. This may either affect transcription of the genes through altering the promoter sequence or affect translation of the mRNA by altering the reading frame. Hence, instead of switching between the expression of two alternative genes, as happens in site specific inversions, this mechanism could also be used to switch between a greater number of protein variants and hence antigenic possibilities. The loss or gain of tandem repeats is thought to occur during the replication of DNA by a process known as slipped-strand mispairing. Single strand breaks may arise as a consequence of the sequence and degree of negative supercoiling in the region. For example single strand breaks can arise in A-T rich sequences when supercoiled. A combination of exonuclease degradation of the single stranded DNA and repair synthesis may lead to a decrease or increase in the number of tandem repeats in the sequence respectively. However, although a compelling hypothesis for explaining how variations in the number of tandem repeats can arise it is by no means proven experimentally. This process appears to be independent of homologous recombination and RecA function in the mechanisms that control opacity protein expression in *Neisseria* and LPS expression in *Haemophilus influenzae* (see below). In other cases RecA may play a role but this remains to be determined experimentally.

The means by which variations in tandem repeats of oligonucleotide can alter the expression of surface antigens in some pathogenic bacteria are detailed below.

Variation of the opacity proteins in Neisseria gonorrhoeae and Neisseria meningitidis

One of the distinctive features of pathogenic *Neisseria* species is the high degree of antigenic variation exhibited in pilin proteins and the surface opacity proteins. In this bacterium there are mechanisms for phase and antigenic variation operating together.

The mechanism by which pilin variation is mediated is discussed below under RecA mediated homologous recombinations between multiple copies of related gene sequences. The opacity proteins (Opas or PII, see Chapter 7) are involved in mediating adherence of the bacterium to epithelial cells and are also a major factor in recognition of the bacteria by polymorphonuclear phagocytes. Hence a number of antigenic variants would be a distinct advantage to the invading bacterium. *N. gonorrhoeae* contains at least 11 and up to 13 intact *opa* genes. These are commonly different variants of the same gene and not all are expressed. However, in *N. meningitidis* and *N. lactamica* (a human commensal *Neisseria* species) there are between two and four equivalent *opa* genes. The possibility of recombination between copies of the *opa* genes as a source of variation will also be discussed below. Genetic studies of the regulation of expression of multiple variants of the *opa* gene led to the conclusion that there was no *trans* acting regulatory mechanism and that regulation was determined in *cis*. *Neisseria* species are unusual in that it is relatively easy to bring about efficient uptake of naked DNA molecules into the cells. This is termed transformation and is accompanied by an efficient RecA mediated homologous recombination process. When Opa⁻ strains of *Neisseria* are transformed with DNA preparations from different Opa⁺ variants the resulting Opa proteins produced by the recipient cells after recombination are the same as in the donor cells. Hence a *cis*-acting controlling sequence accompanies the newly recombined donor *opa* DNA sequence. There appears to be no control at the level of transcription and not all *opa* gene transcripts are translated into a stable and functional Opa protein at the cell surface. A clue to the *cis*-acting translational control mechanism lies in the sequences of the various *opa* genes. The sequence first transcribed in the *opa* genes is a series of pentameric repeats consisting of CTCTT. The number of these short repeats can vary from 7 to 28 units. This part of the *opa* structural gene encodes the hydrophobic core of a transport signal sequence of amino acids which are responsible for locating the Opa protein at the cell surface.

Sequence analysis of the various copies of the *opa* genes shows that there are variable numbers of the CTCTT pentameric repeats present. This means that deletions or additions to the number of pentameric units will lead to the possibility of frameshifts occurring. Hence the same sequence will not always be translated to a functional protein depending on the number of pentameric repeats. Indeed, DNA primer extension experiments using mRNA as template, and designed to determine the sequence of each *opa* transcript present, showed that the number of repeated units correlated with the sequence of each *opa* gene. The expression of Opa corresponds precisely to the number of pentameric repeats transcribed. Extending or deleting the sequence by precisely three pentameric units leads to the production of functional Opa protein as a frameshift does not occur in this case. However, a loss or gain of one or two units leads to loss of Opa expression. Therefore some *opa* gene variants are in the ON state and others in the OFF state. The phase and antigenic variation are generated by the constitutive expression of mRNA from multiple copies of the *opa* genes, which encode different Opa variants. As a result of variation in the number of copies of CTCTT sequences in the leader sequence of DNA only some of the mRNA will be in frame and generate functional protein. The constitutive expression of mRNA is therefore a wasteful process. That the bacterium makes such a commitment to this mechanism suggests that there is a strong selective pressure in favour of the generation of variable Opa proteins. *N. gonorrhoeae* also generates fimbrial variants but by a different mechanism (see below).

An example showing the possible configuration of *opa* genes is shown in Figure 9.18. The process of varying the number of repeat units is very frequent and occurs in approximately 1 in 100 cells. This process is known to be entirely independent of homologous recombination and RecA in *Neisseria*. Direct repeats of DNA sequence are generally unstable in bacterial genomes and one hypothesis is that a process of slipped-strand mispairing occurs during DNA replication. Essentially this means that the replicase complex somehow misses one or more repeats out and jumps to the same sequence repeated downstream on the template thereby deleting the

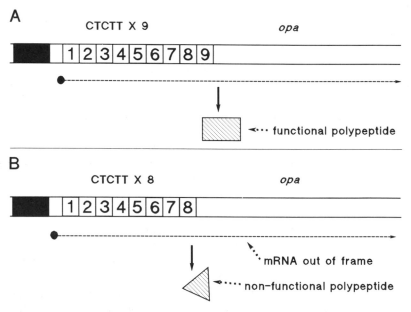

Figure 9.18. Multiple repeats of the pentameric DNA sequence CTCTT control antigenic and phase variation of the opacity protein gene (*opa*) in *Neisseria gonorrhoeae*. In the examples illustrated, 9 repeats (A) leads to a functional Opa protein whereas a deletion to 8 repeats (B) leads to a frameshift and a non-functional polypeptide

intervening sequence. One possibility is that due to a high degree of negative supercoiling there may be regions of triple stranded DNA (known as **H-DNA**) where there are a number of direct repeats of a short sequence. This extra strand of DNA could act as an alternative template for slipped-strand mispairing. Although not finally proven this seems a compelling explanation for deletions arising. However, it does not easily explain how the same mechanism might lead to the insertion or deletion of the repeat sequences.

Lipopolysaccharide antigenic variation in Haemophilus influenzae

Monoclonal antibodies raised to distinct oligosaccharides in the LPS of *H. influenzae* strains have demonstrated extensive antigenic variation. Also reversible loss of specific oligosaccharide subunits occurs at a high frequency. Determining the molecular basis for variation of surface proteins is relatively straightforward when compared to the complexities of determining what controls the expression of polysaccharide components. This is simply due to the fact that for proteins there is one structural gene variant leading to one variant surface protein. In the case of LPS and other polysaccharides, there are many genes which encode the enzymes of the biosynthetic pathway and there is no direct relationship between the gene sequence and the final product. In *H. influenzae* (and other bacteria such as *Neisseria* spp. *Bordetella pertussis* and *Bacteroides fragilis*) the LPS is composed of lipid A, an inner core oligosaccharide and an outer oligosaccharide (see Appendix Figure A11). Extensive variations have been shown to occur in all three main components of the LPS. Although there are no full structural details determined for all of the various LPS variants, the use of monoclonal antibodies raised to some of the variable and specific saccharide components and structures has led to a partial understanding of how switching of antigenic types occurs. In *H. influenzae* there are at least two antigenically distinct lipid A components expressed. Monoclonal antibodies raised against variants in the core oligosaccharide have shown the presence of two antigenically variable structures or epitopes at the terminus of the core namely Gal(α1-4)Gal and Gal(β1-4)GlcNAc. The former epitope cross-reacts with a human blood-group antigen which is coincidentally the receptor for the PapG adhesin of *E. coli*. The epitope is also present in *N. gonorrhoeae* and is indicative of the cross-reactivity that can occur between *H. influenzae* and *Neisseria*. Other monoclonal antibody studies with variants of the whole LPS structure of one serological grouping, *H. influenzae* type b strains, has revealed three major antigenic groups. These have been defined largely by the use of two monoclonal antibodies which bind to two distinct epitopes on different LPS molecules. The genes for the expression of the two LPS types have been mapped to two distinct loci termed *lic1* and *lic2*. Considerable switching and variation has been determined for these loci in cultures, single colonies and even on the surface of individual bacterial cells. The frequency of loss or gain of these epitopes varies but is usually at least 10^{-2} per cell per generation. The situation is clearly very complex as the loss of up to six distinct epitopes can occur concurrently as well as the independent loss of single epitopes. The potential for many combinations leading to diversity in LPS structure is therefore extensive. The *lic1* locus consists of four genes in order, *licA, B, C, D*. Although the functions of the genes in the *lic* loci have not been fully determined, they are clearly involved in LPS expression. Deletions in *lic1* DNA cloned into a *H. influenzae* strain which did not cross-react with antibodies specific for the original type b strain led to a loss of expression of two epitopes. The *lic1* locus also contains a consensus promoter sequence upstream of the first *licA* gene and a *rho*-independent termination sequence downstream of *licD*. Sequence analysis of phase variants has shown that the number of tetrameric CAAT tandem repeat sequences in *licA* determines the phase variation. There are usually about 30 tandem repeats. By fusing the lacZ gene into the *lic1* locus in frame with *licD* it was possible to determine quickly when the *lic* genes were switched on or off as the activity of the β-galactosidase enzyme (β-Gal) encoded by *lacZ* can be detected colorimetrically. Resulting colonies showed highly variable switching between β-Gal⁺ and β-Gal⁻ phenotypes and this process is independent of the action of RecA. When DNA from single colonies was amplified by polymerase chain reaction and individual sequences determined it was clear that expression of the fused β-Gal was correlated with the number of tandem repeats, but not in any simple way. With 29 copies of CAAT repeated the sequence was out of frame but there was either a low level of β-Gal expression or no expression in clones. Clones with 30 copies were not found and with 31 copies the sequence was in frame and clones showed either a high level of β-Gal expression or no expression. The repeats of CAAT appear to determine both the level of expression of the *lic1* genes and antigenic switching and clearly another mechanism or group of mechanisms is operating. Certainly *licD* appears to be expressed from a polycistronic message and is not under the control of an independent promoter. This complexity is confirmed by the discovery of other related loci. By using DNA probes of repeated CAAT sequences, two other *lic* loci have been cloned, *lic2*, which was already determined and an additional *lic3* locus. *lacZ* gene-fusions in the *lic3* locus have shown that there are three possible levels of β-Gal expression depending upon the number of CAAT repeats as well as phase variation. How expression of the *lic* genes from their respective promoters is affected by the number of CAAT repeats remains to be determined.

Surface antigen expression involving dinucleotide repeats

Variation in the numbers of dinucleotide repeat sequences can also determine the switching on or off of surface antigens. The expression of fimbriae in *H. influenzae* is determined by two genes *hifA*, which encodes the structural protein, and *hifB*, another essential protein called a chaperone protein. Switching between fimbriae on and fimbriae off is controlled at the transcriptional level. The *hifA* and *hifB* genes are transcribed on opposite templates in different directions from the promoter region. The spacing sequence between the promoters is filled by a variable number of TA dinucleotide repeats, which overlap with the −35 and −10 sequences of both opposing promoters. The structure is shown in Figure 9.19. The length of the spacing sequence between the −35 and −10 sequences is very important for binding of RNA polymerase. Maximal expression of both genes takes place when there are 10 AT repeats. A greater or lesser number of repeats leads to loss of expression. However, the possible role of RecA in this process has not been determined.

Additions or deletions to homopolymeric repeated DNA sequences

Homopolymeric repeated DNA sequences are long repeats of the same nucleotide. Variations in the length of such sequences have been shown to determine the expression of surface antigens in a number of bacteria. This can take place either through transcriptional control, whereby the efficiency of a promoter is affected, or by translational control, whereby a gene is in frame or not.

In *Bordetella pertussis* there is coordinate regulation of many virulence determinants by the action of gene products from the *bvg* locus (environmental modulation; see below). There is also a genetic switch between virulent and non-virulent types determined by insertions or deletions in 6 cytidines (polyC sequence) within the *bvgS* gene which enco-

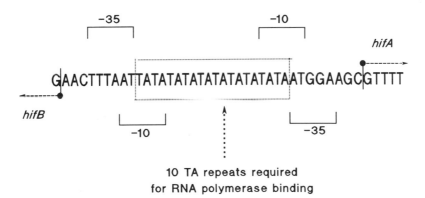

Figure 9.19. The genetic mechanism of fimbrial phase variation in *Haemophilus influenzae*. Variation is determined by the number of TA repeat sequences in the promoters of two of the fimbrial structural genes *hifA* and *hifB*. For optimal expression from the opposing promoters, there must be 10 TA repeats

des one of the key *bvg* regulatory proteins. Additions or deletions cause a frameshift, leading to a non-functional BvgS protein and a change from a virulent to non-virulent state. In addition to this mechanism there is fimbrial phase variation controlled at the level of transcription. Expression of frimbriae is determined by polyC sequences in the promoter regions of the *fim2* (15 cytosines) and *fim3* (13 cytosines) genes. As for the dinucleotide repeats in the promoter region of the *hif* genes of *H. influenzae* (see above), the activity of the promoters is affected. However, in this case, there are no −35 sequences and the length of the polyC sequences, which are located 70 base pairs upstream, determines the distance between the site of an activator protein and the −10 RNA polymerase binding site.

Similarly, in *Mycoplasma hyorhinis*, antigenic variation in the expression of surface lipoproteins encoded on the *vlp* genes is determined at the transcriptional level by the length of a polyA sequence between the −35 and −10 regions of the promoter. With 17 adenines there is efficient transcription, otherwise the genes are switched off. In addition there is evidence that the expression of the Opc opacity proteins in *Neisseria meningitidis* is determined by a 10 to 14 polyC sequence between the −35 and −10 regions of the promoter. This variation is in addition to that in the Opa proteins of this bacterium detailed earlier.

In *N. gonorrhoeae*, *Yersinia pestis* and *Yersinia pseudotuberculosis* the length of polynucleotide sequences determines phase variation through frameshifts and translational control. In the case of the phase variation in the PilC protein of *N. gonorrhoeae*, there is a polyG sequence in the part of the sequence coding for the leader peptide needed for transport of this protein to the outside of the cell and assembly of a pilus. Sequence changes in this region lead to frameshifts and no assembled pili. In *Yersinia* spp. the *yad* (*yopA* or *yop1*) gene encodes an outer membrane protein which is involved in the adhesion of *Y. pseudotuberculosis* prior to its invasion of epithelial cells. Interestingly, Yad expression is switched off in the highly virulent *Y. pestis*. The difference is due to a single base deletion in a 15 nucleotide polyA sequence causing a frameshift. A similar deletion in the polyA sequence of *Y. pestis* reduces its virulence (see Chapter 8).

RecA mediated homologous recombinations between multiple copies of related gene sequences and within single gene sequences

The use of homologous recombination as a mechanism to generate antigenic variation in pathogenic bacteria is widespread. The ability to generate variants is dependent upon there being more than one copy of the genes involved in the same cell or repeated sequences within a single gene. Sequence variations in such genes may arise through point mutation and antigenic drift or through programmed rearrangements. However they arise, recombinations between variants of the genes will lead to further variants. In addition to this general mechanism, not all of the copies of a functional gene need to be expressed and there may be recombinations between non-expressed loci and expressed and fully functional loci. This means that mutations can accumulate within the non-expressed loci without affecting function yet contribute to the variability of functional and expressed loci through homologous recombination.

Variation in the *pil* genes of *Neisseria gonorrhoeae* is a good example of how this can work. There is considerable antigenic variation in the pilins produced by this bacterium despite the fact that pilin is expressed from one gene termed *pilE* (for Expression). The variability is, however, not surprising when it is clear that there are at least 10 different silent *pilS* loci with close sequence homology to the *pilE* gene. These cannot be expressed and are not functional as they lack the largely invariant amino-terminus portion of the protein. Variants can arise because of intergenomic recombination within a single cell; however, this is not the complete story. *N. gonorrhoeae* is very efficient at taking up DNA into its cells by a process of transformation. Hence intragenomic recombinations using DNA from lysed neighbouring cells can also contribute to *pil* variation (Figure 9.20). This process occurs at a frequency of about 1 in 1000 cells per generation. As well as determining antigenic variation this process is also responsible for

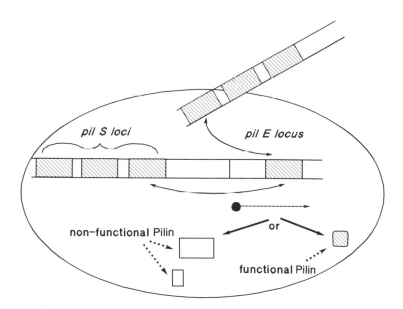

Figure 9.20. Antigenic variation in the Pilin protein of *Neisseria gonorrhoeae*. This is determined by RecA mediated recombinations between silent *pilS* loci and an expressed *pilE* locus. This may involve DNA acquired from other bacteria by transformation

phase variation. Two types of non-pilus variant are produced from the *pilE* locus. The L-variants are long non-functional pili produced by recombinations that lead to tandem repeats of the *pilS* sequence in the *pilE* locus. When these are in-frame, long and unstable pilin proteins are produced. Similarly recombinations can lead to the production of soluble or S pili. These are shortened defective pilin proteins which are not assembled and are secreted into the medium.

Other examples of homologous recombinations contributing to antigenic variability are the M protein variants in group A *Streptococcus pyogenes*, the Vmp lipoproteins of *Borrelia* spp. and the capsular polysaccharide variation in *Haemophilus influenzae*. One of the virulence factors of *Streptococcus* spp. is the M protein on the surface of the bacterium (Chapter 7). These are dimeric molecules which vary considerably. As these proteins are firmly attached to the cell surface, they have been difficult to isolate; however, pepsin digestions have allowed partial proteins to be characterised and their amino acid sequences have enabled the intact gene variants to be cloned and sequenced in *E. coli*. Unlike the *pil* genes of *N. gonorrhoeae* only a single gene copy was found. The *emm6* gene encodes the M6 pepsin fragment of the protein and has been studied in detail. Sequencing of the whole of the *emm* gene has revealed a highly complex repetitive structure. The gene encodes a long leader or signal peptide necessary for export of the protein to the outside of the cell. At the carboxy terminus there is a very hydrophobic region thought to prevent complete transfer of the protein through the membrane. Internal to the *emm* gene there are three regions of tandem repeat sequences: one with five direct repeats of 42 base pairs, another with five repeats of 72 base pairs and another with two repeats of 81 base pairs. These repeats are all multiples of three and additions or deletions retain the transcript in frame. Not surprisingly immunological studies using western blots on isolates from small cultures have revealed that variants with smaller M proteins are produced at a frequency of about 1 in 2000 cells per generation. These are generated by homologous recombination between the extensive repeat sequences within a single gene.

The mechanism by which *Borrelia* spp. undergo antigenic variation is similar to that of *Neisseria gonorrhoeae*. The classical relapsing fever caused by *Borrelia* spp. in the blood, which is transmitted by ticks or lice, was considered to be a useful model for studies of the immune system as long ago as 1887. An initial fever which lasts about 5 days is followed by an apparent recovery of 7 to 9 days and a relapse of fever for 2 to 3 days. This pattern of events may recur. Examination of a mouse relapsing fever, which is caused by *Borrelia hermsii*, revealed that the antigenic variation of variable membrane lipoproteins occurred as a result of the host specific immune response. This bacterium expresses highly variable lipoproteins (Vmp proteins) at its surface. These are encoded by at least 27 genes which are on large linear plasmids. Most of the genes are partial copies, without a promoter, and are not expressed. Recombination between these silent copies and an expressed copy on one plasmid takes place at a frequency as high as 1 in 1000 and leads to the generation of diverse Vmp types.

Production of type b capsules of *Haemophilus influenzae* (see Chapter 7) is determined by genes at the *cap* locus. Cap⁻ variants arise at a high frequency due to a *recA* dependent process. The *cap* locus contains a duplication of approximately 17 kilobase pairs separated by about 1.3 kilobase pairs. Recombinations between the duplicated regions lead to a loss of the intervening sequence and a key gene, *bexA*, required for expression of the type b capsule. The BexA protein appears to be an ATP binding protein similar to those needed for transport across the periplasm. Hence BexA is probably necessary for transport of the capsule to the outside of the cell. Indeed Cap⁻ variants accumulate capsule components which can be detected immunologically by electron microscopy and immunogold labelling within the periplasmic space. As this process leads to the deletion of a key gene it is not surprising that Cap⁻ variants do not revert to Cap⁺. However, as *Haemophilus influenzae* is known to transform DNA relatively easily, the Cap⁻ variants may be able to take up DNA and revert to Cap⁺ again via a *recA* dependent process.

Antigenic variation and DNA methylation

The phase variation of Pap pili in *E. coli* (see Chapter 7) seems to be unique in that the phase switch is determined by adenine methylation at two Dam methylation sites ($GATC_{1028}$ and $GATC_{1130}$) that are upstream of the *papA* gene which encodes the main pilin protein. In the pilin ON state only the $GATC_{1130}$ site is methylated, whereas only the $GATC_{1028}$ site is methylated when in the pilin OFF state. Normally all of the GATC sites are methylated in *E. coli* (see 'Mutations and Genetic Recombination in Bacteria' earlier) and only become transiently hemimethylated as a DNA replication fork passes. This state would normally be expected to last for a few minutes before the Dam methylase completes full methylation. The unusual non-methylation at the *pap* locus appears to be due to protection of one or other of the GATC sites from Dam methylase action. This is mediated by a methylation blocking factor (Mbf) and PapI. In addition to protecting non-methylated GATC sites, these factors must also be able to bind to and protect hemimethylated GATC sites in order to switch from protection of $GATC_{1130}$ to $GATC_{1028}$ during DNA replication. The switch from either ON to OFF or vice versa would theoretically require two rounds of DNA replication. As this mechanism does not rely on a change of DNA sequence it is not surprising that the frequency of switching is affected by nutritional and environmental changes. For example, low growth temperatures favour pilus ON to OFF transitions. The regulation of pilus expression by DNA methylation perhaps lies at the border between the mechanisms responsible for genetically controlled phase switching of virulence determinants and phenotypically controlled switching of virulence determinants. Some of these phenotypic regulatory mechanisms which are controlled by environmental signals are outlined below.

ENVIRONMENTAL REGULATION OF VIRULENCE DETERMINANT EXPRESSION

The expression of a number of specialised virulence genes in a closely coordinated manner is one of the main factors in determining the success of a pathogenic bacterium. The successful pathogen must recognise signals from the host and express key virulence determinants in order to ensure rapid growth in the host environment. It is therefore no surprise that there exist a number of complex regulatory networks that ensure the expression of these key determinants. These are, in turn, linked to environmental stimuli via sensor systems. The environmental stimuli that trigger virulence gene expression are usually associated with conditions within the host. These include temperature, osmotic and pH changes and low levels of iron and calcium ions. These conditions are not usual in laboratory culture media and virulence determinants are often not evident until analysed in the host or under conditions that mimic the host environment. Many virulence determinants need to be expressed as soon as the host environmental conditions are encountered and they may be switched on by a global cellular response. Other determinants, however, may only be required at key stages of infection and more subtle regulatory mechanisms may operate. Only now is it becoming possible to understand the complex changes which take place in the physiology of a pathogen as it moves from the outside environment into the selective environment of the host.

The diversity and interaction of regulons in bacteria

The regulation of gene expression in bacteria is brought about by a wide range of systems which can work at an almost bewildering number of levels. Virtually all of these might be expected to have some impact on the expression of virulence determinants in pathogenic bacteria. Where the expression of a group of genes is under the control of a single regulator gene product the whole system (i.e. the controlled group of genes, regulator gene and its product) is called a **regulon**. One regulon may control a group of unique and related genes required for a particular cellular function. It is also clear that some regulons control a wider range of genes which may be in other regulons. In a regulon where several genes may be controlled by one regulator, expression of some of the genes may also be influenced by another regulator and also be part of that regulon. Bacterial cellular systems are therefore controlled by a network of overlapping regulons and cascades. Control of gene expression may therefore be complex. The main regulons known to operate in bacteria are listed in Table 9.8. Many of these affect expression of virulence genes, but there are in addition a number of specific virulence regulons. Much information has been obtained about how these systems interact by studying bacteria with mutations in the regulator genes and determining which other genes are affected. The more genes that are affected by the mutation the higher up the controlling gene is in the cellular hierarchy of control. Where a regulator controls more than one gene, the control is termed **pleiotropic**. Regulators which affect a large number of genes are high up in the cellular hierarchy of control and are termed highly pleiotropic.

A system of regulons which is very high in the cellular hierarchy, sometimes referred to as **global regulation**, are those which affect DNA topology and DNA supercoiling. These will be considered below in detail since DNA topology and supercoiling regulation appears to affect the expression of many virulence genes as well as associated phase and antigenic variation recombinations.

Catabolite repression and the heat shock response are also high up in the regulatory hierarchy. Good examples of catabolite repression occur in *E. coli* and *S. typhimurium*. The catabolite repressor protein (CRP) which binds to cyclic AMP (cAMP) (sometimes called the cAMP receptor protein) is responsible for negatively regulating at least 200 genes. Since an active catabolite repression system is necessary for the virulence of *S. typhimurium*, it follows that some of these genes are virulence associated. In *E. coli*, fimbrial expression is influenced by catabolite repression (see Chapter 7, Figure 7.3).

In the heat shock response, a family of heat shock or stress proteins is produced in increased amounts by bacteria in response to, amongst other stimuli, increases in temperature. Many of these proteins are termed molecular **chaperonins** in that they assist the folding of other proteins into their

Table 9.8. Examples of bacterial regulons

Catabolite repression
DNA supercoiling
Stringent response to amino acid starvation
SOS response to DNA damage
Osmotic stress response
Oxidative stress response
Heat shock response
Switch to anaerobic growth
Sporulation in some bacteria
Response to nutrient starvation, e.g. iron, phosphate, carbon or nitrogen

correct conformations. Two of these proteins, GroEL and GroES in *E. coli*, are highly conserved in both prokaryotes and eukaryotes. For example the BCGa antigen of *Mycobacterium tuberculosis* and *M. bovis* is 45% identical to GroES. Another heat shock protein from *E. coli*, DnaK, is closely related immunologically to the 71 kDa antigen of *M. leprae* which is also produced after heat shock. The stresses which promote the production of the 'heat shock' proteins include, as well as heat, starvation, oxidative shock and acid treatment. The heat shock proteins are the immunodominant antigens recognised by the host during infection with some intracellular bacteria. It is likely that the stress response is induced by the rigours of intracellular survival. As a result of the similarities in heat shock proteins between pro-karyotes and eukaryotes their production during an infection may play a role in the triggering of some autoimune diseases (see Chapters 3 and 8).

Another well-studied example of pleiotropic control is the Fur system in *E. coli* in which the genes necessary for iron scavenging and other functions are controlled by the *fur* gene product, which is sensitive to iron concen-tration (see Chapter 5).

A number of other regulons which control virulence genes come into the family of two component environmental sensor/gene regulator systems. These are considered below in more detail along with their environmen-tal signals.

The role of DNA topology and DNA associated proteins in the regulation of virulence determinant expression

In order to effectively package DNA into a bacterial cell it is normally supercoiled. This is brought about by the action of enzymes called **topo-isomerases** (see 'The replication of DNA' earlier in this chapter and Figure 9.2). These are enzymes that affect the **topology** of the DNA. When DNA is in a relaxed circular form without any winding it is under little torsional stress. Winding of the DNA in the same rotational direction as the twisting of the duplex strands can be achieved by breaking and rejoining the DNA. This results in **positive supercoiling**. However, all evidence points to bac-terial DNA being **negatively supercoiled**. This is when the circular DNA is wound in the opposite rotational direction to the twist of the duplex DNA. This is the normal state of DNA in most cells and positively superco-iled DNA is rare. Double-strand breaking and rejoining of DNA to intro-duce the negative supercoils is mediated in *E. coli* by the ATP-dependent DNA gyrase. The reverse reaction to remove the negative supercoils is mediated by DNA topoisomerase I which does not require ATP and intro-duces single strand breaks to untwist the DNA. Negative supercoiling imposes considerable **torsional stress** on the molecule and divides or opens up regions of the duplex DNA structure. DNA in this state is energetically more favourable as a substrate for transcription, recombination, tranpsosition and replication. The balance between the actions of DNA gyrase and topoisomerase I is important in maintaining the optimum level of negative supercoiling and torsional stress. Not surprisingly, any change in the level of DNA supercoiling is likely to affect cellular processes through the control of expression of a wide range of genes. The level of transcription from many promoters appears to be greatly affected by the degree of supercoiling; however, this is not a general effect. Some promoters express at a higher level from relaxed DNA, others from negatively coiled DNA and others do not seem to be affected by supercoiling. Although most of the DNA appears to be supercoiled within the bacterial cells, there is also strong evidence that some of the DNA is affected by the binding of a range of histone-like proteins that also affect the topology of the DNA in the region of binding. Examples of proteins that affect DNA topology are listed in Table 9.9. The role of the histone-like HU, FIS and IHF proteins in the recombinations involved in phase and antigenic variations has been outlined earlier under

Table 9.9. Some proteins that affect DNA topology and expression of virulence genes

Protein (gene)	Function	Effect on virulence gene expression
Topoisomerases		
DNA gyrase (*gyrA/B*)	Promotes −ve supercoiling	Affects phase transitions/recombinations
Topoisomerase I (*topA*)	Relaxes −ve supercoiling	As above
Topoisomerases III (*topB*) and IV (*parC/E*)	Promotes chromosome partitioning	No known effect
Histone-like proteins		
IHF (*himA/D*)	Bends DNA	Affects phase transitions/recombinations
FIS (*fis*)	Bends DNA	As above
HU (*hupB/A*)	Wrapping of DNA	As above
HNS/H1a (*hns/osmZ*) (also in *Salmonella typhimurium*)	Compacts DNA	Affects *ompC, ompF* and *pap* expression in *E. coli*
VirR (*virR*)	As *osmZ/hns*	Regulates *virB* and invasin gene expression in *Shigella flexneri*
YmoA (*ymoA*)	As *osmZ/hns*	Regulates *virF* and *yop* genes in *Yersinia enterocolitica*
AlgP (*algP*)	Uncertain	Regulates *algD* and alginate production in *Pseudomonas aeruginosa*

'Mechanisms of Antigenic and Phase Variation'. In addition to modifying rates of recombination through bending DNA, IHF protein is also required for transcription of the fimbrial protein gene *fimA* and the outer membrane protein genes *ompC* and *ompF* in *E. coli* (see below). Another protein HNS (often called H1) is present in three isomeric forms, H1a, b and c in *E. coli*. H1a is encoded by the *osmZ* gene (renamed *hns*) and is required in stationary-phase cells for tight compaction of the DNA. However, mutations in *osmZ* are highly pleiotropic and many genes are deregulated in its absence. This gene is present in both *E. coli* and *S. typhimurium*. Mutations in *osmZ* were originally discovered as **osm**otic-stress response variants of both *E. coli* and *S. typhimurium* and it is now clear that supercoiling and compaction of DNA is important in the response of cells to osmotic shock. The osmotically inducible *proU* operon is derepressed in *osmZ* mutants as are the *pap* pilus, *ompC* and *ompF* genes. The *ompF* and *ompC* genes encode outer membrane proteins called **porins**. These are trimeric structures which enable the passage of small molecules across the outer membrane. Normally the outer membrane protein OmpF is produced in low osmotic strength conditions which are found in external environments. This porin has a larger pore size and will allow larger molecules into the cell. OmpC is required under high osmotic strength conditions which are found in the human gut. This porin has a smaller size and prevents harmful solutes such as bile salts from entering the cell. Expression of these two proteins is also under the control of a two component regulon (see below); however, the degree of supercoiling may exert control at a higher level of the regulon hierarchy. Mutations in *ompF* and *ompC* in the same strain attenuate the virulence of *S. typhimurium* as do mutations in the *osmZ* locus. The counterpart to *osmZ* in *Shigella flexneri* is *virR* and in *Yersinia enterocolitica* is *ymoA*. These affect temperature induced regulons; the invasin regulon in *S. flexneri* and the *yop* regulon in *Y. enterocolitica*. In both cases the VirR and YmoA proteins work in conjunction with other regulators. In *Y. enterocolitica* the VirF protein is required for expression of the *yop* genes and outer membrane proteins needed for invasion. Expression of VirF is negatively regulated by YmoA at temperatures below 37 °C. Mutations in *ymoA* or increasing the temperature to 37 °C lead to expression of *virF* and *yop* genes. Similarly, the invasin genes of *S. flexneri* require VirB protein to be expressed and this is negatively controlled by VirR (see Chapter 8, Figure 8.4). DNA supercoiling must therefore play a role in the temperature induction of genes as well as osmotic induction. The level of DNA supercoiling certainly alters in many bacteria with changes in environment. In addition to the effects of osmotic conditions and temperature there are changes associated with growth substrate and anaerobiosis. The mechanisms by which bacterial cells sense these environmental changes and alter their level of DNA supercoiling is largely unknown. It seems likely that different environmental effects are detected by different mechanisms. These may be antagonistic with respect to their effect on DNA supercoiling.

Specific virulence gene regulons

Many environmental signals are passed to the internal cellular systems of bacterial cells via two-component regulators. In these systems a **sensor** protein is located on the outside of the cell cytoplasmic membrane and is responsible for sensing a key environmental change. This protein in turn activates a **regulator** protein, which is associated with the membrane but inside the cell, by phosphorylating it. Examples of such systems known to regulate virulence gene expression by this mechanism are summarised in Table 9.10. With the possible exception of ToxS, all of the sensor proteins appear to be part of a family of histidine protein kinase reponse regulators. These regulatory systems are probably much lower in the cellular hierarchy than catabolite repression and DNA supercoiling. A good example is the expression of OmpF and OmpC under low and high osmotic conditions respectively. These are under the DNA supercoiling regulon as well as the two component EnvZ/OmpR regulon. Under conditions of high osmolarity, EnvZ is autophosphorylated at a histidine site on the protein in the presence of ATP. The phosphate is then transferred to an aspartate site on OmpR. Both the histidine sites and aspartate sites appear to be conserved in this type of regulatory system. There is an increase in the concentration of phosphorylated OmpR (OmpR-P) in the cell. Normally low levels of OmpR-P are bound to a high affinity site near the *ompF* promoter which activates transcription of this gene. Increasing the level of OmpR-P causes binding to a low affinity site in *ompC* and transcription of this gene. Increased binding of OmpR-P to another low affinity site in *ompF* leads to

Table 9.10. Some examples of two-component systems for the regulation of virulence genes

Organism	Sensor	Regulator	Main influence	Virulence genes affected
Salmonella typhimurium	EnvZ	OmpR	High osmolarity	*ompC* and *ompF* expression
Salmonella typhimurium	PhoQ	PhoP	C, N and P starvation	*phoN* (acid phosphatase)
Vibrio cholerae	ToxS	ToxR	Temperature	*ctxA/B* (toxin) operon
Bordetella pertussis	BvgS	BvgA	Temperature	Many genes (e.g. filamentous haemagglutinin, *phu*).

repression of transcription of this gene. Hence, as osmolarity increases, the production of OmpF declines and OmpC increases.

Another member of the histidine protein kinase family of regulators is the *agr* gene of *Staphylococcus* which is known to control a number of virulence determinants including enterotoxin, toxic shock syndrome toxin, haemolysin and staphylokinase (see Chapters 2 and 5).

Increases in temperature appear to be very important in the expression of virulence genes in both *Vibrio cholerae* and *Bordetella pertussis*. Transcription of a number of genes, including the *ctxAB* genes which encode the A and B subunits of the cholera toxin, is determined by ToxR. Unlike the OmpR system described above, ToxR needs to be dimeric and membrane bound to actively promote *ctxAB* operon expression. ToxS, also in the membrane, appears to be the sensor which promotes dimerisation of ToxR (see Chapter 6, Figure 6.5). Although there is close homology between the DNA binding regions of the ToxR and OmpR proteins it appears that ToxR is more closely related to the family of eukaryotic tyrosine kinases. The *toxR* gene is divergently transcribed from a gene *hptG* (*heat shock protein* G), which is normally expressed after heat shock of the cells after modification of the RNA polymerase. This is brought about through the production of new sigma factors which alter the recognition of promoters by the RNA polymerase. Although ToxR dimer binds to a tandemly repeated TTTTGAT sequence upstream of the *ctxAB* operon and promotes toxin expression it does not appear to do the same for other ToxR dependent genes. In these cases, expression appears to be promoted via a cascade involving ToxT.

Bordetella pertussis, which causes whooping cough, is a classic example of a bacterium which reversibly loses the ability to express a whole range of virulence determinants, including pertussis toxin, haemolysin, filamentous haemagglutinin and dermonecrotic toxin, in response to changes in the growth conditions. These were initially described by Lacey in 1960 as the virulent X-mode (for xanthic or yellow coloured colonies) and avirulent C-mode (for cyanic or greenish-blue coloured colonies). It is now known that the *bvg* operon controls this environmental modulation. Sequencing of the *bvg* operon has led to the conclusion that it is also a histidine kinase two-component system; BvgS is the environmental sensor which phosphorylates BvgA. BvgA activates some genes (*virulence activated genes*) and represses others (*virulence repressed genes*). It probably also forms part of a cascade of control of gene expression. The environmental stimuli known to bring about these changes include temperature and changes in the concentration of molecules of nicotinic acid and $MgSO_4$. Superimposed on this environmental modulation (or phenotypic variation) is the genotypic ON/OFF switch mediated by insertions and deletions within the *bvgS* gene (see above in 'Additions or deletions to homopolymeric repeated DNA sequences').

Other examples of two-component systems regulating virulence associated genes include alginate production in *Pseudomonas aeruginosa* and acid phosphatase in *Salmonella typhimurium*. Expression of the *algD* gene in *P. aeruginosa* is necessary for the production of alginate by virulent mucoid strains which cause lung infections in cystic fibrosis sufferers. Nitrogen starvation and changes in osmolarity and oxygen concentration increase the production of alginate. A number of regulons appear to be involved in addition to a two-component system where the regulator gene *algR* and the sensor gene *algQ* have been identified. Indeed the function of *algR* can be replaced by *ompR* in *E. coli*.

The acid *pho*sphatase in *S. typhimurium* is encoded by the *phoN* gene and is expressed upon carbon, nitrogen and phosphorus starvation of the cells as well as low pH conditions. Expression of *phoN* and a number of other genes, including those involved in intracellular survival, is controlled by the PhoP/Q two-component sensor/regulator system (see Chapter 8, Figure 8.5).

The above two-component systems use protein phosphorylation as part of the sensory mechanism. More recently it has become clear that the secretion of a class of low molecular mass compounds called N-acyl homoserine lactones (HSLs) may directly induce the expression of a range of virulence determinants. HSL production by the marine bacterium *Vibrio fischeri* is determined by the *luxI* gene and more HSL is produced as bacterial cell densities increase. The HSL is an autoinducer of *luxI* as well as inducing the *lux* structural genes by binding to the repressor, LuxR which increases bioluminescence by these bacteria. It is likely that many bacteria produce HSLs although the role that they play in virulence gene expression remains to be determined in many cases. Homologues of *luxI/R* are present in many bacteria and have been implicated in gene expression (e.g. elastase production in *Pseudomonas aeruginosa*).

The theory that some pathogenic bacteria might use the production of signalling molecules such as HSLs to induce the expression of virulence determinants when a suitable cell density is attained is an attractive one. Nevertheless, it must be remembered that there are many other environmental conditions affecting the bacteria at the same time. The final outcome of an infection will reflect all of these influences.

CONCLUSION

It is clear that variation in the expression of virulence determinants in bacteria is not only under complex genetic control, but also subject to changes in response to environmental stimuli. There is also the potential for overlap between these two types of control, where environmental stimuli may influence gene rearrangements.

This phenomenal potential to generate variation has many implications for studies of bacterial virulence and for the potential management of bacterial infection. In studies of bacterial virulence, the validity of studying bacteria cultured in laboratory growth media immediately comes into question. The selective pressures of the host may govern the expression of the characteristics of the bacterium which relate to virulence and in the absence of these selective pressures not only may these be absent, but also the genetic information encoding these characteristics may be lost entirely from the population. This underlines the importance of studying fresh clinical isolates in experimental systems which model the natural infection as closely as possible. The presence of a particular characteristic implicated in virulence should also be verified in bacteria taken from clinical material. Without this information it is difficult to make rational choices for vaccine design. In the development of immunodiagnostic clinical tests based on monoclonal antibodies it is again important to be aware of the stability of expression of the epitope of choice. An antigen which undergoes rapid antigenic variation is obviously unsuitable. Also if amplification of DNA by the polymerase chain reaction (PCR) is to be used as a means of identifying bacteria in clinical material it is improtant to be aware of the stability of the target DNA sequence.

In terms of the future management of bacterial disease and the development of 'designer' antibiotics, it is possible to speculate that interfering with the bacterial mechanisms for the generation of variation could prove to be a fruitful area. If these mechanisms are not too similar to the genetic mechanisms of eukaryotic cells, perhaps it might be possible to design antibiotics which permanently switch off the expression of virulence determinants.

FURTHER READING

General

Cairns J. 1963. The Chromosome of *Escherichia coli*. Cold Spring Harbor Symposium on Quantitative Biology 28, 43–46.

Chater K. F., Hopwood D. A. 1989. Genetics of Bacterial Diversity. Academic Press, London, UK.

Dorman C. J. 1994. Genetics of Bacterial Virulence. Blackwell Scientific Publications, Oxford, UK.

Neidhardt F. C., Ingraham J. L., Shaechter M. 1990. Physiology of the Bacterial Cell. Sinaur Associates Inc., Sunderland, USA.

Ogawa T., Okazaki T. 1980. Discontinuous DNA replication. Annual Review of Biochemistry 49, 421–432.

DNA recombination and transposition

Berg D. E., Howe M. M. (Eds). 1989. Mobile DNA. American Society for Microbiology, Washington, USA.

Cox M. M. 1994. Why does RecA protein hydrolyse ATP? Trends in Biochemical Sciences May 19, 217–222.

Kowalczkowski S. C., Eggleston N. K. 1994. Homologous pairing and DNA-strand exchange proteins. Annual Review of Biochemistry 63, 991–1043.
Radding C. M. 1993 A universal recombination filament. Current Biology 3 (6), 358–360.
West S. C. 1992. Enzymes and molecular mechanisms of genetic recombination. Annual Review of Biochemistry 61, 603–640.

Phase and antigenic variation

Foster T. J., O'Toole P. W., O'Reilly M. 1988. Genetic analysis of *Staphylococcus aureus* virulence. In: Immunochemical and molecular genetic analysis of bacterial pathogens (Eds P. Owen, T. J. Foster). Elsevier, NL. Chapter 8.
Glasgow A. C., Hughes K. T., Simon M. I. 1989. Bacterial DNA inversion systems. In: Mobile DNA (Eds D. E. Berg, M. M. Howe). American Society for Microbiology, Washington, USA. Chapter 28.
Moxon R. E., Rainey P. B., Novak M. A., Lenski R. E. 1994. Adaptive evolution of highly mutable loci in pathogenic bacteria. Current Biology 4(1), 24–33.
Robertson B. D., Meyer T. F. 1992. Antigenic variation in bacterial pathogens. In: Molecular Biology of bacterial infection; Current status and future prospects (Eds C. E. Hormaeche, C. W. Penn, C. J. Smyth). Symposia of the Society for General Microbiology 49. Cambridge University Press, UK. pp 61–73.
Robertson B. D., Meyer T. F. 1992. Genetic variation in pathogenic bacteira. Trends in Genetics 8(12), 422–427.
Saunders J. R. 1989. The molecular basis of antigenic variation in pathogenic *Neisseria*. In: Genetics of bacterial diversity (Eds D.A. Hopwood, K.E. Chater). Academic Press, London. Chapter 13.
Seifert H. S., So M. 1988. Genetic mechanisms of bacterial antigenic variation. Microbiological Reviews 52(3), 327–336.

Environmental regulation of virulence determinant expression

Clarke V. L. 1990. Environmental modulation of gene expression in gram-negative pathogens. In: Molecular basis of bacterial pathogenesis (Eds B.H. Iglewski, V.L. Clarke). Academic Press, London. Chapter 6.
DiRita V. J., Mekalanos J. J. 1989. Genetic regulation of bacterial virulence. Annual Review of Genetics 23, 455–482.
Dorman C. J., Ni Bhriain N. 1992. Global regulation of gene expression during environmental adaptation: implications for bacterial pathogens. In: Molecular Biology of Bacterial infection; Current status and future prospects (Eds C. E. Hormaeche, C. W. Penn, C. J. Smyth). Symposia of the Society for General Microbiology 49. Cambridge University Press, UK. pp 193–230.
Dorman C. J., Ni Bhriain N. 1993. DNA topology and bacterial virulence gene regulation. Trends in Microbiology 1(3), 92–99.
Lacey B. W. 1960. Antigenic modulation of *Bordetella pertussis*. Journal of Hygiene 58, 57–93.
Swift S., Bainton N. J., Winson M. K. 1994. Gram-negative bacterial communication by N-acyl homoserine lactones: a universal language? Trends in Microbiology 2(6), 193–197.

Appendix

HOST CELL SURFACE CARBOHYDRATES

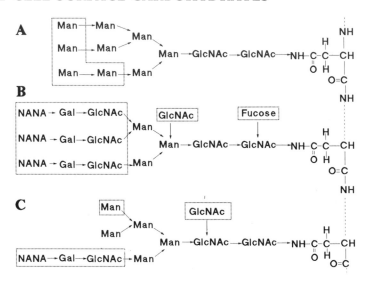

Figure A1. N-linked glycans. Examples of the three major types of oligosaccharide which are linked to glycoproteins via asparagine residues within the consensus sequence; asparagine-X-serine or threonine, where X is any amino acid. A. High-mannose type which consists of only mannose and N-acetylglucosamine residues. B. Complex type with a common pentasaccharide structure known as the trimannosyl core. C. Hybrid type which has features of both the high-mannose and complex type. Boxed regions of the structures indicate areas of the molecule which can be variable. Man, mannose; GlcNAc, N-acetyl glucosamine; Gal, galactose; NANA, N-acetyl neuraminic acid. Glycoproteins with identical peptide chains may carry oligosaccharides which contain different sugars and if there is more than one potential glycosylation site different oligosaccharides may be attached at different sites. Where the different oligosaccharides are attached to the peptide in the one cell type the different glycoproteins are termed glycoforms. For example 30 different oligosaccharides have been identified which may be associated with IgG, although there are more than 30 possible glycoforms as IgG may have more than one glycosylation site. Where the same peptide is produced by different cells (such as Thy-1 which may be synthesised by both brain cells and thymocytes) the different cells will synthesise two different families of glycoforms, called glycotypes. In rats there is no overlap between the brain and thymocyte families of oligosaccharide. Therefore Thy-1 produced by brain cells is essentially a different molecule from Thy-1 produced by thymocytes, although they share a common peptide sequence. The implications of this on studies of the activities of biological molecules which rely heavily on the use of 'recombinant' peptides, either expressed in *E. coli* and therefore not glycosylated, or atypically glycosylated by another type of eukaryotic cell, remain to be determined

---

Figure A2. O-linked glycans. Examples of oligosaccharides which are linked to glycoproteins via either serine or theonine residues found on A. submaxillary mucins and human erythrocytes; B. Human glycophorin, gonadotrophin β-subunit, fetuin, lymphocyte plasma membrane C. Human chorionic gonadotrophin β-subunit, human serum IgA, rat brain glycoproteins D. Bronchial mucin from cystic fibrosis patients. (There is no consensus amino acid sequence for the attachment of O-linked oligosaccharides.)

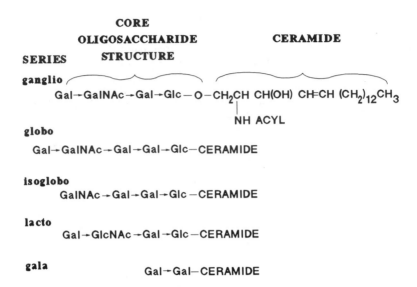

Figure A3. Glycolipids. In mammalian cells glycolipids are generally glycosphingo-lipids in which a hyrophobic moiety, termed ceramide, composed of a sphingosine and fatty acid (ACYL) is attached to the hydrophilic oligosaccharide. These molecules are classified according to the sugar residues which may be present in the core structure of the oligosaccharide

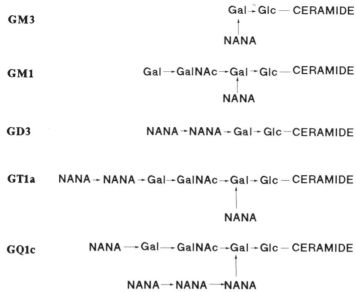

GM3

Gal→Glc — CERAMIDE
↑
NANA

GM1

Gal→GalNAc→Gal→Glc—CERAMIDE
↑
NANA

GD3

NANA→NANA→Gal→Glc—CERAMIDE

GT1a   NANA→NANA→Gal→GalNAc→Gal→Glc — CERAMIDE
↑
NANA

GQ1c   NANA→Gal→GalNAc→Gal→Glc — CERAMIDE
↑
NANA→NANA→NANA

Figure A4. Glycolipids: ganglio series gangliosides. Examples of some gangliosides. The letters M, D, T and Q refer to the numbers of NANA residues (1, 2, 3 and 4 respectively); the following number is the number of uncharged sugar residues (NB: NANA carries a negative charge) subtracted from five; the lower case letter relates to the biosynthetic pathway

NATURAL SIALIC ACIDS

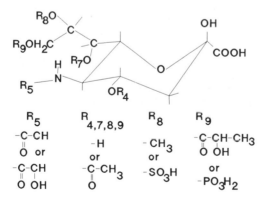

Figure A5. Structure of sialic acid. By substitution of the 9 carbon amino sugar neuraminic acid with different groups (R), 23 different natural derivatives can be formed. These make up the sialic acid family of sugars. Suggested biological roles for sialic acids include: binding and transport of positively charged ions, influence of the conformation of glycoproteins, surface antigens, cell surface receptors and masking of cell surface receptors

BACTERIAL CELL SURFACES AND MOLECULES

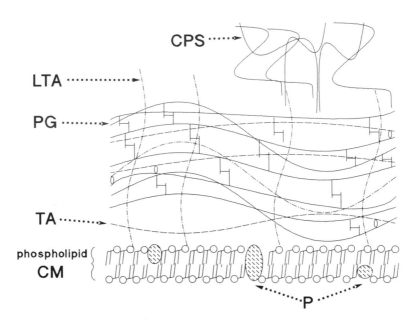

Figure A6. The Gram positive bacterial cell envelope. The envelope or wall of Gram positive bacteria is composed of a complex three-dimensional matrix of surface polymers. Fifty to eighty per cent of the wall is peptidoglycan (PG) which forms the shape of the bacterium; interwoven and convalently attached to the peptidoglycan are polymers such as teichoic acids (TA). Lipoteichoic acids (LTA) are attached to the phospholipid of the cytoplasmic membrane (CM) and extend to the cell surface where they form surface antigens. Capsular polysaccharide (CPS) forms the outermost layer in some bacteria and others have a crystalline surface protein layer (S-layer; not illustrated). A variety of proteins (P) are embedded in the cytoplasmic membrane. Their functions include: transport of molecules out of and into the bacterium, sensing changes in the outer environment, electron transport and oxidative phosphorylation, DNA replication and biosynthesis of the outer layers

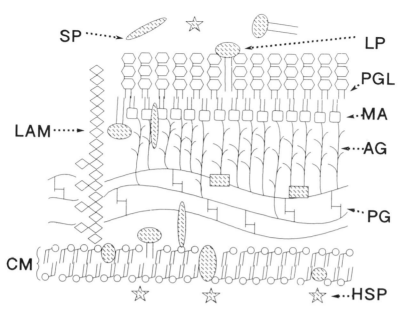

Figure A7. The mycobacterial cell envelope. Schematic representation of the possible organisation of the envelope of *Mycobacteria*. Outside the cytoplasmic membrane (CM) there are three layers. 1. The peptidoglycan layer. 2. A loosely defined
outer membrane attached to the peptidoglycan through arabinogalactan (AG) and
composed of mycolic acid (MA) and phenolic glycolipid (PGL) which have fatty
acid chains of 30–34 carbons. These are sometimes referred to as the waxes of the
mycobacterial envelope. 3. The outermost layer, sometimes called the polysaccharide layer, thought to be composed of the triglycosyl chain (hexagons) of the phenolic
glycolipid and the outermost region of the lipoarabinomannan (LAM) which
extends from the cytoplasmic membrane to the outside of the envelope. A number
of proteins (oval shapes) and lipoproteins (LP) are associated with the cytoplasmic
membrane and the envelope. Some of these may be secreted from the bacteria (SP)
while other proteins are strongly associated with the envelope (rectangle). The heat
shock proteins (HSP; star) are generally present in the cytoplasm but can also be
detected in the supernatant during exponential growth. Freund's complete adjuvant
is a crude preparation of killed mycobacteria and it is the bacterial envelope which
possesses the adjuvant properties. Using staining techniques the mycobacterial cell
envelope is classified as acid fast as red carbol-fuchsin stain is retained within the
bacterial cell when it is treated with acid, whereas it is washed out of Gram positive
and Gram negative bacteria

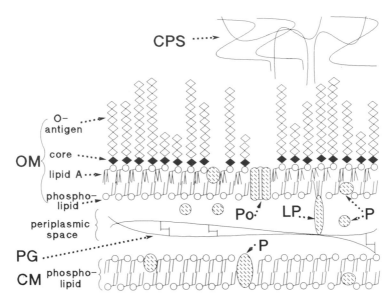

Figure A8. The Gram negative bacterial cell envelope. This envelope is more complex than that of the Gram positive bacterium in that it has an outer membrane which effectively creates a second compartment in the Gram negative bacterium outside the cytoplasmic membrane (CM), the periplasmic space. Peptidoglycan (PG) is not a major component of the Gram negative envelope, although it forms the shape of the bacterium and acts as an anchor for the outer membrane (OM) through attached lipoproteins (LP). The outer membrane is not symmetrical and has an inner phospholipid leaflet and an outer leaflet of lipopolysaccharide. Lipopolysaccharide has three distinct regions 1. the lipid A; 2. the core oligosaccharide; and 3. the O-antigen which can extend outwards from the cell for up to 30 nm. Proteins (P) involved in the movement of molecules across both the outer and cytoplasmic membranes are embedded in the membranes. Porin proteins (Po) are trimers which form channels in the outer membrane through which passive non-specific diffusion of low molecular weight molecules occurs. The periplasmic space contains a number of proteins involved in the translocation of molecules out of and into the bacterium, the biosynthesis of surface components and the destruction of antibacterial molecules which pass through the outer membrane. The cytoplasmic and outer membrane can join together directly to form adhesion points (see Figure 5.4) and molecules may be secreted without passing through the periplasmic space. It is likely that these adhesion points are the vulnerable points at which the host's defences, such as the membrane attack complex of complement, act. Capsular polysaccharide (CPS) forms the outermost layer in some bacteria, others may have a crystalline protein surface layer (S-layer; not illustrated)

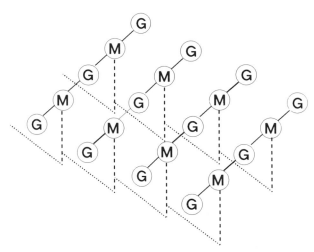

Figure A9. Structure of peptidoglycan. Polysaccharide chains of alternating N-acetyl glucosamine (G) and N-acetyl muramic acid (M) are cross-linked by short peptide chains. N-acetyl muramic acid is unique to peptidoglycan. The amino acids in the cross-links vary amongst different species of bacteria and include D-amino acids (most naturally occurring amino acids are of the L-form). Four amino acids (dashed line) are attached to the muramic acid. Depending on the bacterial species, these may be linked directly with the fourth amino acid of one chain linking to the third amino acid of the other chain. Alternatively, five lysine residues may form a linking bridge (dotted line)

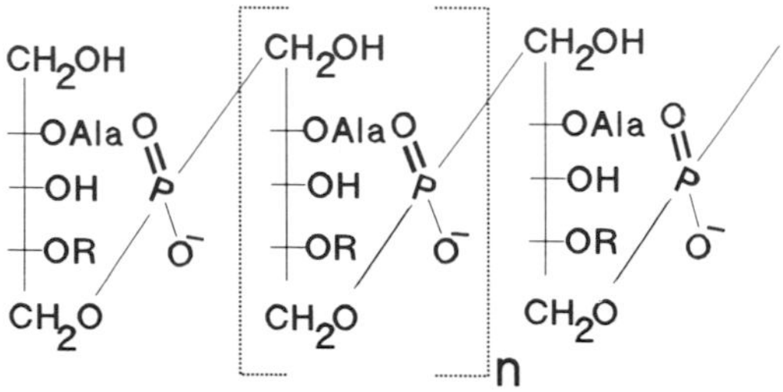

Figure A10. Teichoic acid. Teichoic acids are phosphate containing polymers found in Gram positive bacteria in the walls, membranes and capsules. Examples of peptidoglycan associated teichoic acids include polyglycerol phosphate (A), polyribitol phosphate (B) and polymers of glucose phosphates. Polyribitol and glycerol phosphate may have attached amino acids (e.g. Ala = D-alanyl) or sugars (e.g. R = N-acetyl glucosaminyl). Polyglycerol phosphate may also be associated with glycolipids of the cytoplasmic membrane, thus forming a lipoteichoic acid. Teichuronic acids are wall polymers of Gram positive bacteria with similar properties to teichoic acids. They are linear polysaccharides in which uronic acids, rather than phosphate groups, confer the negative charge. Examples include repeating alternating units of glucuronic acid and N-acetyl glucosamine or N-acetyl mannosaminuronic acid and glucose. Some bacteria will change from production of teichoic acids to teichuronic acids under phosphate nutrient limitation

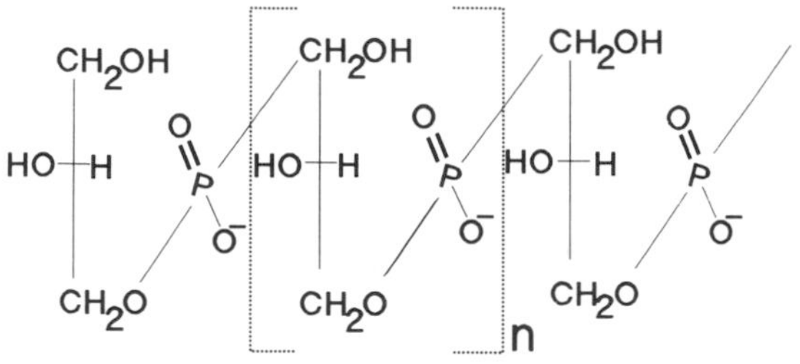

Figure A11. (*opposite*) Lipopolysaccharide (LPS) forms the outer leaflet of the outer membrane of Gram negative bacteria. The three regions of the lipopolysaccharide molecule are: 1. The lipid A (A and dotted box in B) which can have variable numbers and chain lengths of fatty acids which are attached to phosphorylated diglucosamine (GluN). 2. The core oligosaccharide which is usually linked to the lipid A via the sugar 2-keto-3-deoxymanno-octonic acid (also called 3-deoxy-D-manno-2-octulosonic acid) (KDO). The sugar constituents of the core vary amongst and within bacterial species, although most have an inner core of KDO and heptose. 3. The O-side chain polysaccharide (or O-antigen) which is composed of variable numbers of repeating oligosaccharide units of between 2 and 6 sugars. The sugar components of the O-antigen can vary considerably amongst different strains of bacteria. The O86 antigen of *E. coli* is illustrated (box). This variation in the sugar components gives rise to a large number of antigenically different LPS. Bacteria which produce a complete core and O-antigen are termed smooth, because of the appearance of the bacterial colonies on agar plates; mutant bacteria which synthesise a complete core but are not able to polymerise the oligosaccharide units are termed semi-rough; and mutant bacteria which cannot synthesise the O-antigen are termed rough

A

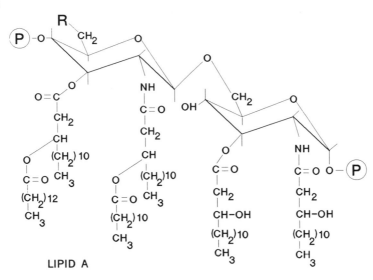

LIPID A

B

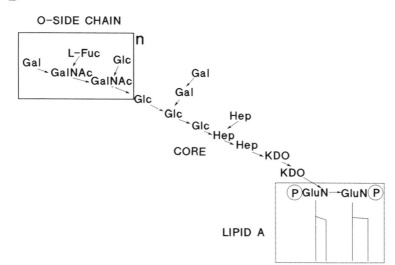

THE HOST CELL PLASMA MEMBRANE

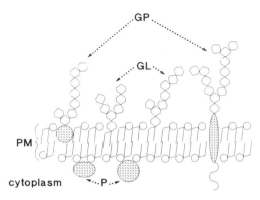

Figure A12. The plasma membrane (PM). The host cell membrane consists of a phospholipid bilayer. Glycoproteins (GP) may either be embedded in the outer leaflet or traverse the membrane. The oligosaccharide moieties (see Figures A1–4) of the glycoproteins and glycolipids (GL) extend out from the cell surface. Cytoplasmic proteins (P) may be associated with the inner side of the membrane

STRUCTURE OF HUMAN IMMUNOGLOBULINS

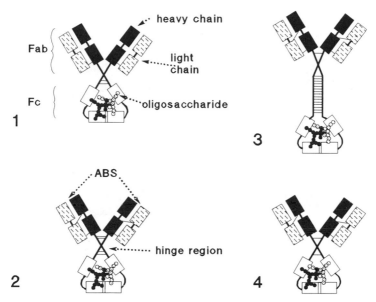

Figure A13. Human immunoglobulin G. Immunoglobulin G (IgG) is produced in four different subclasses or isotypes, designated 1–4. The isotype is determined by the nature of the high molecular weight heavy chain. One of two possible types of light chain (κ or λ) are bound to the heavy chains by disulphide bonds (narrow solid lines). Proteolytic cleavage at the hinge region of IgG produces two identical antigen binding fragments (Fab) and one crystallizable fragment (Fc). The isotypes differ in the number and position of the disulphide bonds which join the heavy chains together and the light chains to the heavy chains. The region of the IgG which varies between different clones of B-cells contains the antigen binding site (ABS), the rest of the molecule has a conserved amino acid sequence. The heavy chain has a flexible region termed the hinge region. This flexibility allows independent positioning of the two ABSs. There is a conserved N-glycosylation site in the Fc region near to the hinge region (white and black circles). IgG may also be N-glycosylated in the variable region if the asparagine-X amino acid-serine or threonine amino acid sequence is generated (see Figure A1)

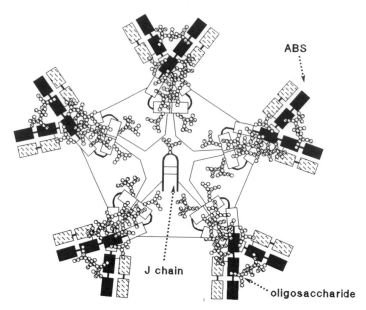

Figure A14. Human immunoglobulin M. Immunoglobulin M is usually a pentamer composed of individual units each with two heavy and light chains, similar in structure to IgG, joined with disulphide bonds. A peptide chain, the J chain, is also involved in holding the molecule together. The heavy chain of IgM is more heavily glycosylated than IgG. ABS, antigen binding site

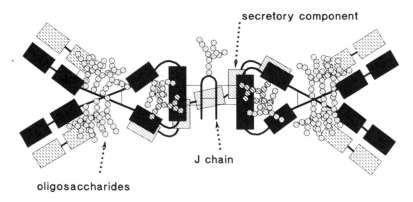

Figure A15. Human secretory immunoglobulin A. Secretory immunoglobulin A consists of a dimer joined by disulphide bonds and a J chain similar to that of IgM. The secretory component is part of the IgA epithelial cell receptor which remains associated with the IgA as it passes through epithelial cells during secretion into the gut lumen

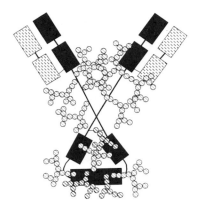

Figure A16. Human immunoglubulin D. Immunoglobulin D is similar in organisation to IgG, but with a larger number of oligosaccharide units

PERIODATE OXIDATION OF POLYSACCHARIDES

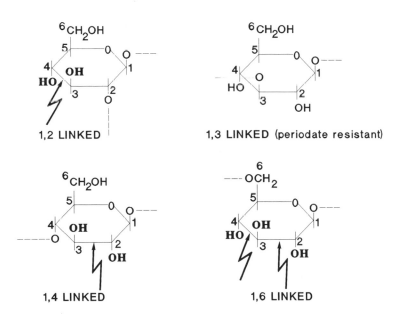

Figure A17. Periodate oxidation. Sodium metaperiodate selectively oxidises unsubstituted hydroxy groups to carbonyl groups where the hydroxy groups are on adjacent carbons in the sugar ring structure (zigzag arrow). This breaks the ring. Some sugars will resist periodate oxidation as in the 1-3 linkage

FURTHER READING

Host Cell Surface Carbohydrates

Feizi T. 1989. Glycoprotein oligosaccharides as recognition structures. In: Carbohydrate recognition in cellular function. Ciba Foundation Symposium 145. J Wiley, Chichester. pp 62–67.

Fukuda M. 1992. Cell surface carbohydrates and cell development. CRC Press, USA.

Raedmacher T. W., Parekh R. B., Dwek R. A. 1988. Glycobiology. Annual Review of Biochemistry 57, 785–838.

Sharon N., Lis H. 1993. Carbohydrates in cell recognition. Scientific American January.

Natural Sialic Acids

Acheson A., Sunshine J. L., Rutishauser U. 1991. NCAM polysialic acid can regulate both cell–cell and cell–substrate interactions. Journal of Cell Biology 114, 143–153.

Schauer R. 1985. Sialic acids and their role as biological masks. Trends in Biochemical Sciences September, 357–360.

Bacterial Cell Surfaces and Molecules

Hammond S. M., Lambert P. A., Rycroft A. N. 1984. The bacterial cell surface. Croom Helm, Beckenham, UK.

Hancock I., Poxton I. 1988. Bacterial cell surface techniques. J Wiley, Chichester.

Index

Note: Page references in *italics* refer to Figures; those in **bold** refer to Tables

Index compiled by Annette Musker